STUDY GUIDE

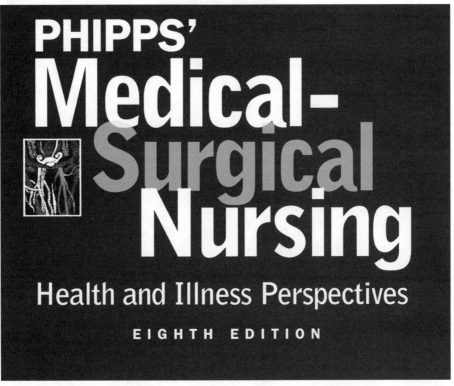

PHIPPS'
Medical-Surgical Nursing

Health and Illness Perspectives

EIGHTH EDITION

MONAHAN • SANDS • NEIGHBORS • MAREK • GREEN

STUDY GUIDE

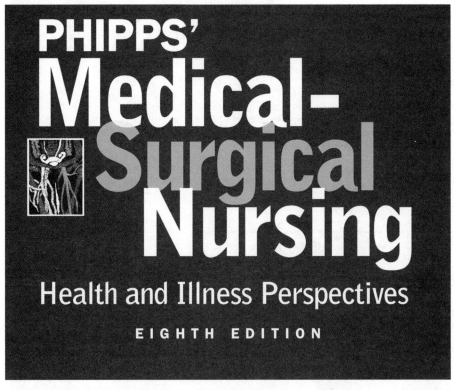

PHIPPS'
Medical-Surgical Nursing
Health and Illness Perspectives
EIGHTH EDITION

MONAHAN • SANDS • NEIGHBORS • MAREK • GREEN

Carol J. Green, PhD, RN
Professor of Nursing
Johnson County Community College
Overland Park, Kansas;
CAPT, Nurse Corps
United States Navy

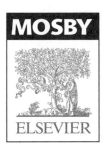

MOSBY

ELSEVIER

MOSBY
ELSEVIER

11830 Westline Industrial Drive
St. Louis, Missouri 63146

Study Guide for
Phipps' Medical-Surgical Nursing: Health and Illness
Perspectives, Eighth Edition

ISBN-13: 978-0-323-03171-4
ISBN-10: 0-323-03171-4

Copyright © 2007, 2003 by Mosby, Inc.

Notice

Knowledge and best practice in this field are constantly changing. As new research and experience broaden our knowledge, changes in practice, treatment and drug therapy may become necessary or appropriate. Readers are advised to check the most current information provided (i) on procedures featured or (ii) by the manufacturer of each product to be administered, to verify the recommended dose or formula, the method and duration of administration, and contraindications. It is the responsibility of the practitioner, relying on their own experience and knowledge of the patient, to make diagnoses, to determine dosages and the best treatment for each individual patient, and to take all appropriate safety precautions. To the fullest extent of the law, neither the Publisher nor the Author assumes any liability for any injury and/or damage to persons or property arising out or related to any use of the material contained in this book.

The Publisher

ISBN-13: 978-0-323-03171-4
ISBN-10: 0-323-03171-4

Executive Editor: Michael Ledbetter, Tom Wilhelm
Senior Developmental Editor: Laurie Gower, Jill Ferguson
Publishing Services Manager: Deborah L. Vogel
Project Manager: Katherine Hinkebein
Senior Book Designer: Amy Buxton
Marketing Manager: Tricia Schroeder

Printed in the United States of America

Last digit is the print number: 9 8 7 6 5 4 3 2 1

Working together to grow
libraries in developing countries

www.elsevier.com | www.bookaid.org | www.sabre.org

ELSEVIER   BOOK AID International   Sabre Foundation

Preface

In a climate of continual health care change, nursing shortages, and increased nursing responsibilities in all areas of health care, it is imperative that nurses be prepared to assume the roles of manager, collaborator, consumer advocate, teacher, decision maker, and problem solver. Consequently, a comprehensive understanding of adult health care concepts and principles and the ability to think critically are basic to assuming these responsibilities.

It is the aim of this study guide to provide varied learning exercises that promote critical thinking and facilitate learning in order to meet the challenge of producing capable, thinking nurses. The exercises are designed to enhance analytical reasoning, divergent thinking, reflection, problem solving, and decision making. Case studies, recognition and correction of false statements, analogies, and compare and contrast exercises are some of the methods used to facilitate higher order thinking and maintain student interest.

I hope that students find this challenging study guide beneficial in reinforcing knowledge and transferring that knowledge to various patient situations. Although many of the exercises in this study guide are not considered easy, I hope that students will accept them with an open mind and a willingness to learn. I also hope that students will find this type of learning challenging, exciting, and enjoyable.

Carol J. Green

1 Scope of Medical-Surgical Nursing

1. Identify each organization or program related to medical-surgical nursing.

_____ a. Tests four domains of practice: biophysical and psychosocial, pathophysiology of body systems, patient care issues, and issues and trends.

_____ b. Mechanism for recognizing excellence in practice.

_____ c. Examination focuses on the care of acutely ill, hospitalized adult patients.

_____ d. The mission is to enhance clinical expertise, professionalism, and leadership of nurses caring for adults.

_____ e. Awards credentials based on the applicant's educational level.

_____ f. Describes the responsibilities for which practitioners are accountable.

_____ g. Entitles the practitioner to use the credential Certified Medical-Surgical Registered Nurse.

2. Explain how certification differs from registered nurse licensure.

1

3. Identify several factors that are currently influencing medical-surgical nursing practice.

4. Correct any false statements about evidence-based practice (EBP).
   a. EBP grew out of efforts to improve patient care through a process of problem-based investigation.

   b. The result of EBP is improved patient compliance and positive health outcomes even though economic outcomes are not improved.

   c. Increasing consumer demands to understand and make informed health care choices was one factor that contributed to the acceptance of EBP.

   d. Translating evidence-based knowledge into clinical practice is perceived by the Institute of Medicine (IOM) as being the easiest aspect of EBP.

   e. EPB is the same as research or research-based practice.

   f. EPB requires that practitioners acquire new skills, including efficient literature searching and application of rules of evidence when evaluating clinical literature.

   g. The ACE Star Model of the Cycle of Knowledge Transformation identifies five stages: discovery, evidence summary, translation, implementation, and revision.

   h. The Agency for Healthcare Research and Quality refers to evidence summaries as systematic reviews.

5. What is the goal or mission of NANDA International?

6. Write a nursing diagnosis (other than the one listed in the text) and label the parts as diagnostic label, descriptor axis, and health status axis.

7. Differentiate between Nursing Interventions Classification (NIC) and Nursing Outcomes Classification (NOC).

2 The Aging Population

1. Explain how the primary and secondary changes of aging differ.

2. Identify potential secondary changes in older adults related to:
   a. Reduced cough reflex

   b. Vertebral disk shrinkage

   c. Decreased production of digestive enzymes

   d. Loss of arterial compliance

3. Identify nursing activities for older adults related to their:
   a. Activities of daily living

b. Spiritual well-being

c. Sexuality

d. Family

e. Nutrition

f. Cognitive function

g. Sensory perception

4. Correct any false statements.
   a. Most senses and sensations, such as pain, vision, taste, and touch, are dulled by aging.

   b. Older adults may need to take supplements because their diets generally lack sufficient calcium, vitamins A and C, iron and zinc.

c. Keeping older adults oriented to the present and discouraging them from useless discussions about their past is important to prevent confusion.

d. If blinds or curtains are left open so that older adults can see sunshine, they are less likely to become confused.

e. Touching older adults is discouraged because they cannot always recognize the person who is doing the touching.

5. What are the four reasons why assessment of the older adult for alcohol, medication, and drug use is essential?

6. Correct false statements about Alzheimer's disease (AD).
   a. Known risk factors for AD are primary age-related changes and family history.

   b. Amyloid plaques and neurofibillary tangles are found in the brains of those with AD.

   c. AD is subtle, progressive, and frequently diagnosed during the early stages.

   d. Medications, such as the statins, may reduce deterioration and slow the progression of AD.

   e. Keeping the person with AD safe is one of the most important aspects of caregiving.

   f. The majority of AD caregivers are able to maintain strong family ties and meaningful interactions.

7. **Case Study:** A 72-year-old man who resides in a long-term care facility is alert and oriented. He is able to ambulate with the assistance of another person or a walker and has no history of falls. He wears glasses and a hearing aid. He takes a daily diuretic to control his hypertension. Score the man's risk for falls based on the Risk for Falls Assessment Tool.

8. **Case Study:** A 77-year-old woman is admitted to an acute care facility for penumonia. She becomes confused at night and has gotten out of bed on more than one occasion. When assessing the woman, the nurse notes that she is oriented to person and place but not to time. The woman can articulate her needs and make herself understood, but she cannot concentrate very long on what others are saying to her, partly because she is hard of hearing. What further information is needed to accurately assess the woman's cognition and state of confusion?

9. A 76-year-old man is scheduled to undergo a bowel resection for removal of a mass. Other than the abdominal mass, the patient has no health problems. Explain why the man is a greater surgical and postoperative risk than a man who is 30 years younger.

10. **Case Study:** An 85-year-old woman is being discharged from an acute care facility to home. She is alert and oriented but tends to forget details. She is on a decreasing dose of prednisone (a glucocorticoid medication), which consists of 2 tablets for 4 days, 1 tablet for 4 days, then 1 tablet every other day for 4 days. Plan a method or activity to help the woman remember how and when to take her prescribed medication.

3 Healthy Lifestyles

1. Analyze your own health-related behaviors. Identify any unhealthy behaviors you may have and describe how they may interfere with your nursing role.

2. A 65-year-old woman reports insomnia. She states that she has difficulty falling asleep and wakes up frequently throughout the night.
   a. Write several questions that you need to ask the woman to assess the possible causes of her insomnia.

   b. Identify several strategies that may help promote sleep.

3. Label each type of prevention as either primary (P), secondary (S), or tertiary (T).

   _____ a. Blood pressure screening

   _____ b. Smoking cessation classes

   _____ c. Cholesterol screening

   _____ d. Immunizations

   _____ e. Cardiac rehabilitation

_____ f. Mammography

_____ g. Aerobic exercise classes

_____ h. Diabetes management classes

_____ i. Fecal occult blood testing

_____ j. Dietary classes for individuals with hypertension

4. Correct any false statements.
   a. Many of the health indicators in *Healthy People 2010* are directed at behaviors that can significantly decrease morbidity and mortality.

   b. Regular exercise decreases the proportion of high-density lipoproteins and subsequently reduces the risk for coronary artery disease.

   c. Rest is required to replenish the pool of adenosine triphosphate because it cannot be stored.

   d. Diet indirectly affects the development of major disease processes.

   e. Approximately 50% of adults older than 20 years and 64% of persons younger than 20 years are overweight or obese in the United States.

   f. Nicotine is one of the most powerful of the known addictive substances.

   g. Inhaling cigarette smoke causes hypoxia, impairs vision and thinking, and increases the incidence of atherosclerosis.

   h. Sexually transmitted diseases tend to be a more serious problem in men because men tend not to seek medical attention in a timely manner.

i. The hectic pace of contemporary lifestyles often reduces restorative rest and sleep and may contribute to violence and injury.

5. **Case Study:** A 49-year-old mother of three teenage children works full time and has difficulty meeting monthly financial obligations. She is too tired to cook and buys TV dinners and fast food as a matter of convenience. The children get home from school at different hours and are generally hungry. Identify barriers that this woman perceives as prohibiting a change in the family's eating habits. Suggest strategies to help her improve the nutritional status of her family.

6. **Case Study:** A 30-year-old woman weighs 150 pounds and is 5 feet tall. On an average day she consumes approximately 2000 calories. She is a secretary, sits 8 hours per day, and is only moderately active at home. After an evaluation of her diet, you determine the following:
    Protein intake = 30 g/day
    Carbohydrate intake = 1 fruit, 1 vegetable, 2 grains
    Fat intake = 50% of total daily calories
What recommendations can you make to help this woman move toward meeting dietary guidelines and weight reduction?

7. A 41-year-old registered nurse has a history of obesity. At age 20 years, she began smoking one pack of cigarettes per day to control her weight after many unsuccessful attempts at weight loss. Both of her parents, who were former smokers, have recently been diagnosed with cancer. The nurse wants to stop smoking but finds quitting difficult because she does not want to regain her lost weight. Identify factors that may be contributing to the nurse's difficulty with smoking cessation.

4 Complementary and Alternative Therapies

1. Discuss ways in which complementary and alternative therapies (CAT) fit into the holistic philosophy of nursing.

2. Identify your own personal strengths and limitations regarding your ability to address the spiritual needs of patients. How can you best respect patients' individual religious practices, taking into account your own belief system and comfort level?

3. Identify three reasons CAT is gaining popularity in the United States.

4. **Case Study:** A patient with a chronic illness has decided to use an herbal remedy along with traditional therapy for her disease.
   a. Discuss the possible benefits of combining such therapies.

   b. Discuss possible problems related to combining therapies.

   c. What is the most important nursing action for this patient?

5. Match the interventions with the appropriate classification of CAT.

_____ a. Acupressure

_____ b. Meditation

A. Alternative medical systems
B. Mind-body interventions
C. Biologically based treatments
D. Manipulative/body-based methods
E. Energy therapies

_____ c. Massage

_____ d. Ginger root

_____ e. Acupuncture

_____ f. Spinal manipulation

_____ g. Music therapy

_____ h. Therapeutic touch

_____ i. Prayer

_____ j. Echinacea

_____ k. Biofeedback

_____ l. Reflexology

_____ m. Vibration

_____ n. Hypnosis

Chapter **4** **Complementary and Alternative Therapies**

6. Correct any false statements about CAT.
   a. Research evidence indicates that pharmacologic interventions are by far the most effective for the relief of pain.

   b. Most individuals are reluctant to use and report use of alternative therapies to their physicians.

   c. Women who are pregnant should not receive acupuncture.

   d. The homeopathic philosophy is based on the principle of self-treatment.

   e. Two major concerns regarding herbal products are multiple ingredients and the lack of dosage standards.

   f. Research on herbal products is unreliable.

   g. Herbal products are safe because they are naturally occurring nutrients.

   h. Massage therapy involves the manipulation of tissues to enhance healing and health.

   i. The Alexander technique focuses on postural or antigravity reflexes.

Chapter **4 Complementary and Alternative Therapies**

5 Genetics and Disease

1. Correct any false statements regarding basic molecular biology and the role of genetics in health and illness.

   a. The first step in identifying specific genes and their functions relative to protein production is knowing the sequence of base pairs.

   b. Amino acid molecules are a major source of human variation in health and disease.

   c. Autosomal-dominant inheritance occurs when a person receives an affected gene from two carrier parents.

   d. Knowing their genetic profiles allows individuals to decrease their risks and susceptibilities to disease.

   e. Predispositional testing provides an individual with information about the likelihood of being a carrier of a genetic disorder.

   f. Gene therapies are divided into three categories: somatic, chromosomal, and germline.

   g. In the future, adverse drug reactions may be reduced or eliminated on the basis of genetic tests.

2. Design a three-generation display for your family. What tendencies, if any, can you identify?

3. List the primary benefit of predisposition testing and list two diseases that could be altered by knowledge of the predisposition.

4. Why is the nursing intervention of decision-making support important for the nursing diagnosis of *decisional conflict* related to genetic testing?

5. List the four goals of genetic counseling.

6. Identify the single most important barrier to genetic testing. Justify the answer.

7. **Case Study:** Because of her family history, a woman wishing to become pregnant undergoes genetic testing to determine if she is a carrier for the neurologic disorder Huntington's disease. She learns that she is a carrier.
   a. What type of inherited trait does this represent if only one parent is a carrier?

   b. What dilemma(s), if any, may knowledge of this information cause for the woman and her partner?

   c. Consider whether, and under which circumstances, you would choose to be genetically tested.

6 Infectious Diseases and Bioterrorism

1. Match the terms to the correct descriptors.

_____ a. Resident flora

_____ b. Transient flora

_____ c. Endogenous infection

_____ d. Exogenous infection

_____ e. Endotoxin

_____ f. Exotoxin

_____ g. Pathogenicity

_____ h. Invasiveness

A. Ability to cause disease or damage
B. Water- or soil-induced infection
C. Released when cell wall is disrupted
D. Adapts to life within the human body
E. Pathogen's ability to penetrate target tissues
F. Reside in body for weeks to months
G. Protein secreted by bacteria
H. Contamination of tissue by normal flora

2. Identify each process involved in the chain of infection.
   a. Respiratory tract

   b. Human asymptomatic carrier

   c. Direct contact with caregiver's hands

   d. An infectious or pathogenic microbe

e. Person with compromised defense mechanisms

f. Someone with an acute clinical infection

g. Insect or rodent

h. Open lesion on the skin

3. Complete each sentence pertaining to the pathophysiology of infections.

   a. An _____ period occurs before the appearance of

      _____.

   b. The second period of infection is the _____ period,

      characterized by the onset _____ symptoms.

   c. Infections during the acute period may be _____ or

      _____.

   d. The final phase of infection is _____, during which time

      _____ occurs and _____ disappear.

   e. _____ bacteria require _____ to grow

      whereas _____ bacteria do not.

   f. Once a _____ gains entrance into the host cell, it transforms

      that cell's _____ _____ into a

      _____ producing cell.

   g. Localized _____ infections, known as _____,

      typically occur on the _____, _____ or

      _____.

   h. _____ are not likely to be transmitted from person to person, but

      _____ transmission has been reported.

   i. _____ and _____, the primary _____

      that infect human beings, invade _____ tissues and reside within

      the _____ _____ until _____.

4. List at least three consequences related to the emergence and reemergence of infection.

5. Give an example of how each condition or factor is contributing to the emergence of infections.
   a. Human behavior

   b. Demographics

   c. Economic development

   d. Global travel

   e. Food distribution

   f. Medical technology

g. Ecologic changes

h. Microbial evolution

6. Correct any false statements about new and reemerging infections.
   a. Typhoid is acquired from ingesting raw or undercooked eggs, beef, poultry, or milk.

   b. *Campylobacter jejuni* is an infrequent bacterial cause of gastroenteritis that produces severe watery diarrhea.

   c. Hanta pulmonary virus is transmitted to human beings through inhalation of aerosolized urine, droppings, and saliva from infected rodents.

   d. Although rare, West Nile virus produces a deadly febrile disease with a 50% mortality rate.

   e. *Borrelia burgdorferi* can produce a localized or disseminated disease known as Dengue fever.

   f. Creutzfeldt-Jakob disease is transmitted to human beings by prion proteins, which produce neuronal death, rapidly progressive dementia, and death in human beings.

   g. Methicillin-resistant *Staphylococcus aureus* infections are the leading cause of nosocomial bacteremia, urinary tract infections, and surgical wound infections.

7. Explain how each of the following measures helps prevent or control infectious diseases.

   a. Immunization programs

   b. Hand washing

   c. Avoiding artificial nails in patient care areas

8. Differentiate between airborne and droplet precautions.

9. Identify each agent that can be used as a biologic weapon.

   _____ a. Without treatment, the mortality rate from inhalation is nearly 100%.

   _____ b. A potent protein that is highly toxic when ingested, inhaled, or injected.

   _____ c. A zoonotic disease that follows exposure to tissues or body fluids of infected animals or tick or mosquito bites.

   _____ d. Infection occurs from inhaling a small amount of the virus that travels from the lungs to regional lymph nodes and replicates.

_____ e. Inhalation of spores produces a paralytic illness and respiratory failure that constitutes a medical emergency.

_____ f. A disease, transmitted by fleas, that causes high fever, malaise, and painful lymph nodes.

10. Contrast the actions and treatment for nerve agent exposure to that for vesicants.

11. Indicate the correct order of the emergency responder's actions when caring for a person who has been exposed to radiation.

_____ a. Remove the victim's clothing.

_____ b. Move the victim away from the source of contamination.

_____ c. Don protective clothing, masks, and gloves.

_____ d. Use soap and water to remove surface contamination.

12. **Case Study:** The infection control nurse noticed an unusual incidence of *Staphylococcus aureus* infections among infants in the newborn nursery. After meticulous monitoring of equipment and personnel, the nurse determined that a nursery nurse was infecting the newborns.
a. Explain how the nurse can be infecting infants while showing no signs or symptoms of infection.

b. On the basis of your understanding of nosocomial infections, what conclusions can you draw about preventing such infections as a whole?

13. **Case Study:** Several patients present to the emergency department over the course of 8 hours with similar symptoms: chills, fatigue, headache, backache, and vomiting. Each has a fever of at least 103.5° F (39.7° C). Two patients have small red lesions in the oropharyngeal area. List at least three priority actions that you should take on the basis of the data.

7 Rehabilitation and Chronic Illness

1. Fill in the blanks with the correct word referring to rehabilitation.

   a. _____ hospital stays for _____ problems and

      the _____ population with its related _____

      _____ have greatly _____ the need for

      _____ programs and facilities.

   b. Rehabilitation can occur in _____, _____

      _____, or _____ settings.

   c. Rehabilitation is focused on supporting the patient's _____

      _____ through _____,

      _____, and the use of _____

      _____.

   d. Rehabilitation nursing requires a _____ knowledge base to

      tailor care to patients' _____ and _____.

   e. Allowing the patient to master a skill a _____ at a time is a

      _____ used to build the patient's _____.

   f. The Level of Rehabilitation Scale includes _____ items that yield

      a general _____ of the patient's _____ ability.

2. Explain how chronic illness differs from acute illness. Give examples of each.

3. How does each of these factors affect chronic illness?
   a. Age

b. Race/ethnicity

c. Culture

d. Personal costs of disability

4. Describe the stages involved in the natural history of a disease.

5. Match the description with the correct theory.

_____ a. Homeostasis reflects the family's striving to maintain equilibrium in the face of internal or external changes.

A. Family systems theory

B. Family stress theory

_____ b. The stress event can be either external or internal to the family.

_____ c. The family's view of the event's seriousness constitutes the family's perception of the crisis.

_____ d. Rules are the family's expectations about family how each person's role relates to other members.

_____ e. Family resources may include social support, coping skills, or financial resources.

_____ f. Two of the family's most important internal resources are adaptability and cohesion.

6. Identify the phases of chronic illness.

_____ a. Downward spiral with profound physiological and psychologic changes.

_____ b. Symptoms are not well controlled but the patient is not acutely ill.

_____ c. Returning to a satisfactory life after a crisis of a chronic condition.

_____ d. Disabilities intensify as efforts to control them fail.

_____ e. Symptoms are controlled and the disease is considered to be in remission.

7. List at least two nursing actions for people with chronic illnesses that help:
   a. Limit disability

   b. Promote self-care

   c. Build self-esteem or confidence

   d. Support coping skills

8. Correct any false statements.
   a. Many factors influence a person's ability to carry out a prescribed treatment regimen.

   b. Goals of care for those with progressive, chronic illnesses are similar to goals for those with nonprogressive illnesses, but they take longer to achieve.

   c. Nurses have a responsibility to inform the disabled about their rights under the law.

   d. Nurses can advocate for the chronically ill by helping articulate their needs to the general public.

   e. The ability of the individual family to pay its own way is determined by the type of illness the family member develops.

   f. Epidemiology examines the causes of various diseases within specific geographic areas.

   g. Verbalizing fears and concerns does little to help families cope with a member's chronic illness.

   h. Spouses are more concerned than adult children about family, time, and emotional conflicts when a member is chronically ill.

9. Two patients have similar progressive chronic illnesses. One family adapts well and is quite supportive of their ill family member. The other family can neither adapt to the family member's illness nor provide adequate emotional support. On the basis of your reading, offer an explanation for the differences between these two families.

10. **Case Study:** An older man is diagnosed with a chronic illness that requires numerous dietary restrictions. Before his wife's death, she cared for him and prepared all his meals. Now he shows a general disinterest in learning how to plan or prepare his meals. Before his discharge from the acute care facility, the nurse sees the man eating potato chips, which are not allowed on his prescribed diet.

    a. Should the nurse assume that the patient is noncompliant because he does not care about his own welfare?

    b. What other explanation is possible for the man's behavior?

    c. Identify ways in which the nurse may intervene.

11. In what ways can the care of one person with a chronic illness be generalized to the care of all persons with chronic illnesses?

8 Palliative and End-of-Life Care

1. Correct any false statements about palliative care.
   a. Palliative care is whole person care based on interdisciplinary medical advances that prolong life to the extent possible.

   b. The nurse's primary role in palliative care is the coordination of care across all disciplines and health care settings.

   c. Advance care planning is limited to discussions regarding a person's living will and durable power of attorney for health care.

   d. Any verbal statement made by the patient may serve as an advance directive as long as it is documented in the medical record.

   e. Patients who are unable to pay for pain medications are more likely to be cared for at home.

2. Identify the category of collaborative management for patients at the end of life that each action addresses.
   F = Functional dependence and rehabilitation
   C = Comorbid disease management
   S = Symptom management

   _____ a. Monitoring of pain, dyspnea, and changes in level of consciousness.

   _____ b. Assessing the home for safety.

   _____ c. Ruling out underlying, reversible causes of dysfunction.

   _____ d. Providing close coordination with health care specialists.

   _____ e. Managing side effects of medical treatments.

_____ f. Using off-label drugs.

_____ g. Reviewing medications on an ongoing basis.

_____ h. Assessing family coping and behaviors.

_____ i. Helping the patient understand the benefit versus burden of treatment.

_____ j. Completing a whole patient assessment.

3. Complete the table related to pain in patients at the end of life.

Type of Pain	Descriptors	Effective Treatments
Visceral nociceptive		
Neuropathic		

4. How does intractable nausea and vomiting differ from nausea and vomiting in general? Who are the patients most likely to have intractable nausea and vomiting?

5. Identify at least one nursing action for patients receiving palliative care who have:
   a. Anorexia

   b. Constipation

c. Mental status changes

6. **Case Study:** A patient's family is grieving over the pain their loved one is experiencing. One family member is requesting palliative sedation, but another is concerned that palliative sedation is assisted death. How would you explain palliative sedation to the concerned family member?

7. Fill in the blanks of statements about the peri-death period.

   a. The underside of the body becomes _____ and skin

   _____ as _____ _____ is

   reserved for _____ _____ and is

   _____ to the body's extremities.

   b. _____ is thought to be the last sense to be _____,

   even though no evidence supports this belief.

   c. _____ sounds occur because of the inability of the patient to

   _____ up normal _____.

   d. Breathing becomes _____ and _____ with

   periods of no breathing, which is known as _____

   _____ breathing.

   e. Throughout the dying process the nurse must be aware of _____

   and _____ _____, _____,

   and _____ of the patient and family.

8. Explain how spirituality and religiosity differ as they pertain to dying and death.

9. Explain the mnemonic BREATH AIR.

10. Discuss strategies that can help nurses cope with the loss of their patients.

11. Differentiate between active, passive, voluntary, and involuntary euthanasia.

12. Why is death so difficult to define?

9 Emergency Care

1. Using the four color–coded disaster triage system, triage each of these emergency patients. Provide rationales for the triage assignments.
   a. A 28-year-old man fell from a roof while working. He has a wrist fracture, several small lacerations, and a swollen ankle. He is awake, alert, and reporting pain.

   b. A 3-year-old bit through her lower lip when she fell off her tricycle. Her lip is swollen but the bleeding is controlled. She is frightened and crying.

   c. A 62-year-old man has had an acute myocardial infarction. Emergency personnel defibrillated him at home for ventricular fibrillation. His blood pressure is 100/60 mm Hg, and he is diaphoretic, pale, and experiencing severe chest pain.

2. Explain the differences between level I, II, and III trauma centers on the basis of function and specialist availability.

3. Identify potential problems that the nurse may encounter when trauma patients present with the following physical findings.
   a. Unequal pupils

b. Substernal retractions

c. Confusion

d. Decreased urinary output

e. Decreased level of consciousness

f. Respiratory stridor

g. Decreased peripheral sensation

4. A nurse is present at a race track when a man collapses. The nurse renders cardiopulmonary resuscitation until emergency personnel arrive. Explain why the nurse can or cannot be held liable for his actions.

5. While playing outside, a 6-year-old child is hit by a motorcyclist traveling at a high rate of speed. A nurse is the first to arrive at the scene. The child is sitting up, alert, and crying. How should the nurse respond?

6. A 27-year-old rape victim is brought into the emergency department. She is very frightened and withdrawn.
   a. What subjective and objective data are important to obtain from the woman?

   b. How can the nurse provide emotional support to the woman?

   c. What actions need to be taken when planning the woman's discharge from emergency care?

7. **Case Study:** A 24-year-old man is brought to the emergency department after a gunshot wound to his abdomen. He has been drinking heavily, is thrashing about, and is belligerent. The nurse is chastising the man for his behavior while leaning over his chest to restrain him.
   a. Evaluate the nurse's approach to the patient.

   b. What can be done to deescalate the situation?

8. An elderly woman is admitted to the emergency department after a fall in her bathroom. The nurse quickly assesses the woman's ability to breathe, lung sounds, pulse rate, blood pressure, peripheral circulation, and neurologic status. What important assessment parameters still need to be assessed, if any?

10 Critical Care

1. Identify four or five characteristics that a critical care unit should ideally have to maximize care for critically ill patients.

2. **Case Study:** An adult patient is being cared for in a critical care unit. He has multiple monitoring lines and infusion pumps and requires hourly assessments throughout the day and night. How will the nurse know if the patient is experiencing sleep deprivation?

3. Suggest at least two nursing measures that may help decrease acute confusion in a patient being cared for in a critical care environment.

4. Compare the role of the critical care nurse with that of the nurse on a general medical or surgical unit. What characteristics of their roles differ?

5. Explain how the critical care nurse can obtain a history and perform a physical assessment on a critically ill patient that does not further compromise the patient's condition.

6. What information is provided by these monitoring procedures, and what are the primary nursing responsibilities for each?

   a. Intraarterial monitoring

   b. Pulmonary artery monitoring

   c. Intracranial pressure monitoring

   d. Continuous airway pressure monitoring

7. List at least two nursing activities that:

   a. Encourage the critical care patient and family to express their feelings.

   b. Keep the critical care patient informed about treatments and interventions.

   c. Prepare the patient for transfer out of the critical care unit.

8. Identify the patient outcome that each nursing activity addresses.
   a. Raise or lower the shades or open or close the window curtains to simulate a normal day/night pattern.

   b. Encourage family members to touch the patient or hold his or her hands despite the presence of equipment, dressings, etc.

   c. Provide explanations of procedures and offer emotional support to the critically ill patient.

   d. Place a wall calendar and clock in easy view.

   e. Avoid excessive conversation within the critically ill patient's hearing.

   f. Initiate teaching regarding rehabilitation and health maintenance.

9. A critical care unit's visiting hours, which are 10 minutes at the beginning of each hour, are strictly enforced. A patient in the critical care unit will probably not survive the night. The family wishes to stay with the patient during her final hours. How can the nurse best handle this situation?

11 Community-Based Care

1. A 75-year-old man with several chronic health conditions frequently forgets to take his prescribed medications. Identify some techniques that may help him remember when to take his medications.

2. A 34-year-old woman being treated for cancer had a peripherally inserted central catheter (PICC line) placed 2 months ago so that she could receive chemotherapy at home. Her husband, who is her primary caregiver, calls the home care nurse when his wife develops a fever of 101° F. What additional information does the nurse need?

3. A 62-year-old man with cancer takes 60 mg of MS Contin every 6 hours but continues to have severe, unrelenting pain. As a result, an epidural catheter was placed and he was discharged to home. He is receiving fentanyl at 4 mg/hr. His wife calls the nurse case manager stating that her husband is lethargic. What information does the case manager need to further assess the situation?

4. **Case Study:** A 92-year-old man with a newly created colostomy is being visited biweekly by a home health nurse who performs skin care and changes the skin barrier. Medicare coverage only pays for a weekly home visit, and he is worried that his financial resources are dwindling. The colostomy is functioning properly, but an excoriated area surrounding the stoma is present. The client lives alone but has a neighbor who occasionally helps him with simple chores. He has two sons, each living more than 200 miles away. They plan to alternate visits every other week. Analyze this situation and develop several alternative solutions that may address the patient's concern about the cost of home care.

5. **Case Study:** A 76-year-old woman was diagnosed with a progressive debilitating disease 8 months ago. She is weak and becoming confused. During the early stage of her illness she expressed her desire to remain at home and currently states that she does not want to go to a nursing home. She requires intravenous medications and assistance with feeding and all activities of daily living. Her husband is her primary caregiver but he, too, has physical disabilities. Even so, he plans to manage his wife's care with the help of their daughter, who is a registered nurse. The patient's health care insurance pays for limited home care.

   a. Discuss the discharge planning needs of this family.

   b. As the patient's condition declines, the husband and daughter struggle with the issue of continued therapy. Identify potential or actual nursing diagnoses related to this family situation.

6. **Case Study:** A 55-year-old man with chronic pancreatitis requires antibiotic therapy every 6 hours, total parenteral nutrition therapy at night, and central line care. His wife works part time, his son lives nearby, and his daughter lives approximately 20 minutes away. The patient is no longer able to assume his responsibilities around the house, such as lawn care and home maintenance tasks.

   a. Identify teaching needs for this family.

b. Discuss a teaching plan that addresses risk factors evident in managing the patient's care.

c. Identify factors that could contribute to situational depression for the client and caregivers if not addressed.

d. Plan strategies to help reduce the possibility of caregiver role strain.

7. **Case Study:** A 56-year-old woman with an infected leg ulcer caused by type 1 diabetes mellitus requires daily dressing changes, intravenous antibiotic therapy, fingerstick blood sugar analysis, and insulin administration. When able, her primary activity is baking cookies for neighborhood children who frequently visit. She insists that her care be provided in her kitchen because she spends the majority of her time there. Her daily care is becoming a financial drain. A friend who is a retired nursing assistant lives next door.

a. Identify factors that affect care planning for this woman.

b. How can these factors be addressed to reduce home care expenses?

c. Identify questions to ask the woman to assess her expectations regarding home care.

12 Long-Term Care

1. Correct any false statements about long-term care.
   a. Residents of long-term care facilities are most commonly between the ages of 65 and 85 years.

   b. Medicare funds acute care and long-term care for people who are financially destitute.

   c. Diagnosis-related groups are part of a prospective payment system initiated by Congress to control escalating Medicare expenditures.

   d. Less than 3% of certified long-term care facilities are government owned.

   e. Nursing homes have the option of participating in either Medicaid, Medicare, both programs, or neither program.

   f. The minimum data set is a lengthy screening tool that provides information about how to care for residents.

   g. A complete clinical record contains an abbreviated history of the actual experiences of a resident.

2. Identify the requirements that were set when the Nursing Home Reform Act was enacted.

3. List the four components of a standard survey for long-term care facilities.

4. What is the primary objective of the standard survey for long-term care facilities?

5. What were the major findings of the Institute of Medicine's "Improving the Quality of Care in Nursing Homes" report?

6. List several factors that are contributing to the shortage of nurses and nursing assistants in long-term care facilities.

7. What is the proposed education and training requirement for nurses working in long-term care?

8. Complete the following sentences.

a. The long-term care _____ is accountable for conforming with all relevant _____ and _____.

b. The _____ _____ _____ has by far the most employees, making up _____% of all nursing home personnel.

c. The long-term care _____ is responsible for compliance with all _____, _____, and _____ laws and regulations and for keeping the facility ready for _____ at all times.

d. Nursing services must be sufficient to provide supportive _____ care that allows each resident to attain and maintain the highest practicable _____, _____, and _____ well-being.

e. Long-term care facilities must serve _____ no more than _____ hours after the _____ meal was served.

f. Federal law requires a(n) _____ program to enhance the _____ of _____ for each resident.

g. The three plagues of _____, _____, and _____ account for most of the _____ in a human community.

h. _____ services must ensure _____ handling of soiled linens to protect _____ workers.

9. **Case Study:** Family members must admit their 78-year-old mother to a long-term care facility. The woman has a progressive chronic illness that has left her unable to assist with her own care. She is aware that she can no longer live at home. The family is concerned and grieving about their inability to care for their loved one.
   a. How can the nurse help ensure a smooth transition for the resident and her family?

b. What factors will be considered when determining the resident's ADL dependence?

c. Within what time frame must a comprehensive plan of care be developed for the resident?

d. Who will participate in developing the plan that will guide the resident's care?

13 Preoperative Nursing

1. What is the Perioperative Nursing Data Set, and what are the four elements it provides?

2. Correct any false statements about the preoperative phase of the surgical process.
   a. Contemporary perioperative nursing is more task oriented than patient centered.

   b. The preoperative phase begins as soon as the patient is scheduled for surgery.

   c. Most surgical procedures are given names that describe the site of the surgery and the type of surgery performed.

   d. Minor surgeries, although simple in nature, require the use of general anesthesia in most cases.

   e. Procedures requiring fiberoptic endoscopies are usually classified as minimally invasive surgeries.

   f. An advantage of open surgery is that patients have less postoperative pain and a shorter recovery period.

   g. Ablative surgery is performed to excise tissue that is contributing to the patient's pain or medical condition.

   h. Planned, nonessential surgical procedures are classified as elective surgeries.

3. Identify at least one fear that may be expressed by patients undergoing the following surgeries, other than the fear of the surgery itself or the fear of anesthesia.
   a. Emergency surgery

   b. Diagnostic surgery

   c. Cosmetic surgery

   d. Palliative surgery

   e. Curative surgery

4. A patient signed a consent form for surgery. Has the patient given informed consent? Why or why not?

5. Match the medications or medication classifications with their potential adverse effect(s) on anesthesia or surgery.

   _____ a. Potentiates effects of muscle relaxants

   _____ b. Decreases effectiveness of glucocorticoids

   _____ c. Can result in K$^+$ imbalance

   _____ d. May delay wound healing

   _____ e. Decreases platelet aggregation

   _____ f. Potentiates central nervous system depression

   A. Antihistamines
   B. Aspirin
   C. Antihypertensives
   D. Ephedra sinica
   E. Anticoagulants
   F. Glucocorticosteroids
   G. Diuretics
   H. Echinacea
   I. Antibiotics

_____ g. Bronchodilator

_____ h. Can cause hypotension

_____ i. Possible allergic reaction

6. Identify priority assessments (physical and laboratory) that need to be completed before surgery for each patient.
   a. A 45-year-old man with a 25-year history of cigarette smoking is scheduled for a lung resection to remove a malignant tumor.

   b. A 27-year-old woman with type 1 diabetes mellitus complicated by renal insufficiency is scheduled to undergo a laparoscopic cholecystectomy in the morning under general anesthesia.

   c. A 28-year-old woman is going to have a tonsillectomy. She has a history of asthma and will receive a general anesthetic.

7. Which of the above patients has the highest ASA score according to the Physical Status Classification of the American Society of Anesthesiologists?

8. Identify at least two potential complications for which the following patients are at risk during or after their surgeries.
   a. A 45-year-old man who is 50 pounds overweight and has a 20-year smoking history.

55

b. A 74-year-old woman who has dry oral mucous membranes, an elevated Na⁺ level, and preoperative diarrhea.

c. A 35-year-old woman scheduled for an appendectomy with noticeable scoliosis (curvature of the spine).

d. A 64-year-old man who has type 2 diabetes and inflammatory bowel disease with associated chronic diarrhea.

9. Explain how each action will help minimize the potential for postoperative wound infection in the patient undergoing open abdominal surgery.
   a. The administration of an oral laxative followed the next morning by a cleansing enema

   b. Assessment of the surgical site followed by cleaning and application of an antimicrobial agent

10. **Case Study:** A patient is scheduled to undergo abdominal surgery in the morning. She has a 30 pack-year history of smoking and leads a sedentary lifestyle. This is the first time she has undergone surgery, and she is anxious.

a. List two preoperative nursing activities to help minimize the woman's anxiety before surgery.

b. List two nursing activities to reduce the woman's risk for atelectasis or pneumonia and thrombophlebitis postoperatively.

c. Why should the woman's preoperative charting be accurate and thorough?

14 Intraoperative Nursing

1. Who are the persons directly and indirectly responsible for patient safety during the intraoperative phase of surgery?

2. When donning scrub attire, what area of the body is covered first, and why?

3. When a technician calls in ill the nursing supervisor sends a nursing assistant to sterile services to help prepare supplies and instruments for the next day's surgeries. Was this a good decision? Explain.

4. You are teaching a new scrub nurse about surgical hand antisepsis. Which procedure is acceptable to use in place of the traditional hand scrub? What are the essential components of this procedure? Why may this procedure be superior to the traditional hand scrub?

5. Identify each type of anesthesia.

   _____ a. Drug-induced depression of consciousness

   _____ b. Anesthetic injected through the intervertebral space into the space around the dura mater in the spinal column

   _____ c. Anesthetic agent injected by local infiltration or field block

_____ d. Anesthetic agent administered into the venous system of an exsanguinated extremity

_____ e. Anxiolytic that allows patient to remain responsive

_____ f. Anesthetic agent injected into the cerebrospinal fluid in the subarachnoid space

6. The nurse anesthetist is preparing to deliver a balanced anesthetic to a patient. What combination of drugs and anesthetics will the patient receive?

7. Identify the stage of anesthesia during which each of the following occurs or may occur.

_____ a. Extubation of the endotracheal tube

_____ b. Administration of intravenous agents in combination with oxygen and anesthetic gas

_____ c. Laryngospasm

_____ d. Uncontrolled reflex movement

_____ e. Endotracheal intubation

_____ f. Patient positioning

8. Match each of the following physiologic stress responses to surgery or anesthesia with its corresponding effect(s).

_____ a. Antidiuretic hormone secretion

_____ b. Aldosterone secretion

_____ c. Norepinephrine secretion

_____ d. Glucocorticoid secretion

A. Peripheral vasoconstriction
B. Maintenance of blood volume
C. Protein catabolism for energy
D. Decreased gastrointestinal activity
E. Maintenance of blood pressure
F. Fluid retention with possible fluid overload
G. Susceptibility to infection
H. Elevated platelet count

9. List at least two clinical manifestations of, and priority nursing activities for, the following complications related to surgery or anesthesia.
   a. Malignant hyperthermia

   b. Unplanned hypothermia

10. What are the possible consequences of latex exposure to a person who has a latex allergy?

11. How does each nursing activity ensure the safety of patients undergoing surgical procedures?
   a. Placing gel pads under the patient's heels and elbows

b. Placing a warm blanket over the patient when transferred into the operating suite

c. Placing a grounding pad on the patient's thigh before using an electrical cautery machine

d. Placing a wet towel on the surgical field when using a laser

e. Counting needles and knife blades before closing the surgical incision

f. Administering a prophylactic antibiotic

g. Placing a drain within a wound cavity

h. Placing a sterile dressing over a surgical incision

12. List at least four desired outcomes for the patient during the intraoperative period that can be achieved through appropriate nursing care.

13. A 48-year-old patient receives Demerol 75 mg IM and Versed 1.0 mg IV while in the surgery holding area. As the circulating nurse prepares to move the patient to the surgical suite, the patient reports beginning to feel nauseated and lightheaded. What should the nurse do first in response to the patient's symptoms and why?

14. A 78-year-old woman is scheduled to undergo a colon resection to remove a tumor. She has been in relatively good health until recently, when she was diagnosed with adenocarcinoma of the sigmoid colon. Why is the patient at increased risk for complications related to anesthesia?

15. Correct any false statements regarding nursing care of the patient during surgery.
    a. The cardiovascular system is the system most influenced by body positioning during surgery.

    b. Surgical positioning of extremities must not exceed a 90-degree angle to the body.

    c. The use of electricity in the operating room introduces hazards of electric shock, power failure, and fire to patients.

    d. Sponges, sharps, and instruments are counted before the surgical procedure and after the patient leaves the operating room.

e. Core body temperature is measured before and after all surgical procedures.

f. Intraoperative documentation includes all measures taken, equipment used, and patient responses to treatment.

g. Blood can be suctioned from the surgical wound, drapes, or sponges and be used for autotransfusion.

h. Procedures considered at high risk for potential infection include coronary artery bypass graft, colon surgery, hip and knee replacement, and eye surgeries.

15 Postoperative Nursing

1. Identify the three phases of postanesthesia care based on activities that occur in each phase.

   _____ a. Patient's level of consciousness returns to baseline.

   _____ b. Continues until the patient is ready to resume activities of daily living.

   _____ c. Encompasses the care of the patient emerging from anesthesia.

   _____ d. Patient achieves manageable pain status.

   _____ e. Protective reflexes and motor function return.

   _____ f. Patient is transferred to nursing division or short-stay unit.

   _____ g. Continues until the patient no longer needs one-to-one care.

2. A postoperative patient's oxygen saturation is 88% even though she is receiving oxygen. What is a plausible explanation for the patient's decreased oxygen saturation, and what should the nurse do to correct the problem?

3. Evaluate the adequacy of the following report given to the PACU nurse by the operating room nurse. Identify any missing data.

The patient is a 62-year-old woman who had a colon resection under general anesthesia for colon cancer. The entire tumor was removed, and no complications were encountered. Fentanyl was used as a muscle relaxant, and no antagonist drug was necessary. One gram of cefazolin (Ancef) was administered in the operating suite. The patient had an estimated blood loss of 280 ml. She received a total of 750 ml of lactated Ringer's solution in the operating suite. Her preoperative vital signs were temperature, 98.6° F; blood pressure, 150/88 mm Hg; pulse, 84 beats/min and regular; and respirations, 24/min. On leaving the operating suite, her vital signs were temperature, 97.9° F; blood pressure, 138/82 mm Hg; pulse, 88 beats/min and regular; and respirations, 28/min.

4. Correct any false statements about the immediate postoperative assessment of patients after surgery.
   a. Wound complications are the leading cause of morbidity and mortality in the immediate postoperative period.

   b. Hypoxemia may occur from hyperventilation, which increases the exchange of oxygen between the alveoli and atmosphere.

   c. Aspiration of gastric contents can cause pneumonitis and increased risk for secondary infections.

   d. The most common cause of hypotension during the immediate postoperative phase is increased preload secondary to hypovolemia.

   e. Hypoxia, respiratory acidosis, pain, or hypothermia can precipitate cardiac dysrhythmias in the recovering patient.

   f. Bradycardia, shivering, and decreased respiratory rate are indicators of hypothermia.

   g. If hydration is adequate, patients generally void within 6 to 8 hours after surgery.

5. Complete the following sentences pertaining to complications that can occur during the postoperative period.

a. Emergence _____ is an alteration in level of

_____ that most commonly occurs in _____,

the _____, and persons with a history of _____

_____ or _____ disorders.

b. The most common postoperative respiratory complications are

_____, _____, and _____

_____.

c. Common presenting clinical manifestations of atelectasis are _____

and _____, which may be accompanied by

_____, _____, or diminished

_____ _____.

d. Assessment for pulmonary _____ is challenging because

symptoms are _____ and _____.

e. Postoperative blood clots often form in the _____ of the

_____, _____, _____, or

_____.

f. _____ and _____ prolong

_____ time, _____ length of stay and

hospital costs, and increase postoperative _____.

g. Acute _____ dilation may result in _____;

_____, _____, _____

pulse; and _____, which indicate _____.

h. _____ syndrome occurs when increased _____

causes _____ and compromises the _____

of _____ within the space.

i. Prolonged _____ leading to urinary _____

may contribute to postoperative urinary tract _____.

6. What advantage or disadvantage does each of these patients have in regard to their wound-healing potential?

   a. An 8-year-old boy who recently underwent an appendectomy

   b. A patient recovering from a mastectomy who takes glucocorticoid steroids as part of her cancer treatment

   c. A nurse in a hurry does not wash her hands before changing the dressing on a patient's abdominal incision

   d. A patient who is a vegetarian takes multiple vitamins and minerals daily, but her protein intake is very low

   e. An 82-year-old man who has just returned to his room after a skin graft for a pressure ulcer, which was a complication of diabetes mellitus

7. Correct any false statements.

   a. The first actions taken by the nurse when wound evisceration is identified are calling the physician and preparing the patient for return to surgery.

   b. A patient with malaise is not necessarily experiencing a complication; malaise commonly occurs after any type of surgical procedure.

68

c. The device collecting bloody drainage from a surgical wound should be marked with the time and amount of drainage so that the amount and rapidity of bleeding can be assessed at frequent intervals.

d. Prescribed antimicrobial therapy should be taken by the patient for up to 2 weeks after surgery to decrease the likelihood of developing resistant strains of pathogens.

e. Tachycardia, cold clammy skin, a change in blood pressure, and vague reports of uneasiness from the patient may indicate the presence of postoperative hemorrhage.

f. Direct irradiation of a wound postoperatively may slow wound healing because it interferes with the development of blood vessels throughout the wound.

g. Pus and purulent material must be removed when cleaning a postoperative wound because pus contains enzymes that can irritate healthy skin.

h. Breathing exercises, early ambulation, and adequate fluid intake make the patient feel better but do little to prevent postoperative complications.

8. Which complication does each nursing action detect or prevent? Explain how the action will detect or prevent the complication.
   a. Placing a warm blanket, hyperthermia pad, or warming light over patients

   b. Reminding patients that they are not alone, that the surgery is over, and that they are in the recovery room

   c. Assessing pupils for equality and responsiveness to light

d. Administering oxygen by mask, catheter, or blow-by procedure

e. Placing patients in side-lying or semiprone positions, with their heads tilted back and jaws supported forward

9. **Case Study:** A 60-year-old patient underwent colon surgery to relieve a bowel obstruction. This is her third postoperative day. She has a nasogastric tube in place, which is attached to low suction. She has an intravenous infusion of 0.9% normal saline infusing at 100 ml/hr and an indwelling urinary catheter attached to dependent drainage. She has a patient-controlled analgesia pump, and is receiving meperidine (Demerol) for pain control. The evening nurse finds the patient disoriented to person, time, and place. Her skin is moist and pale. After further assessment and review of the patient's laboratory data, the nurse notes that her serum sodium and serum potassium levels are below normal.

a. Which complication(s) should the nurse suspect on the basis of the patient's data?

b. What is the most likely cause of the patient's fluid alteration?

c. Calculate the woman's daily fluid requirements.

d. What factor(s) contributed to the patient's loss of potassium?

e. The patient staggers and reports feeling dizzy when assisted in getting up to ambulate. What is most likely causing the patient to feel this way?

f. While ambulating, the woman confides in the nurse that she is afraid to use the patient-controlled analgesia pump because she fears she will become addicted to pain medication. How should the nurse respond to the patient's concerns?

16 Pain

1. A man is working with tools in his garage. When he tries to hammer a nail into a piece of wood, he accidentally hits his thumb. Trace the pathway of his pain sensation from his thumb to his brain, where interpretation of the pain occurs.

2. A young woman who is frightened of bees is stung while working in her flower garden.
   a. Explain her response to pain based on:
      (1) The affect theory of pain transmission
      (2) The specificity theory of pain transmission
      (3) The pattern theory of pain transmission

   b. How could the girl's pain perception be altered based on the gate control theory of pain transmission?

3. Two women in the same hospital room are both first-day postoperative after abdominal surgery for cancer. Patient-controlled analgesia infusion pumps are available for both patients. The patient in bed 1 has been receiving visitors and has used an average of 2 mg/hr of morphine sulfate. The patient in bed 2 is restless and crying out in pain despite using an average of 4 to 6 mg/hr of morphine sulfate. Compare these two patients by discussing possible factors that may be influencing their perception and response to pain.

4. A woman has just returned to her room from postanesthesia recovery after a total hysterectomy. She is awake and reporting severe pain. Select three pain modalities other than medication that might be considered in the pain management plan for this patient.

5. Each of the following patients is experiencing pain. Classify each as either acute (A) or chronic (C).

_____ a. Low back and leg pain of 2 years' duration

_____ b. Insomnia related to toothache and jaw pain

_____ c. Intermittent severe pain of 8 months' duration

_____ d. Sudden left knee pain persisting for 1 month

_____ e. Left arm pain of 48 hours' duration

_____ f. Intermittent migraine headaches over the past 3 years

_____ g. Abdominal cramping; vital signs within normal limits

_____ h. Off-and-on chest pain for 3 months

6. **Case Study:** A 59-year-old woman admitted for abdominal pain rates her pain as 3 on a numeric scale of 0 (no pain) to 10 (worst pain). Her vital signs are normal and no behavioral signs of discomfort are visible. The nurse concludes that the patient is fairly comfortable and in no serious distress at the present time.

   a. Is there any faulty logic in the nurse's conclusion? If so, discuss and make corrections.

   b. Is the rating scale alone sufficient to assess the patient's pain experience adequately? Why or why not?

7. **Case Study:** An 86-year-old patient is being treated for severe bone pain. Below are alternative pain management selections for this patient, who is rating his pain as 8 on a scale of 0 to 10. Discuss the advantages and disadvantages of each intervention in this situation.

   a. Demerol 50 mg with Phenergan 25 mg q6h IM prn

   b. Morphine sulfate 10 mg q4h IV prn

   c. Aspirin gr $\times$ PO q4h prn

   d. Heat and cold applications q2h

e. Toradol 30 mg IM q6h prn

f. Morphine sulfate 1 mg/hr per continuous PCA infusion

g. Decadron 10 mg q6h PO

8. Critique the following nursing care plan for a patient in pain. Give reasons for any additions, deletions, or changes.

Subjective data: "My incision really hurts. I'd say on a scale of 0 to 10, it's about a 10."

Objective data: Blood pressure, 170/90 mm Hg; pulse, 100 beats/min; respirations, 32/min; first day postcholecystectomy; grimacing on movement; holds body rigid; skin diaphoretic

Nursing diagnosis: Chronic pain related to abdominal incision secondary to surgery

Expected outcome: The patient will be pain free second day postoperatively.

Nursing interventions/rationales:

• Encourage the patient to report pain when moderate to severe. *Severe pain is more amenable to treatment and relief with analgesics, especially narcotics.*

• Use pain relief measures that the patient believes will work. *Attitude toward pain relief measures can provide a placebo response.*

• Administer analgesics on a prn basis for the first 48 hours postoperatively, *which will decrease the potential for addiction to opioids.*

• Explain to the patient and family that getting out of bed the first few times will cause increased pain. Instruct on splinting techniques. *Advising the patient of pain before it occurs decreases anxiety and increases a sense of control.*

17 Fluid and Electrolyte Imbalance

1. Match the following terms with their correct definition.

_____ a. Diffusion

_____ b. Osmosis

_____ c. Osmolarity

_____ d. Hydrostatic pressure

_____ e. Colloid osmotic pressure

_____ f. Hypertonic solution

_____ g. Hypotonic solution

A. The movement of molecules from an area of higher to lower concentration of molecules

B. The expression of the concentration of particles in 1000 ml of solution

C. The movement of water from an area of higher to lower water concentration

D. Pressure caused by blood pressing against the walls of blood vessels

E. Pressure required to overcome the pull of proteins in the blood

F. Solutions that exert a lower osmotic pressure than that of the cell

G. Solutions that exert a greater osmotic pressure than that of the cell

2. Correct any false statements about fluid and electrolyte compartments, distribution, and function.
   a. Plasma is the largest constituent of the body, accounting for 45% to 75% of body weight.

   b. Precise concentrations of electrolytes are vital to osmolarity, body pH, and overall homeostasis.

   c. The body expends a great deal of energy moving potassium back into the cell because the intracellular fluid can tolerate the presence of only small amounts.

   d. Plasma osmolarity is the main regulator of the release of antidiuretic hormone.

77

e. Vascular osmotic pressure drops and fluid leaves the vascular space if large amounts of protein leave the capillary.

f. Edema is the same as overhydration.

g. Inflammatory mediators that cause dilation of arterioles can increase capillary fluid pressure.

h. Antidiuretic hormone controls sodium reabsorption and aldosterone controls water reabsorption.

i. Prostaglandin is secreted in response to decreased blood fluid volume to increase systemic blood pressure and restore renal perfusion.

j. Inappropriate ADH secretion occurs when normal physiologic stimuli for antidiuretic hormone release are absent.

k. Vomiting results in the loss of bicarbonate, whereas diarrhea causes a loss of sodium.

3. Identify the fluid imbalance for each patient situation described. The patient may be at risk for more than one imbalance, so think in terms of "water" (hypoosmolar or hyperosmolar) and "saline" (isotonic) imbalances. Use these labels:
   SD = Saline deficit (isotonic volume deficit)
   SE = Saline excess (isotonic volume excess)
   WD = Water deficit (hyperosmolar deficit or dehydration)
   WE = Water excess (hypoosmolar excess or overhydration)

_____ a. An 80-year-old confused patient needs assistance eating and drinking.

_____ b. A 33-year-old woman compulsively drinks tap water.

_____ c. A patient is hemorrhaging from traumatic wounds.

_____ d. A poststroke patient has aphasia, paralysis, and difficulty swallowing.

_____ e. A young adult has third-degree burns over 60% of his body.

_____ f. A diabetic patient has a serum glucose level of 600 g/dl.

_____ g. A 70-year-old patient received three tap water enemas in preparation for a colonoscopy.

_____ h. An athlete runs 6 miles in 90° F weather.

_____ i. A 78-year-old woman has a history of congestive heart failure and is receiving prednisone.

_____ j. An elderly patient is receiving high-protein tube feedings without adequate water intake.

_____ k. A critically ill patient is receiving albumin and plasma expanders.

_____ l. A 45-year-old patient has just returned to his room after extensive abdominal surgery.

_____ m. A 55-year-old man has severe nausea and vomiting after chemotherapy.

_____ n. A 90-year-old man is receiving diuretic therapy.

_____ o. A middle-aged adult with oat cell carcinoma of the lung has syndrome of inappropriate excretion of antidiuretic hormone.

_____ p. A postoperative ileostomy patient has excessive watery stool output.

4. The physician has ordered "force fluids" for a patient with a diagnosis of dehydration. The nurse must make a judgment as to the desirable amount because no standard or specific amount is prescribed. Identify any additional data needed for the nurse to make the best possible decision regarding the patient's fluid intake.

5. An elderly patient is taking a loop diuretic for hypertension. The visiting nurse notes that fewer pills are left than should be, indicating that the patient has taken more than prescribed. Outline the potential fluid and electrolyte problems this situation creates and create a brief teaching plan for the patient and/or caregiver.

6. A 75-year-old man who was already malnourished contracted gastroenteritis and has been vomiting for several days. On admission to the hospital, his chemistry profile indicates a serum albumin level of 2.2 mg/dl. Identify factors important for assessing calcium balance in this patient. List data needed to confirm the patient's calcium status.

7. **Case Study:** A 69-year-old man is hospitalized with a diagnosis of congestive heart failure. Clinical manifestations include 3+ pitting edema; alert and oriented; blood pressure, 190/90 mm Hg; pulse, 110 beats/min and bounding; shortness of breath; weakness; and urine specific gravity, 1.002.
   a. Which of the patient's manifestations suggest fluid excess?

b. Explain why extracellular fluid excess is a common fluid imbalance in congestive heart failure.

c. Three days after admission the patient exhibits a 10-pound weight gain and his pitting edema advances to 4+. Lung sounds indicate crackles in the bases. The patient's blood pressure drops on standing, and urine output has decreased. These clinical signs indicate a fluid volume deficit. Explain how the patient can gain weight and yet show signs of extracellular fluid volume deficit.

d. Identify abnormal laboratory values and state the cause of each imbalance, if present.
Chloride: 90 mEq/L
Potassium: 3.1 mEq/L
Sodium: 136 mEq/L

e. Explain why a measurable increase in the serum sodium level is not evident (normal value of 136 mEq/L) despite the patient's fluid overload.

8. **Case Study:** A 72-year-old woman is hospitalized with a diagnosis of fever of unknown origin and diarrhea. On admission she exhibited: temperature, 101° F; serum sodium level, 150 mEq/L; skin flushed and diaphoretic; urine dark in color, and urine specific gravity, 1.038. Her husband states that she has been very confused.

a. Identify the signs and symptoms indicative of dehydration.

b. Which of these symptoms occur early on and are most indicative of cellular dehydration?

c. Because of her confusion, the patient is unable to eat adequately. A feeding tube is placed, and she is given high-protein tube feedings. What effect could the tube feedings have on her fluid and electrolyte status? Explain.

d. The physician orders 0.45% NaCl at 100 ml/hr followed by 5% dextrose and 0.45% NaCl with 20 mEq KCl. Discuss the rationale for these solutions and any precautions the nurse needs to take during their administration.

e. List at least three priority nursing actions appropriate for this patient.

9. **Case Study:** A 67-year-old woman has a 4-week history of diarrhea and a medical history of CHF. She takes digitalis and furosemide (Lasix) daily. She complains of extreme muscular weakness and is lethargic and apathetic. Her respirations are slightly depressed at 12/min; BP 100/66, pulse irregularly irregular; and serum sodium is 142 mEq/L. The nurse suspects hypokalemia.

a. Identify the cues that led the nurse to suspect hypokalemia.

b. The serum potassium is 1.8 mEq/L. Identify nursing actions that need to be taken immediately. Explain.

c. The physician orders 40 mEq of KCl to be given IV push. Should the nurse comply with this order? Why or why not? Give the rationale for your decision.

18 Acid-Base Imbalance

1. Match each acid-base imbalance with the correct descriptor.

_____ d. Results from hyperventilation

_____ b. Compensatory response involves
increased respirations

_____ c. Administer sodium bicarbonate

_____ d. Can occur from potassium depletion

_____ e. Assess for signs and symptoms of
potassium depletion

_____ f. Caused by retention of acid or loss of
bicarbonate

_____ g. Produced by hypoventilation

_____ h. Tetany and convulsions can be a consequence

_____ i. May be associated with hyperkalemia

_____ j. May be evidenced by Kussmaul respirations

A. Respiratory acidosis
B. Respiratory alkalosis
C. Metabolic acidosis
D. Metabolic alkalosis

2. Indicate whether the values of pH, $PaCO_2$, and HCO_3 are high (Hi), low (Lo), or normal (N) and the type of acid-base imbalance.

a. ___ pH 7.30, ___ $PaCO_2$ 50 mm Hg, ___ HCO_3 24 mEq/L _____

b. ___ pH 7.50, ___ $PaCO_2$ 40 mm Hg, ___ HCO_3 30 mEq/L _____

c. ___ pH 7.47, ___ $PaCO_2$ 32 mm Hg, ___ HCO_3 20 mEq/L _____

d. ___ pH 7.32, ___ $PaCO_2$ 30 mm Hg, ___ HCO_3 18 mEq/L _____

e. ___ pH 7.31, ___ $PaCO_2$ 52 mm Hg, ___ HCO_3 20 mEq/L _____

f. ___ pH 7.48, ___ $PaCO_2$ 48 mm Hg, ___ HCO_3 38 mEq/L _____

Make some generalizations about the direction of the pH, $PaCO_2$, and HCO_3 values.

3. Based on the example, analyze each set of arterial blood gases.

Example: pH, 7.25; $PaCO_2$, 55 mm Hg; HCO_3, 24 mEq/L

Acidic	Normal	Alkaline
pH	HCO_3	$PaCO_2$
Respiratory acidosis	No compensation	

a. pH, 7.48; $PaCO_2$, 48 mm Hg; HCO_3, 28 mEq/L

Acidic	Normal	Alkaline

b. pH, 7.22; $PaCO_2$, 50 mm Hg; HCO_3, 30 mEq/L

Acidic	Normal	Alkaline

c. pH, 7.22; $PaCO_2$, 33 mm Hg; HCO_3, 16 mEq/L

Acidic	Normal	Alkaline

d. pH, 7.46; $PaCO_2$, 38 mm Hg; HCO_3, 32 mEq/L

Acidic	Normal	Alkaline

e. pH, 7.39; $PaCO_2$, 31 mm Hg; HCO_3, 20 mEq/L

Acidic	Normal	Alkaline

4. Each patient is at risk for an acid-base disturbance. Identify the acid-base imbalance and outline a brief teaching plan focused on preventing the acid-base imbalance.
   a. A 48-year-old patient with chronic bronchitis

   b. A 40-year-old patient with acute pain and anxiety

c. A 20-year-old newly diagnosed patient with diabetes

d. A 75-year-old patient who frequently abuses laxatives

5. By applying what you know about each of the four acid-base disturbances, determine the acid-base imbalance for which the patient is at greatest risk. Write a nursing diagnosis for each patient.
   a. A 55-year-old man with a head injury

   b. A 22-year-old woman with asthma

   c. A 78-year-old man resuscitated following cardiac arrest

   d. An 18-year-old woman who is anorexic with persistent vomiting

6. Correct any false statements about assessment and management of patients with acid-base imbalances.

   a. If $PaCO_2$ is greater than 25 to 50 mm Hg, the patient may require intubation and mechanical ventilation.

   b. Changes in level of consciousness, lethargy, or coma may indicate progression of respiratory acidosis.

   c. Rebreathing into a paper bag is an effective treatment for severe symptoms of metabolic alkalosis.

   d. Intravenous sodium bicarbonate is highly recommended for severe metabolic acidosis.

   e. Monitoring for dysrhythmias is important because they can occur as a consequence of metabolic acidosis.

19 Shock

1. Correct any false statements about the etiology and pathophysiology of shock.
   a. The heart, large blood vessels, and brain function interdependently to maintain adequate cardiac output and tissue perfusion.

   b. Cardiac output is the amount of blood ejected by the ventricle with each heartbeat.

   c. The amount of ventricular stretch at the end of diastole determines the pressure on the walls of the ventricles.

   d. Systemic vascular resistance influences right ventricular afterload.

   e. Extrinsic control of peripheral blood flow is mediated by the central nervous system.

   f. Oxygen consumption refers to the amount of oxygen used by the tissues each minute.

   g. Oxygen delivery depends on blood flow and the percentage of arterial oxygen hemoglobin saturation.

   h. The oxygen extraction ratio provides an estimate of the balance between tissue oxygen consumption and supply.

2. Three patients are being cared for in the critical care unit. One patient is recovering from hypovolemic shock, the second is experiencing cardiogenic shock, and the third is seriously ill from septic (distributive) shock.
   a. Compare the three types of shock on the basis of their primary defects and characteristics.

b. What conclusions can be drawn about all types of shock, regardless of their cause?

3. Summarize the basic difference between compensatory, progressive, and refractory shock.

4. What is the significance of each clinical finding? During which stage of shock is it most likely to occur initially, and what additional assessments are needed in each case?
   a. Urinary output 5 ml/hr

   b. Periorbital edema

   c. Narrowed pulse pressure

   d. Tachycardia

e. Pulmonary rales and rhonchi

f. Lethargy and altered sensorium

g. Bleeding at injection sites

5. What is the primary desired effect of each drug when used for patients in shock?
    a. Epinephrine

    b. Nitroprusside

    c. Dopamine

6. A patient has been ordered to receive an intravenous vasoactive drug. What nursing activities related to this procedure will need to be implemented?

7. What is the primary benefit of these mechanical supports when used to treat shock?
    a. Intraaortic balloon counterpulsation

    b. Ventricular assist device

c. Pneumatic antishock garment

8. Match the solutions with their correct definition, use, or example.

_____ a. Produces rapid expansion of plasma
volume

A. Whole blood
B. Albumin
C. Dextran
D. Packed red blood cells
E. Hespan
F. Ringer's solution

_____ b. Most commonly used for initial fluid
replacement

_____ c. May produce circulatory overload in
patients with severe congestive heart failure

_____ d. Does not contain lactate; it can therefore be
given to patients with hypoperfusion

_____ e. Advantageous because of low incidence of
anaphylactic reactions

_____ f. Increases oxygen-carrying capacity of blood

_____ g. May precipitate congestive heart failure after rapid
infusion

_____ h. Inadequate for volume replacement or correction
of hypovolemia

_____ i. Provides additional potassium and calcium

9. **Case Study:** A 28-year-old woman was admitted to the critical care unit with suspected sepsis and septic shock. She is receiving oxygen, an intravenous infusion of lactated Ringer's solution at 250 ml/hr, and intravenous antibiotics. Her skin is flushed, warm, and dry. Her rectal temperature is 104° F (40° C), heart rate is 124 beats/min, respirations are 36/min, and blood pressure is 80/40 mm Hg.

   a. What are the four primary pathophysiologic changes that occur with septic shock?

   b. Based on the woman's clinical manifestations, what phase of shock is she most likely in?

   c. Why is the pulse pressure widened during this early phase of septic shock?

   d. Why is the woman receiving such large volumes of intravenous fluids if she has lost no fluids from bleeding or other means?

10. **Case Study:** A 37-year-old man is admitted to the critical care unit, having collapsed after a bee sting. He is severely dyspneic, flushed, diaphoretic, and anxious. Intravenous epinephrine has been administered, and he is receiving oxygen.

   a. What are the primary defects occurring during anaphylaxis?

   b. Why does shock follow anaphylaxis if it is not treated?

c. Why are compensatory mechanisms unable to reverse or retard anaphylactic shock?

11. A 60-year-old man is being treated for hemorrhagic shock from injuries received during an automobile crash. Cite at least two nursing activities that address each of the following categories of care.
   a. Cardiac support

   b. Respiratory support

   c. Preventing infection

   d. Promoting comfort and rest

20 Assessment of the Immune System

1. In your own words, describe the differences between innate and adaptive immunity. Give examples of each.

2. Correct any false statements about the inflammatory response.
   a. Eosinophils and basophils are phagocytic cells, whereas neutrophils and monocytes protect by releasing vasoactive chemicals.

   b. Basophils are the most efficient and responsive of the phagocytic cells.

   c. Once the inflammatory response is initiated, eosinophils are the first cells to migrate to the site of infection or injury.

   d. Macrophages capture and destroy foreign antigens found in the fluids of their environment.

   e. Basophils degranulate and release vasoactive mediators that act on smooth muscle and blood vessel walls.

   f. Natural killer cells secrete interferons that enhance macrophage ability to kill microbes.

   g. Complement serves to accentuate or complete the action of phagocytic cells.

97

3. Explain the importance of serum complement and interferon to the immune system.

4. Differentiate between localized and systemic inflammation.

5. Use an analogy to explain cellular and humoral immunity.

6. Identify at least one primary function of each immune cell.
   a. Macrophages

   b. Antibodies

   c. T4 helper (inducer) cells

   d. T8 suppressor cells

   e. Delayed T cells

f. Cytotoxic T cells

g. Memory cells

7. Explain the major differences between the primary and secondary responses.

8. What changes occur in the immune system as a result of aging that may leave a 70-year-old at greater risk for infection than a 30- or 40-year-old?

9. What additional assessments or history is needed when any of the following problems are noted on initial assessment of a patient?
   a. Wheezing

   b. Localized area of increased skin temperature around a joint

   c. Periorbital edema

d. Masklike facies

e. Cough producing thick yellow or green sputum

f. Reports of pain when lymph nodes are palpated

10. Explain the significance of each patient's data.
    a. A 78-year-old man has a white blood cell count of 4200/cm^3.

    b. A 47-year-old woman has a lymphocyte count of 52%.

    c. A 32-year-old woman has an elevated erythrocyte sedimentation rate.

    d. A patient's differential count demonstrates a shift to the left.

e. A 28-year-old woman has a CH50 of 138 mg/dl.

11. Which immune cells are affected in each situation? How are they affected?
    a. Allergic asthma

    b. Acute exacerbation of an autoimmune disease

    c. Chemotherapy

    d. Antigen-antibody reaction (e.g., acute glomerulonephritis)

    e. Intestinal parasites

12. Identify the condition(s) for which these diagnostic tests are indicated, and give the name of the involved cell or antibody as applicable.
    a. Rheumatoid factor

b. Antinuclear antibodies

c. Indirect Coombs' test

d. Enzyme-linked immunosorbent assay

e. LE cells

13. You have just given a patient an intradermal skin test for histoplasmin. After explaining that you will read his skin test at 24, 48, and 72 hours, he asks you why three readings are necessary and if a positive test means he has histoplasmosis. What is the best answer to the patient's question?

14. **Case Study:** A 67-year-old woman has been admitted for fatigue and loss of appetite. While returning to bed, she reports pain in her knees and back. Assessment reveals a scaly, reddened rash over her upper trunk. Her temperature is 101° F, pulse is 86 beats/min, respirations are 30/min, and blood pressure is 146/86 mm Hg.

a. Which finding suggests that she has an infection?

b. What further information is needed to confirm the presence of infection?

21 Immunologic Problems

1. A patient has just completed his second round of chemotherapy for lung cancer. Another patient is being treated for severe combined immunodeficiency disease.
   a. What are the major similarities between these two patients?

   b. What are the primary differences in their conditions?

2. What type of immunosuppression is produced by each of the following therapies?
   a. Radiation therapy

   b. Weekly injections of specific antigens

   c. Prednisone (glucocorticosteroid) therapy

   d. RhoGAM administration

3. In what ways are monoclonal and polyclonal gammopathies different?

4. **Case Study:** A 47-year-old woman has been admitted to the acute care facility for suspected early-stage multiple myeloma. She has mild spinal cord compression without paraplegia or quadriplegia. She is in renal insufficiency. A complete blood count and differential, urinalysis, and beta 2 microglobulin test have been completed.
   a. Which laboratory values will be abnormal if the patient has multiple myeloma?

   b. List measures to protect the patient's spinal stability and explain why such measures are necessary?

   c. Why is multiple myeloma considered an immune disorder?

5. Match the hypersensitivity reaction with the correct descriptor.

_____ a. Wheal and flair appear within 30 minutes

_____ b. Skin graft rejection

_____ c. Results from IgE attachment to mast cells

_____ d. Produces erythema and edema within
        3 to 8 hours

_____ e. Causes release of histamine and kinins from
        mast cells

_____ f. Involves IgG, IgM, and complement

_____ g. Hemolytic disease

_____ h. Produces erythema and edema within 24 to 48 hours

_____ i. Causes inappropriate stimulation of the target cell

_____ j. "Hay fever" and allergies

_____ k. Involves primarily polymorphonuclear neutrophil leukocytes

_____ l. Produces direct cytotoxic destruction of cells

_____ m. Tuberculin reaction

_____ n. Autoantibodies bind to target cell surface antigens

_____ o. Serum sickness

_____ p. Systemic anaphylaxis

A. Type I: immediate
B. Type II: cytotoxic
C. Type II: immune complex
D. Type IV: cell mediated
E. Type V: stimulatory

6. A 25-year-old man lived in a hot, damp climate most of his life without ever contracting serious illnesses or requiring antibiotics. After moving to a warm, dry climate, he developed an upper respiratory tract condition that progressed to pneumonia. He was treated with a broad-spectrum penicillin. Within 20 minutes of the first injection of penicillin, he developed systemic anaphylaxis. Explain how this is possible.

7. One patient has an atopic hypersensitivity. Another patient has a nonatopic hypersensitivity. How do allergy reactions differ for these patients?

8. **Case Study:** A 43-year-old man is receiving two different intravenous antibiotics for severe infection secondary to abdominal trauma. Within minutes after the third dose of antibiotic was started the patient starts having difficulty breathing. He is restless, pale, cool to the touch, diaphoretic, short of breath, and wheezing.
   a. List nursing actions that take priority in this situation.

   b. If the patient is hypersensitive to the antibiotic, why did he not react to the first dose of medication?

   c. Several hours after the reaction, the patient's blood pressure is 132/82 mm Hg, heart rate is 96 beats/min, and respirations are 26/min. His urine output is between 30 and 45 ml/hr, and he has no signs of peripheral edema. He is breathing normally. Are these assessment findings adequate to determine that a positive outcome has been achieved?

108

d. What is the most effective treatment for this patient's hypersensitivity, and how can it be accomplished?

9. A 31-year-old man with type O, Rh-negative blood is being treated for massive blood loss from a bleeding ulcer. Can this patient be treated with any Rh-negative blood type? Why or why not?

10. **Case Study:** A patient is receiving an infusion of whole blood. Approximately halfway through the infusion, she reports getting colder. Her oral temperature is 101.6° F.
   a. Which two reactions may the patient be experiencing?

   b. How can you differentiate between the two possibilities when they both cause fever and chills?

   c. What collaborative care measures will be taken for either of these conditions?

11. In what ways are delayed hemolytic reactions similar to graft-versus-host disease?

12. Identify several nursing measures to prevent or detect an immunologic blood reaction when administering blood or blood products.

13. A patient has no history of exposure to the *Mycobacterium tuberculosis* bacillus, yet her skin test was highly positive. Explain how this is possible.

14. Explain the concept of autoimmunity as you would to a patient with a newly diagnosed autoimmune condition.

15. In what ways may a "fatigue diary" be useful to a person with chronic fatigue syndrome?

22 HIV Infection and AIDS

1. Explain the differences between HIV infection and AIDS.

2. A young adult patient was exposed to the HIV virus 4 weeks ago. The enzyme-linked immunosorbent assay test is negative for antibodies to HIV.
   a. What conclusions can be drawn from this finding?

   b. Does any follow-up need to be considered? If so, what?

3. What is the single most important principle nurses must follow when caring for patients with AIDS or any bloodborne pathogen?

4. Explain why diagnosing the opportunistic infection *Mycobacterium avium* complex is sometimes difficult. Which assessment findings are most definitive?

111

5. List several nursing diagnoses that are appropriate for the patient with AIDS who has a *Cryptococcus* infection.

6. Identify the similarities between *Candida,* toxoplasmosis, and *Cryptosporidium* infections.

7. A patient with cryptosporidiosis has been admitted to the hospital for total parenteral nutrition. What ongoing assessments need to be made on this patient? Why?

8. A man has had AIDS for more than a year. He lives alone with his two cats. He is able to care for himself with occasional assistance from his sister, who visits regularly. What precautions must the patient take in regard to his cats and why? Should he be advised to give up his pets?

9. What conclusions can be drawn about opportunistic infections as a whole?

10. A 35-year-old man is very ill with AIDS. His parents are visiting from another state and do not know that he has AIDS. He confides in the nurse that he told his parents he has leukemia and he does not want them to know he has AIDS. How should the nurse respond?

11. A patient with AIDS has Kaposi's sarcoma. Because this infection is a malignant neoplasm, why does it generally go untreated?

12. Why should nurses who specialize in the care of older adults learn about HIV infection and AIDS?

13. Give an example of how any one of the *Healthy People 2010* objectives relating to HIV infection may be met.

14. Match the drugs with the opportunistic infections for which they are most commonly used.

_____ a. Azithromycin

_____ b. Toxoplasmosis

_____ c. Pentamidine isethionate

_____ d. Amphotericin B

_____ e. Rifampin

_____ f. Nystatin

_____ g. Streptomycin

_____ h. TMP-SMX

_____ i. Pyrimethamine

_____ j. Ethambutol

_____ k. Clindamycin

A. *Pneumocystis carinii*
B. *Cryptosporidium*
C. *Toxoplasmosis gondii*
D. *Candida albicans*
E. *Mycobacterium avium* complex

15. **Case Study:** A 25-year-old woman is being treated for AIDS. She has pneumocystis pneumonia, cytomegalovirus retinitis, and cryptosporidiosis. Her CD4 T-cell count is 250 mm^3. She is fatigued, anorexic, unable to perform ADLs, and occasionally disoriented. She has bilateral lung crackles, watery diarrhea, and a fever (101° F orally). Her heart rate is 96 beats/min, respirations are 32/min, and blood pressure is 118/82 mm Hg. She is 5 feet 6 inches tall and weighs 94 pounds. Her older sister, who is her primary support person, visits frequently and is well informed about the patient's medical history, current condition, and prognosis. The patient is being treated symptomatically and with combination antiretroviral therapy.

a. Categorize the patient's stage of HIV infection.

b. What changes have occurred in the patient's immune system as a result of her infection with HIV? Of what consequence are those changes?

c. Which assessments take priority for this patient?

d. List several nursing diagnoses appropriate for this patient.

e. Identify the patient's most obvious asset. Of what importance is that asset?

f. What teaching will the sister need if the patient's condition stabilizes and she is able to go home?

115

16. **Case Study:** A 29-year-old patient is being monitored every 6 months for HIV infection. He has generalized lymphadenopathy and is 10 pounds below his ideal weight. He is and has been free of opportunistic infections. His CD4 T-cell count is 500 mm^3, and his HIV RNA level is 10,000 copies/ml.

    a. What inferences can be made about the patient on the basis of his laboratory findings?

    b. According to the Centers for Disease Control and Prevention, which medications are appropriate for the patient at this time?

    c. What are the advantages and disadvantages of this drug regimen?

    d. What is the goal of antiretroviral therapy?

17. **Case Study:** A 47-year-old woman is being treated for AIDS. She was hospitalized 2 days ago for low-grade persistent fever, weight loss, nausea, and vomiting. This morning she vomited 250 ml of bile-appearing liquid containing a thick white substance. She has numerous yellowish patches surrounded by erythema in her mouth.

    a. What conclusions can be drawn about your findings?

    b. What treatment measures will most likely be instituted if the infection is limited to her mouth?

c. If blood cultures demonstrate systemic infection, how may her treatment protocols change?

d. For which problems will the patient be monitored if she is placed on intravenous drug therapy for her infection?

23 Cancer

1. Correct any false statements about the etiology and risk factors for cancer.
   a. The actual number of deaths from cancer continues to increase because of an aging and expanding population.

   b. The incidence of breast and colon cancer in women continues to decrease, but these decreases have slowed in recent years.

   c. Older adults are diagnosed with cancer more frequently than are younger adults because they participate in prevention and screening programs.

   d. African-American women have the highest cancer incidence, but caucasian women have the highest cancer mortality rate.

   e. Genetic differences among populations are why international variations in cancer exist.

   f. The three discrete stages of cancer development are invasion, propagation, and progression.

   g. Sixty percent of all diagnosed cases and 70% of deaths occurring in persons ages 65 years and older are caused by cancers.

   h. Breast cancer and ovarian cancer associated with the *BRCA1* and *BRCA2* genes are examples of hereditary cancer syndromes.

   i. Oral contraceptives have carcinogenic potential for breast cancer but exhibit a protective effect against ovarian cancer.

   j. Skin cancer occurs more frequently in persons who are directly exposed to sunlight than in those who receive ultraviolet radiation by artificial sources.

k. Tobacco contains 30 carcinogens that are present most often in mainstream smoke.

l. A higher intake of red meat appears to be associated with higher incidences of breast and prostate cancer.

2. What is the meaning of each term or phrase as it relates to the pathophysiology of cancer?
   a. Contact inhibition

   b. Cell cycle

   c. Differentiation

   d. Dysplasia

   e. Neoplasia

   f. Benign tumor

   g. Metastasis

3. Classify each tumor as malignant (M) and or benign (B).

   _____ a. Neuroma

   _____ b. Adenocarcinoma

   _____ c. Osteosarcoma

   _____ d. Fibroma

_____ e. Squamous cell carcinoma

_____ f. Lipoma

_____ g. Glioma

_____ h. Fibrosarcoma

_____ i. Meningioma

_____ j. Glioblastoma

_____ k. Multiple myeloma

4. Identify each of the diagnostic tests for cancer based on the description.
   a. Establishes a histologic diagnosis and identifies important cytologic features of a tumor

   b. Used to identify cancer in an asymptomatic person, precancerous lesions, or noninvasive cancer

   c. Allows visual inspection of the interior of the cavity being examined

   d. Radiologic examinations used in the diagnosis of cancer

5. Discuss the ethical implications of biotherapy.

6. What are each of these biotherapy agents and what is the primary function of each?
   a. Interferons

121

b. Interleukins

c. Growth factors

d. Monoclonal antibodies

7. Identify one reason why these cancer treatments may offer an advantage over other types of cancer treatments.
   a. Gene therapy

   b. Molecular targeted therapies

   c. Bone marrow or peripheral stem cell transplantation

8. Outline the major responsibilities of the home health nurse for primary and secondary prevention and early detection of cancer.

9. Identify preventive measures that may help these individuals decrease their risk factors for cancer.
   a. A 25-year-old woman with a light complexion and red hair is a radiology technician. She and her friends frequently sunbathe on the beach.

   b. A 54-year-old farmer uses fertilizers extensively in his farming operation. He and his family raise cattle, and their diet is typically high in animal fat. He thinks his father died of colon cancer.

   c. A 60-year-old woman with diabetes, hypertension, and obesity is married without children and began menopause 1 year ago.

10. Correct any false statements about radiotherapy for cancer.
   a. The most radiosensitive tissue in the body is the brain.

   b. Completely avoiding injury to normal tissue during radiotherapy is impossible.

   c. The time interval required for a radioactive substance to be dissipated by half is called its half-life.

   d. An individual who stands 2 m away from the source of radiation receives half as much exposure as when standing only 1 m away.

   e. Permanent hair loss occurs in any area treated with radiotherapy.

   f. Skin care includes keeping the radiation field moist by applying mild lotions or soothing ointments.

11. Two male patients with cancer are in their mid 40s. Radiation treatments are being planned for patient A before his surgical tumor removal. Patient B is scheduled to undergo surgical removal of his cancerous tumor. Radiation therapy will follow patient B's surgery. Provide a possible explanation for why the treatment approach for these patients is different.

12. Review the medication profile for a patient with cancer. Discuss the benefits and potential complications of the drug-to-drug-to-herb interactions.
   Paclitaxel (Taxol)

   Dexamethasone

   Filgrastim (Neupogen, G-CSF)

MS Contin

Ondansetron

Ginseng

13. **Case Study:** A 40-year-old woman with cancer is being discharged with a newly inserted central line (Hickman Broviac) for chemotherapy administration.
   a. Outline a teaching plan for home care.

   b. Discuss the advantages and disadvantages of having a long-term centrally placed venous access catheter.

14. Write an appropriate nursing diagnosis that addresses the chief problem for each patient situation.
   a. A patient has a platelet count of 10,000 mm^3.

   b. After chemotherapy a patient's neutrophil count falls to 600 mm^3.

   c. Identify nursing activities appropriate for both patients.

15. How might a nurse intervene to help cancer patients solve problems and make decisions regarding continuing treatment or pursuing unproven therapies?

16. **Case Study:** A 60-year-old man is in the terminal stages of cancer and is experiencing severe pain. Discuss how the nurse should begin planning care for this patient.

24 Assessment of the Respiratory System

1. Compare the terms ventilation, respiration, and breathing.

2. Think of an analogy to explain the term compliance. For example, draw a likeness to some common object.

3. Create an analogy to depict the mechanics of inspiration, expiration, and gas exchange.

4. A patient with chronic obstructive pulmonary disease is having difficulty breathing. The physician orders low-oxygen therapy to relieve the patient's dyspnea. Explain the paradox suggested by administering low-oxygen levels to this patient.

5. A nurse practitioner is performing a wellness examination on a 71-year-old man. During assessment, what respiratory changes can be anticipated on the basis of the patient's age?

6. Can chest pain of a pulmonary origin be readily differentiated from chest pain of a cardiovascular origin? Why or why not?

7. Compare nursing care for patients undergoing bronchoscopy, mediastinoscopy, and laryngoscopy, respectively.

8. Identify the method of physical examination (inspection, palpation, percussion, auscultation) that reveals each assessment finding.

_____ a. Crepitation

_____ b. Jugular venous distention

_____ c. Egophony

_____ d. Hyperresonant sounds

_____ e. Fremitus

_____ f. Central cyanosis

_____ g. Whispered pectoriloquy

_____ h. Asymmetrical chest expansion

_____ i. Diaphragmatic movement

_____ j. Rhonchi

9. **Case Study:** When obtaining a history and performing an assessment on a 57-year-old man with dyspnea, the nurse collected the data below. Analyze the data, decide if relevant data are missing and, if so, what. Explain the importance of collecting the additional data.

   Onset of symptoms occurred approximately 1 month ago and has continued daily.
   No complaints of chest pain but patient does complain of fatigue.
   Color is pink.
   Respirations are 28/min.
   Auscultation: diminished breath sounds in the bases with expiratory wheezing.

10. **Case Study:** A 65-year-old woman admitted with pneumonia exhibits the following signs and symptoms: medium-pitched breath sounds heard on inspiration and expiration between the scapulae; loud, clear auscultation of whispered "1, 2, 3"; increased fremitus; dull percussion; and bronchial breath sounds heard over left lower lobe.

    a. What is the significance of medium-pitched breath sounds heard between the scapulae?

    b. Auscultation of voice sounds can be elicited by what two methods?

c. How are the findings of whispered pectoriloquy, fremitus, and dull percussion in this patient interpreted?

d. What is the significance of bronchial breath sounds heard over the left lower lobe?

11. Correct any false statements related to diagnostic tests for respiratory abnormalities.
   a. Sputum specimens are best collected as the patient awakens in the morning.

   b. Special radiologic views such as the oblique, lordotic, or pronated may be obtained to visualize specific parts of the chest.

   c. Computed tomography is a technique used to observe movement in the area being visualized by radiography while the specific study is in progress.

   d. Magnetic resonance imaging is superior to computed tomography scanning in detecting lesions of the chest wall.

   e. Ventilation/perfusion lung scans provide a visual image of the pulmonary vascular system and are used to detect ventilation/perfusion patterns.

   f. Pulmonary function tests are used to evaluate the patient's disease progression and response to therapy.

   g. Thoracentesis is generally performed at the bedside with local anesthesia.

   h. Indirect laryngoscopy may be used for tumor biopsy or removal of a foreign object.

   i. A lung needle biopsy uses a lengthy needle inserted through the chest wall to remove a sample of lung tissue.

130

12. Match the pulmonary function tests with their appropriate definitions.
    Tidal volume (TV)
    Inspiratory reserve volume (IRV)
    Expiratory reserve volume (ERV)
    Residual volume (RV)

_____ a. Volume of gas inspired and expired with a normal breath

_____ b. Maximal volume that can be inspired from the end of a normal inspiration

_____ c. Maximal volume that can be exhaled by forced expiration after a normal expiration

_____ d. Volume of gas left in the lung after maximal expiration

25 Upper Airway Problems

1. A patient had endoscopic sinus surgery 3 days ago for chronic sinusitis. During the postoperative telephone assessment he tells the nurse he has reddish drainage. What questions should the nurse ask in response to the patient's statement?

2. Below are postoperative care measures for persons after sinus surgery. Provide the scientific rationale for each.
   a. Monitor for increased swallowing.

   b. Check visual acuity.

   c. Encourage fluids.

   d. Teach the patient to avoid nose blowing for 48 hours after packing, report increased pain, and expect tarry stools.

3. A 42-year-old patient has streptococcal pharyngitis. The patient also has a history of endocarditis. Why should the patient be taught to complete all the prescribed antibiotic therapy?

4. Develop a teaching plan that addresses the nutritional needs of the patient after nasal surgery.

5. Six days after a tonsillectomy, a patient notices an increase in throat pain and calls the office nurse. Identify questions that the nurse should ask to further assess the patient's status. What additional information should be provided by the nurse?

6. A patient is admitted to the hospital for diagnostic tests related to persistent hoarseness. Laryngoscopy confirms cancer of the larynx, and a biopsy indicates stage III: T3, N0, M0. Interpret this TNM classification.

7. Try to imagine having a tracheostomy and being unable to speak. You are in an intensive care unit and hear the sounds of a ventilator and other unfamiliar noises. What expectations might you have of the people caring for you in terms of alleviating your fears and anxiety?

8. How is patient care different when an individual has a radical neck dissection in conjunction with a laryngectomy compared with a laryngectomy alone?

9. Imagine that you have had a total laryngectomy. The surgeon has discussed the three speech methods that are available. Consider each one and identify factors that help you decide which may be best for you.

10. **Case Study:** A 67-year-old retired high school counselor is diagnosed with a maxillary sinus tumor. He is gregarious, enjoys social events, and has six grown children who live within 100 miles of his home. At the age of 31 he lost his left foot in a mowing accident but has adjusted to his prosthesis well. He is scheduled for a maxillectomy and left orbital exenteration. Discuss the emotional implications of these procedures and offer strategies for helping this patient.

11. **Case Study:** A 55-year-old patient who had a radical neck dissection 3 months ago communicates easily with his family regarding his needs. He has quit smoking but has not yet made an appointment with the speech therapist to begin vocal instruction. He is feeling well after the surgery, and his wife reports no problems with stomal care. During an office visit, the nurse notes that his color is pink, and he smiles and nods as his wife talks to him. He appears comfortable and is wearing a colorful ascot around his neck. Interpret the patient's behavior. Is he making a positive adjustment to his physical and vocal changes?

12. A patient with a tracheostomy tube receives a mechanically soft diet for lunch. Should the patient's tracheostomy tube cuff be inflated or deflated while eating? How will the decision to inflate or deflate the cuff be made?

26 Lower Airway Problems

1. Label each of the pulmonary disorders as obstructive (O), restrictive (R), or pulmonary vascular disease (P).

   _____ a. Pneumonia

   _____ b. Emphysema

   _____ c. Adult respiratory distress syndrome

   _____ d. Lung cancer

   _____ e. Pulmonary embolism

   _____ f. Chronic bronchitis

   _____ g. Pleural effusion

   _____ h. Pulmonary infarction

   _____ i. Asthma

2. Correct any false statements regarding restrictive lung disorders.
   a. Acute bronchitis is typically bacterial, but viral pathogens can cause bronchitis either as a primary or secondary infection.

   b. When administered early in the disease process, amantadine or rimantadine may minimize symptoms of *Staphylococcus pneumoniae* infections.

c. The mortality rate for persons with community-acquired pneumonia ranges from less than 1% among outpatients to 30% among those requiring hospitalization.

d. Hospital-acquired pneumonia occurs with aspiration of endogenous oropharyngeal bacteria into the lower respiratory tract.

e. A significant number of nursing home residents with pneumonia can be treated successfully with oral antibiotics.

f. Studies have repeatedly demonstrated that approximately 45% of the medication dose is delivered by a metered-dose inhaler, dry powder inhaler, or nebulizer.

g. Dehydration results in thick, tenacious secretions unless adequate fluid intake is ensured.

h. The patient with hypoxemia may not be cyanotic because cyanosis does not occur until deoxygenated hemoglobin level has reached 15 g or more.

i. The atypical presentation of pneumonia in older adults may delay diagnosis and treatment.

3. Discuss the advantages of using a spacer when delivering aerosol preparations by a metered-dose inhaler.

4. Identify current social, cultural, and economic trends and factors that may be influencing the increasing prevalence of tuberculosis in the United States.

5. Evaluate the effectiveness of tuberculosis skin testing, chest radiograph findings, and bacteriologic studies in the diagnosis of tuberculosis.

6. A 42-year-old patient is placed on isoniazid, rifampin, and pyrazinamide for an active tuberculosis infection. Discuss the implications of this three-drug regimen regarding side effects.

7. How are the diseases histoplasmosis, coccidioidomycosis, and blastomycosis similar?

8. A patient with a history of lung cancer is 2 days post left thoracotomy. The patient has anterior and posterior chest tubes with bloody drainage. The nurse decides to strip the tubing.
   a. Evaluate the nurse's action.

   b. At the beginning of the nurse's shift the water seal chamber was fluctuating. At the end of the shift 11 hours later, the fluctuation has stopped. What should the nurse do, if anything?

139

9. a. Compare nursing care for patients after left thoracotomy and left pneumonectomy.

   b. The night shift nurse decides to withhold morphine from the patient with the thoracotomy because his respirations are 10/min. The patient is rating his pain as 8 on a scale of 0 to 10. Evaluate the nurse's decision.

10. Provide a rationale for each intervention for the patient with acute lung injury/acute respiratory distress syndrome.
    a. Administering monoclonal/polyclonal antibodies

    b. Administering supplemental oxygen at the lowest concentration to stabilize ventilation

    c. Maintaining positive end expiratory pressure

    d. Placing the patient in the prone position

    e. Administering inhaled nitric oxide

    f. Securing endotracheal tube in place

    g. Monitoring pulmonary capillary wedge pressure for value below established range

140

11. **Case Study:** A 66-year-old patient is admitted to the critical care unit for a pulmonary embolism. The physician orders a heparin IV bolus of 10,000 U, followed by a continuous infusion at 1000 U/hr. The pharmacy sends a bag of 500 ml of D5 one-half normal saline with 20,000 units of heparin.

   a. How fast should the solution be administered in milliliters per hour with an infusion pump?

   b. On the second day of anticoagulant therapy, the patient's partial thromboplastin time is 55 seconds. What are the nursing implications of this laboratory finding?

12. What physical assessment finding helps differentiate closed, open, or tension pneumothorax from flail chest?

13. **Case Study:** A 58-year-old patient with a right pneumothorax has a chest tube set to 20 cm of suction (Pleur-Evac system). The suction control bottle is bubbling continuously.

    a. What nursing measures should be taken and why?

    b. During morning rounds, the nurse notes that the water seal compartment of the Pleur-Evac is constantly bubbling. What nursing measures should be taken and why?

141

27 Chronic Respiratory Problems

1. A 65-year-old man recently diagnosed with chronic obstructive pulmonary disease (COPD) is admitted to the hospital with symptoms of dyspnea and inability to do simple daily activities such as dressing. Blood gas analysis reveals a P_{O_2} of 52 mm Hg and a P_{CO_2} of 67 mm Hg. He is started on 2 L of oxygen by nasal cannula. Explain the rationale for placing the patient on low-dose oxygen therapy even though he has dyspnea.

2. Describe a food plan for an older adult patient with longstanding COPD who is extremely short of breath and finds eating difficult because of his dyspnea.

3. Differentiate between an acute asthmatic attack and status asthmaticus.

4. **Case Study:** A 22-year-old woman is diagnosed with asthma. She has a 4-year history of smoking. During hospitalization she is placed on a regimen of albuterol sulfate by inhaler and prednisone 40 mg daily. Two days after she is discharged from the hospital she calls the nurse with a report of chest tightness and severe shortness of breath. She is having difficulty speaking over the phone. She wants to know what she should do.

   a. What additional data does the nurse need to determine the severity of the patient's asthmatic episode?

   b. What instructions should the nurse give the patient?

   c. The patient does not improve, and the nurse instructs her to go to the hospital. She arrives by ambulance and is started on IV Solu-Medrol 125 mg every 6 hours. A loading dose of aminophylline 6 mg/kg over a 30-minute period is initiated, followed by a continuous infusion of 0.5 mg/kg per hour. The patient weighs 122 pounds. How much aminophylline should the nurse administer for the bolus?

   d. How much for the continuous infusion?

   e. The pharmacy sends 1 g aminophylline in 500 ml of D5 one-half normal saline. At what rate (milliliters per hour) should the continuous infusion be administered?

   f. When preparing to administer an intravenous antibiotic the nurse realizes that the antibiotic and aminophylline are incompatible. The nurse turns the aminophylline drip off for the 40-minute infusion. Evaluate the nurse's decision.

144

5. A 32-year-old woman with cystic fibrosis is single and lives with her parents. She was diagnosed at age 14 years and has had multiple hospitalizations for respiratory and gastrointestinal complications. What moral and ethical considerations will nurses face when caring for individuals like this patient, whose life expectancy has increased as a result of medical advances?

6. Identify at least two nursing responsibilities or actions for patients after lung transplantation.

7. **Case Study:** A 60-year-old patient is hospitalized for pneumonia secondary to COPD and started on intravenous antibiotics and low-dose oxygen therapy. Three days after admission the patient reports shortness of breath. The nurse notes a temperature of 101° F orally and auscultates fine crackles throughout both lung fields. The physician orders arterial blood gases, which reveal a Pao_2 of 48 mm Hg, a $Paco_2$ of 30 mm Hg, and a pH of 7.48. The patient is immediately transferred to the critical care unit and intubated. Chest radiograph findings confirm respiratory failure, and the physician orders positive end expiratory pressure.
   a. The patient needs to be suctioned. The nurse has the option of using a closed-system suctioning apparatus or a traditional suction catheter requiring disconnection from the ventilator. Which option is best? Why?

   b. The ventilator alarm sounds, but after a thorough inspection of the patient and equipment no reason for the alarm is identified. What should the nurse do?

c. The patient becomes restless, breath sounds are barely audible in the right lung fields, and color is slightly cyanotic. What additional assessment data does the nurse need to gather?

8. The pressure alarm sounds on a volume-cycled mechanical ventilator. What should the nurse do?

9. An 81-year-old patient with longstanding COPD has become ventilator dependent. He chooses to have the ventilator removed. What nursing actions are appropriate for this patient and his family?

28 Assessment of the Cardiovascular System

1. Use an analogy to describe the structure and function of the heart and major vessels in terms that can be easily understood by health care consumers.

2. A 36-year-old and a 69-year-old are being interviewed and assessed for cardiac health. How will assessments of these two individuals differ?

3. Compare the concept of preload to something familiar, explaining how preload affects stroke volume and cardiac output.

4. Which patients are exhibiting clinical manifestations most reflective of cardiac disease? Explain.
   a. A 50-year-old who reports difficulty "getting his breath" and a productive cough

   b. A 55-year-old who reports shortness of breath at rest and uses two pillows for sleep

   c. A 58-year-old who awakes suddenly with extreme dyspnea approximately 4 hours after going to bed and also experiences sweating and wheezing

5. A 49-year-old patient reports chest discomfort that he first noticed when he was mowing the lawn. It began suddenly and lasted approximately 5 minutes. He states that he had to stop mowing because his chest hurt so badly. What additional data does the nurse need to collect to correctly evaluate the patient's pain?

6. Place these events in the correct sequence as they relate to the cardiac cycle and impulse transmission.

_____ a. Atrioventricular node depolarization

_____ b. Impulse travels along Purkinje network

_____ c. Depolarization of left atrium

_____ d. Impulse travels down right and left bundle branches

_____ e. Ventricular walls are depolarized

_____ f. Depolarization of right atrium

_____ g. Impulse travels to bundle of His

_____ h. Impulse initiated from sinoatrial node

_____ i. Impulse spreads through internodal tracts

_____ j. Ventricular septum is activated

_____ k. Ventricular muscles are depolarized from endocardium to epicardium

148

7. Match the phases of the cardiac cycle with the appropriate descriptor.
   Phase 0
   Phase 1
   Phase 2
   Phase 3
   Phase 4

_____ a. Return of cell to negative resting potential

_____ b. K$^+$ moves out of the cell, and Na$^+$ influx stops

_____ c. Fast Na$^+$ channels open

_____ d. Plateau phase of depolarization

_____ e. Sodium pump moves Na$^+$ out and K$^+$ into the cell

_____ f. Na$^+$ rushes into the cell, creating a positive membrane potential

_____ g. Prolonged state of depolarization

_____ h. Cells rapidly become more negative

_____ i. Final stage of repolarization

_____ j. Cells are refractory to stimuli

8. Identify the effect on cardiac output as a positive/increased effect (+) or negative/decreased effect (0).

_____ a. Increased afterload

_____ b. Pain and fever

_____ c. Peripheral edema

_____ d. Administration of epinephrine

_____ e. Hypertension

_____ f. Administration of intravenous calcium

_____ g. Ventricular hypertrophy

_____ h. Increased peripheral vascular resistance

_____ i. Right ventricular failure

9. Identify the clinical manifestations that are strongly associated or diagnostic of cardiovascular disease with either a yes or no. Explain.

_____ a. Increased creatine phosphokinase MB in serum

_____ b. Central cyanosis

_____ c. Peripheral cyanosis

_____ d. Jugular vein distention

_____ e. S_3 heart sound

_____ f. Increased respirations

_____ g. S_4 heart sound

_____ h. Decreased hair on lower extremities

150

_____ i. Clubbing of nails

_____ j. Fatigue

_____ k. Pulsus paradoxus

_____ l. Palpable thrill

_____ m. Proteinuria

_____ n. Split S_1 heart sound

_____ o. Split S_2 heart sound

_____ p. Bounding pulse

10. The nurse notes that a patient being treated for a recent acute myocardial infarction has a central venous pressure within normal range but that it is gradually rising. She consults a co-worker who believes that this finding is not abnormal and advises the nurse to do nothing. Being concerned, the nurse consults the charge nurse who notifies the physician. Which nurse intervened appropriately? Why?

11. **Case Study:** A 52-year-old man is scheduled for a cardiac catheterization because of a 2-week history of exertional chest pain relieved by rest. The patient and his wife are extremely anxious.
    a. How can the nurse approach teaching to diminish the couple's anxiety? Include specific statements that demonstrate appropriate communication techniques.

b. After cardiac catheterization, the patient is instructed to remain flat with the head of the bed elevated no more than 30 degrees. The nurse notes that the patient's blood pressure is 140/80 mm Hg on return to his room from the catheterization procedure. A sandbag is in place over the right femoral area. Identify data needed to complete this postprocedural assessment.

12. A 63-year-old man is fairly active around the house and has no prior history of cardiac disease, with the exception of mild hypertension. He is moderately overweight and often reports heartburn after eating a heavy meal. His wife states that he sweats a lot at night and that his feet are ice cold. He reports increased fatigue and his shoes feel tight. Before coming to the emergency department the patient was moving some heavy boxes and began feeling pain in his chest. He stopped immediately and sat down on the porch to catch his breath, but the pain continued. He reported feeling dizzy and that his heart felt like it was beating fast in his chest. His wife immediately called 911. Identify the cardinal clinical manifestations of altered cardiovascular status depicted in this situation.

29 Coronary Artery Disease and Dysrhythmias

1. Correct any false statements about coronary artery disease (CAD) and its associated risk factors.
   a. Nonmodifiable risk factors for CAD include age, hypertension, sex, and race.

   b. The use of hormone replacement therapy is recommended for women in an effort to prevent heart disease.

   c. Adults with diabetes mellitus have heart disease rates approximately two to four times greater than adults without diabetes.

   d. Pipe and cigar smokers have the highest incidence of CAD.

   e. Obese persons are more prone to glucose intolerance and elevated triglyceride levels than nonobese persons.

   f. Homocysteine is believed to contribute to vascular disease because it activates the inflammatory response.

   g. The accumulation of mast cells within the vessel walls produces a fibrous streak that protrudes into the lumen of the artery, impeding circulation.

   h. Plaque rupture may leave a residual fibrous clot that extends into the lumen, partially obstructing the artery.

   i. Myocardial infarctions are classified according to their anatomic location.

   j. Patients having an acute myocardial infarction describe their pain as "mild indigestion," "tightness," "aching," or "stabbing."

k. The most common complications of CAD are heart failure, dysrhythmias, and pericarditis.

2. Identity the diagnostic tool for CAD based on the descriptor.

_____ a. Levels rise within 3 to 9 hours and return to normal in 1 to 3 days

_____ b. Pharmacologic agents may be used to simulate exercise response

_____ c. White blood cell count may elevate to 12,000 to 15,000/mm^3 in response to cardiac injury

_____ d. Serial tests or continuous monitoring

_____ e. Levels increase within 1 hour and return to normal within 24 to 36 hours

_____ f. May include both angiography and ventriculography

_____ g. Composed of three proteins; levels normally undetectable

_____ h. Elevations may be associated with increased risk for adverse outcomes in persons with acute coronary syndromes

3. What are these agents and how are they used to prevent or treat CAD?
   a. Aspirin

   b. Clopidogrel (Plavix)

   c. Reteplase (Retavase)

   d. Tirofiban (Aggrastat)

e. Heparin

f. Nitroglycerin

g. Beta-blockers

h. Verapamil (Calan)

i. Angiotensin-converting enzyme inhibitors

j. Morphine

k. Statins

4. Match the treatment for CAD with its correct descriptor.

_____ a. Remain in coronary artery as a scaffold and become
        infiltrated with endothelial cells over a period of weeks

A. Intraaortic
   balloon pump
B. Percutaneous
   transluminal
   coronary
   angioplasty
C. Stents
D. Enhanced external
   counterpulsation
E. Transmyocardial
   laser
   revascularization
F. Coronary artery
   bypass graft

_____ b. Balloon filled with radiopaque dye and saline
        is inflated at pressures great enough to
        reconfigure the arterial blockage

_____ c. Bypasses the obstruction by grafting an artery
        or vein to the coronary artery beyond the blockage

_____ d. Augments early diastolic pressure and coronary artery perfusion

_____ e. Cuffs around patient's calves and lower thighs inflate during diastole,
        thereby increasing coronary perfusion pressure and venous return

_____ f. By using laser energy, channels are created through the left ventricular wall
        into the ischemic myocardium to stimulate angiogenesis and increase
        collateral blood flow

155

5. Provide a rationale for nursing actions included in the care plan for a patient with CAD.
   a. Initiate oxygen administration.

   b. Prepare to administer thrombolytic agents within 4 to 6 hours of symptom onset.

   c. Monitor patient's anxiety and administer anxiolytics as needed.

   d. Include patient's sexual partner in teaching sessions regarding resumption of sexual activity after an acute coronary syndrome.

   e. Monitor for bleeding in patients receiving thrombolytic agents.

6. The QRS complex represents depolarization of the ventricles and is normally measured at 0.05 to 0.10 seconds. What is the implication of a wide QRS complex?

7. Discuss the similarities and differences between sinus tachycardia and sinus bradycardia on the basis of etiology, onset, clinical manifestations, and treatment.

8. An 80-year-old man with a history of sick sinus syndrome is hospitalized for diabetes and pneumonia. The nurse notes that the patient is becoming confused. How can the nurse differentiate among possible causes of this patient's confusion?

9. A 52-year-old man who recently had an acute myocardial infarction is having occasional premature ventricular beats. His hospital roommate is a 73-year-old man with no history of cardiac disease who is also having occasional premature ventricular beats. Identify the significance of each dysrhythmia in these two patients.

10. Identify three NANDA diagnoses that are appropriate for patients with any type of dysrhythmia.

11. Explain how a pacemaker functions by interpreting the three-letter code of VDD.

12. Transtelephonic monitoring determines that the patient's pacemaker is not sensing. What does this mean, and how did the interpreter know this? What are the possible consequences to undersensing, and what intervention should be taken?

13. Match the dysrhythmias with their appropriate drug therapy or treatment. Answers may be used more than once.

_____ a. Sinus bradycardia
              A. Diltiazem
              B. Lidocaine
              C. Digoxin

_____ b. Sinus tachycardia
              D. CPR
              E. Procainamide
              F. Amiodarone

_____ c. Atrial fibrillation
              G. Cardioversion
              H. Pacemaker
              I. Atropine

_____ d. Ventricular tachycardia
              J. Defibrillation
              K. Epinephrine
              L. Reduce caffeine intake

_____ e. Ventricular fibrillation

_____ f. Complete third-degree atrioventricular block

14. A 56-year-old man admitted to the emergency department is pale and weak. He has been receiving chemotherapy for colon cancer and has a history of hyperthyroidism. His complete blood count reveals a hemoglobin level of 8.6 mg/dl. Identify his dysrhythmia.

Rate/rhythm: Atrial _____ Ventricular _____

PR interval: _____ seconds

QRS duration: _____ seconds

Unique characteristics: _____

Interpretation: _____

Major cause(s): _____

Treatment: _____

15. A 69-year-old woman is being monitored while being digitalized. The patient's alarm sounds. The nurse goes to the patient's room immediately and finds the patient slumped over on the stool in the bathroom. Interpret the patient's monitor strip.

Rate/rhythm: Atrial _____ Ventricular _____

PR Interval: _____ seconds

QRS duration: _____ seconds

Unique characteristics: _____

Interpretation: _____

Major cause(s): _____

Treatment: _____

16. A 46-year-old man begins to feel dizzy and weak while driving to his job. He decides to go to the emergency department. He has no cardiac history, is normotensive, and does not smoke. He drinks beer on the weekends. Interpret his monitor strip.

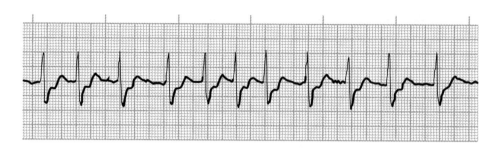

Rate/rhythm: Atrial _____ Ventricular _____

PR interval: _____ seconds

QRS duration: _____ seconds

Unique characteristics: _____

Interpretation: _____

Major cause(s): _____

Treatment: _____

17. A 75-year-old man reports that he feels "like my heart is skipping beats." He has mild congestive heart failure and is receiving diuretic therapy. Does he have a dysrhythmia? If so, which one?

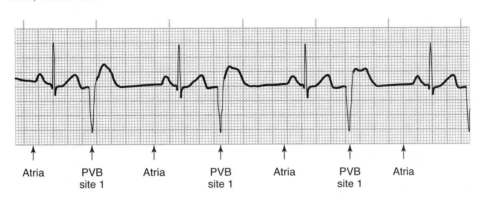

Atria   PVB   Atria   PVB   Atria   PVB   Atria
         site 1   site 1   site 1

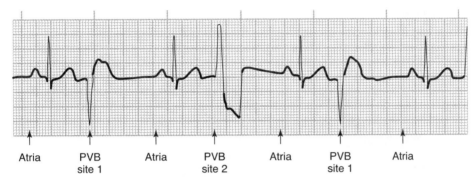

Atria   PVB   Atria   PVB   Atria   PVB   Atria
         site 1   site 2   site 1

Rate/rhythm: Atrial _____ Ventricular _____

PR interval: _____ seconds

QRS duration: _____ seconds

Unique characteristics: _____

Interpretation: _____

Major cause(s): _____

Treatment: _____

Chapter **29   Coronary Artery Disease and Dysrhythmias**

18. A patient is found unresponsive and without spontaneous respirations or pulse. Upon attaching a cardiac monitor, the rhythm is noted. What is it?

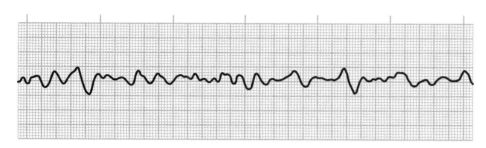

Rate/rhythm: Atrial _____ Ventricular _____

PR interval: _____ seconds

QRS duration: _____ seconds

Unique characteristics: _____

Interpretation: _____

Major cause(s): _____

Treatment: _____

19. A patient with a history of severe coronary artery disease and multiple admissions for chest pain is admitted to the emergency department 2 weeks after his third angioplasty. Interpret the patient's monitor strip.

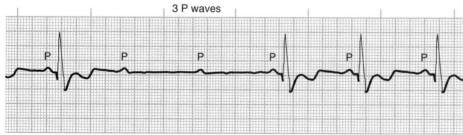

3:1 block

Rate/rhythm: Atrial _____ Ventricular _____

PR interval: _____ seconds

QRS duration: _____ seconds

Unique characteristics: _____

Interpretation: _____

Major cause(s): _____

Treatment: _____

20. Answer the multiple-choice items related to dysrhythmias, pacemakers, and cardiopulmonary resuscitation.
   a. The nurse finds a patient unconscious and without a pulse. The bedside monitor
      shows ventricular fibrillation. What does the nurse do first?
      1. Prepare the patient for pacemaker insertion.
      2. Administer intravenous epinephrine.
      3. Run for the crash cart.
      4. Begin CPR.

   b. The nurse understands that during treatment of atrial dysrhythmias with cardio-
      version the shock is
      1. Timed to hit the T wave
      2. Synchronized with the R wave
      3. Delivered during the refractory period
      4. Initiated anywhere during the cardiac cycle

   c. The nurse notes that a patient's ventricular heart rate suddenly drops to 38 beats/
      min and the patient loses consciousness. The nurse's first action is to
      1. Determine the cause of the syncopal episode.
      2. Administer atropine as ordered.
      3. Call a code blue.
      4. Initiate CPR.

d. The purpose of a demand pacemaker is to
   1. Establish normal heart rate and rhythm when no QRS is sensed.
   2. Obtain baseline data during exercise.
   3. Establish normal atrioventricular synchrony.
   4. Prevent dysrhythmias.

e. Which nursing action is most appropriate immediately after insertion of a pacemaker?
   1. Promotion of activity to prevent thrombophlebitis
   2. Assessment of heart rate, rhythm, and vital signs
   3. Administration of anticoagulants to prevent clot formation
   4. Provision of a quiet environment to avoid extraneous stimuli

f. The effectiveness of patient teaching for home care of the pacemaker can be determined when the patient states that she or he will
   1. Follow a low-sodium diet.
   2. Monitor apical pulse daily.
   3. Monitor blood pressure daily.
   4. Avoid using electrical equipment.

g. The first step in basic life support is to
   1. Open the airway.
   2. Restore breathing.
   3. Provide drug therapy.
   4. Initiate external cardiac compressions.

h. Which is the most common cause of respiratory obstruction in the unconscious patient?
   1. Food
   2. Vomitus
   3. Dentures
   4. The tongue

i. The safest first approach to opening the airway of an individual with a suspected neck injury is
   1. The head tilt
   2. The jaw thrust
   3. The head tilt/chin lift
   4. Turning the head to the side

j. CPR may be discontinued if which condition occurs?
   1. The rescuer believes that the patient is dead.
   2. The rescuer is unable to access help.
   3. Pupils are dilated and fixed.
   4. Another rescuer takes over.

k. Epinephrine is commonly given during resuscitation because it
   1. Causes vasodilation
   2. Has a negative inotropic effect
   3. Reduces myocardial contractility
   4. Enhances the effects of compressions and defibrillation

l. The most common complication of external cardiac massage is
   1. Fractured ribs
   2. Pneumothorax
   3. Torsades de pointes
   4. Pericardial tamponade

30 Heart Failure, Valvular Problems, and Inflammatory Problems of the Heart

1. Match the cardiac condition with its correct descriptor or necessary patient teaching.

_____ a. May occur from drug hypersensitivity, toxicity, or infection.

    A. Myocarditis

    B. Endocarditis

    C. Infective endocarditis

_____ b. Penicillin is the drug of choice for acute episodes and prevention of recurrence.

_____ c. Pericardial pain is the most common symptom during the acute phase of illness.

_____ d. Produces valvular vegetation.

_____ e. Inflammation may involve the lining of the heart or valves.

_____ f. Symptoms may include arthralgia, arthritis, low back pain, or hemoptysis.

_____ g. Inform your dentist of your disease history so that prophylactic antibiotics can be administered before invasive procedures.

_____ h. You will need to know the early warning signs of heart failure so that they can be reported immediately.

_____ i. Avoid excessive fatigue and stop activity immediately if you experience lightheadedness, dizziness, or chest pain.

_____ j. You should avoid the use of nonsteroidal antiinflammatory drugs until medically cleared by your primary care provider.

_____ k. You should avoid persons with infections.

2. Identify each of the valvular diseases by their definitions.

_____ a. The prolapse of one or more valve leaflets into the left atrium during systole

_____ b. Obstructs the flow of blood from the right atrium to the right ventricle

_____ c. Permits the return of blood from the aorta to the left ventricle during diastole

_____ d. Obstruction caused by adhesions between leaflets, which is attributable to calcification, loss of mobility, or fibrosis

_____ e. Causes obstruction of the systolic ejection of blood from the left ventricle into the ascending aorta

_____ f. Regurgitation of blood from the left ventricle to the right atrium during ventricular systole

3. Three patients have different inflammatory heart conditions. One has acute pericarditis, another has chronic pericarditis, and the third has myocarditis. How do these three patients differ based on pathophysiology and collaborative management?

4. Describe the different types of heart failure in your own words.
   a. High-output heart failure

b. Low-output heart failure

c. Left heart failure

d. Right heart failure

e. Backward heart failure

f. Forward heart failure

5. **Case Study:** The nurse notices that a patient being treated for heart failure has audible wheezing and is restless, irritable, and pale. His heart rate is 140 beats/min, and he is gasping for air.
   a. How should the nurse respond?

   b. What is the probable cause of the patient's clinical manifestations?

   c. What are the treatment goals for this patient?

6. Give an example of each class of medication, and list at least one advantage of using this type of medication for treating heart failure.
   a. Diuretics

   b. Vasodilators

Chapter **30** **Heart Failure, Valvular Problems, and Inflammatory Problems of the Heart**

c. Angiotensin-converting enzyme inhibitors

d. Inotropics

e. Beta-blockers

f. Calcium channel blockers

7. Identify at least one nursing action that addresses each of the following problems encountered by patients with heart failure.
   a. Impaired gas exchange

   b. Imbalanced fluid volume

   c. Activity intolerance

   d. Decreased cardiac output

   e. Deficient knowledge

8. **Case Study:** A 73-year-old woman is hospitalized for treatment of heart failure. Her medications include digitalis, Lasix, and Synthroid. The day before discharge she develops frequent ectopic heart beats and diarrhea. She reports headache and double vision. Her laboratory data indicate that her digitalis level is too high, her blood urea nitrogen and serum creatinine levels are slightly elevated, and her potassium and magnesium levels are too low. All other tests are within normal limits.
   a. Speculate about the cause of the patient's elevated digitalis level because she is on a standard dose of digitalis.

   b. Explain the relation between heart failure and renal compromise.

c. Identify several nursing actions for the patient in heart failure.

9. The nurse suspects that a patient is developing pulmonary edema. The presence of which clinical manifestations will help support the nurse's suspicion?

10. Identify the valvular diseases that can result from these cardiac conditions.
    a. Rheumatic fever

    b. Congenital heart defect

    c. Syphilis

    d. Genetic factors

    e. Autosomal dominant disorder

    f. Atrial tumor

    g. Coronary heart disease

    h. Bacterial endocarditis

11. A patient is scheduled for cardiac valve replacement surgery in the morning. What preoperative teaching is needed for this patient?

12. Correct any false statements related to care of the patient undergoing cardiac surgery.
   a. The patient's alcohol or smoking habits are of little importance preoperatively because the patient will not be allowed to smoke or drink while hospitalized.

   b. The complete blood count, white blood cell count, differential, coagulation profile, and pulmonary function studies will be carefully evaluated before cardiac surgery.

   c. If the patient has lung crackles or wheezes, surgery may be postponed to prevent further respiratory complications.

   d. An electrocardiogram will be considered before cardiac surgery, but cardiac enzymes are of little importance because the surgery will correct cardiac problems.

   e. The patient's perception of his or her illness is less important to consider preoperatively than other factors.

13. A patient scheduled for coronary artery bypass graft surgery voices concern about having open heart surgery and wants to know what the "machine" she will be placed on will do for her. How can the nurse best answer this question?

14. Immediately after cardiac surgery, a patient is placed on intraaortic balloon pump counterpulsation. What can be done to prevent the following complications?
   a. Circulatory insufficiency in the catheterized leg

b. Aortic damage

c. Infection

15. Identify possible complications after cardiac surgery that may be present if the patient develops or demonstrates the following.
   a. Cardiac dysrhythmias

   b. Cold, clammy skin

   c. Shivering

   d. Cessation of chest drainage 1 hour after surgery

   e. Disorientation and restlessness

   f. Increased serum creatinine

16. **Case Study:** A 52-year-old man is waiting for a heart transplant because of restrictive cardiomyopathy.
   a. Describe the relation between cardiomyopathy and heart failure.

   b. How will the patient's care be managed while awaiting a donor heart?

31 Vascular Problems

1. Discuss the relation between atherosclerosis, diabetes, heart disease, hypertension, arterial occlusive disease, and stroke.

2. Place a *P* before conditions that may cause primary hypertension and an *S* before conditions that may cause secondary hypertension.

_____ a. Glomerulonephritis

_____ b. Atherosclerosis

_____ c. Smoking

_____ d. Head trauma

_____ e. Pheochromocytoma

_____ f. Obesity

_____ g. Stress

_____ h. Cushing's disease

_____ i. Renal failure

_____ j. Genetic predisposition

175

3. **Case Study:** A 61-year-old man is diagnosed with essential hypertension. His blood pressure is generally approximately 160/100. He has a history of chronic obstructive pulmonary disease. His physician decides to treat with a step-care approach and begins by prescribing Lasix and nifedipine.

   a. Offer an explanation for why the physician selected a beta-blocker to treat the patient's hypertension.

   b. How do the drugs furosemide and nifedipine differ in action?

   c. Which assessments take priority when considering the potential side effects related to furosemide and nifedipine?

   d. The patient's blood pressure does not improve significantly. The physician prescribes captopril (Capoten). Discuss the action of this drug and how it differs from the other prescribed drugs.

   e. What additional side effects should the patient be taught to monitor for?

   f. Discuss important components of a teaching plan for this patient.

4. A patient just returned to his room after femoral-popliteal bypass graft surgery of the right leg. Discuss priority assessments to detect diminished circulation in this patient.

5. Explain the rationale behind wet-to-dry dressings for ulcer management.

6. Discuss proper positioning of a lower extremity after amputation.

7. Explain how thromboangiitis obliterans, arterial occlusive disease, and Raynaud's disease differ.

8. Compare arterial and venous disease based on (a) risk factors common to both arterial and venous conditions and (b) the etiology and incidence of arterial versus venous insufficiency.

9. Discuss the relation of heart disease to arterial versus venous disease in terms of cause and effect.

10. Correct any false statements about deep vein thromboses.
a. Heparin sodium effectively dissolves existing clots.

b. Streptokinase is an enzyme that thins the blood and prevents clot formation.

c. Careful monitoring of prothrombin levels is required for patients receiving heparin therapy.

d. Patients taking Coumadin require vitamin K supplements.

11. **Case Study:** Patient A is a 51-year-old man with a family history of coronary artery disease and who is approximately 20 pounds overweight. He is 24 hours postoperative radical prostatectomy. He reports sharp pain in his left calf both at rest and during activity. His skin on the lower left extremity is warm to touch; peripheral pulses are 3+ left and 3+ right. Ankle edema and swelling of the entire limb are evident. Vessels in the left thigh are engorged.

Patient B is a 53-year-old man with diabetes, hypertension, and atherosclerosis. He reports an aching, cramping sensation in his right leg that is aggravated by walking and sometimes relieved by putting his leg in a dependent position. The skin on his lower right extremity is cool, dry, and shiny, with sparse hair. His peripheral pulses are 1+ right and 2+ left.
a. Identify subjective and objective data for each patient that support a diagnosis of either arterial or venous occlusion.

b. Does either patient demonstrate limb-threatening ischemia? If not, what assessment data would indicate the presence of limb-threatening ischemia?

c. What additional assessment data will help the nurse differentiate between these two vascular conditions?

d. Write three or four nursing diagnoses that are common to both conditions.

e. Discuss how nursing measures for each of these patients are similar or different.

f. Patient A develops a stasis ulcer, and patient B develops an ischemic ulcer. Describe how these two ulcers differ in appearance and occurrence.

12. **Case Study:** A 62-year-old patient recovering from a recent myocardial infarction is in atrial fibrillation. She suddenly reports a severe pain in her left leg. The nurse notes that pulses are absent and the leg is cool to the touch. On further questioning, the patient states that her leg feels numb.
    a. Given the above data, speculate about a possible problem and cause.

    b. How will nursing care for this patient differ from care given to the patient who has arterial occlusive disease?

c. The patient is started on a heparin drip. The following day a partial thromboplastin time is obtained. Analyze the partial thromboplastin time of 45 seconds (normal = 33 to 45 seconds).

13. **Case Study:** A 58-year-old man with a history of hypertension has a smoking history of two packs per day for 21 years. He was admitted to the emergency department with symptoms of back and chest pain over the past 48 hours. He is dyspneic and has audible wheezing. A computed tomography scan confirms a thoracoabdominal aortic aneurysm. The patient is immediately scheduled for a surgical aneurysm repair with aortobifemoral bypass grafting. The nurse is aware that postoperative complications may include acute coronary syndrome, renal failure, and stroke. Plan one or two nursing interventions for each potential complication.

32 Assessment of the Hematologic System

1. A patient who has no renal function because of disease lost a large amount of blood in an automobile crash. What impact will the patient's renal status have on his recovery?

2. On reviewing a patient's laboratory data before her scheduled surgery, the nurse notes significantly elevated neutrophil and monocyte counts. What is the importance of these findings, and what action should the nurse take, if anything?

3. While being prepared for surgery a patient comments to the nurse that he needs an aspirin for his headache. On further questioning, the nurse learns that the patient has taken aspirin several times during the last week for headaches. Of what significance is this information, and should it be reported to the patient's surgeon?

4. A 33-year-old and a 79-year-old patient have pneumonia from the same causative organism. When you receive laboratory data on these patients, how will their complete blood counts compare?

5. When are the following tests particularly useful to the nurse or primary care provider?
   a. Hemoglobin and hematocrit

   b. Red blood cell indexes

   c. Peripheral blood smear

6. Correct any false statements about the hematologic system.
   a. Fever may be present in hematologic diseases; however, night sweats are much more common.

   b. White specks on nails, coarse hair, and pale nail beds are frequently associated with iron-deficiency anemia.

   c. Enlarged lymph nodes are generally insignificant unless coupled with fever and malaise.

   d. Ascertaining the presence of any inherited hematologic disorders is important when obtaining a history on a patient suspected of having a hematologic disorder.

   e. An abdominal assessment is of little value when establishing a medical diagnosis for the patient suspected of having a hematologic disease.

7. Match each of the blood cell types with their primary function. Answers may be used more than once.

   _____ a. Phagocytosis

   _____ b. Formation of immunoglobulins

   _____ c. Mediate exchange of oxygen and carbon dioxide

   _____ d. Combat parasitic infestations

   A. Erythrocytes
   B. Platelets
   C. Neutrophils
   D. Eosinophils
   E. Basophils
   F. Lymphocytes
   G. Monocytes

_____ e. Promote thrombin formation

_____ f. Transport oxygen

_____ g. Immunologic reactions

_____ h. Participate in allergic responses

_____ i. Neutralize action of heparin

8. Identify the primary use for each of these diagnostic tests.
   a. Activated partial thromboplastin time

   b. Prothrombin time

   c. Fibrin split procedure

   d. Coagulation factor assay

   e. Hemoglobin electrophoresis

   f. Iron studies

   g. Lymphangiography

9. **Case Study:** A patient is scheduled to undergo a bone marrow aspiration to help identify the cause of her persistent anemia. She confides that she does not want to undergo the procedure because she has heard that bone marrow aspirations are quite painful. How can the nurse intervene to help reduce the patient's fears?

Chapter **32** **Assessment of the Hematologic System**

33 Hematologic Problems

1. A nurse is caring for three patients. One has iron-deficiency anemia, another has hereditary spherocytosis, and the third has aplastic anemia.
   a. How are these forms of anemia similar? How are they different?

   b. How does nursing care for these three patients compare?

   c. What can be inferred about the care of all patients with anemia based on the care of these three patients?

2. Identify the type of anemia that best fits the descriptions.

   _____ a. Partial or complete inactivity of all blood-producing elements

   _____ b. Causes decreased red blood cell, hemoglobin, and hematocrit values

   _____ c. Causes a deficiency in vitamin B_{12} or folic acid

   _____ d. A genetic disorder that results in decreased synthesis of hemoglobin chain

   _____ e. May be corrected by dietary supplements

_____ f. May be chemically induced, congenital, or autoimmune

_____ g. Produces red blood cell antibodies on antiglobin or Coombs' test

_____ h. A genetic disorder inherited by an autosomal dominant trait

_____ i. May result from bleeding ulcers or malignancies

3. Correct any false statements about anemia.
   a. Aplastic and blood loss anemias are similar in that both can be acute or chronic.

   b. Cessation of the offending drug is the most beneficial treatment for thalassemia major.

   c. Nursing care for the anemia as a whole involves monitoring for signs of infection from leukopenia and bleeding from thrombocytopenia.

   d. Venipunctures and intramuscular injections should be kept to a minimum when attempting to prevent bleeding in the anemic patient.

   e. Hereditary spherocytosis is an autosomal recessive trait characterized by membrane abnormality that leads to shrinkage of the red blood cells.

   f. People with G6PD deficiency often have unrelenting anemia, which does not respond well to therapy.

   g. Sickle cell anemia is characterized by the presence of hemoglobin S, which may lead to increased blood viscosity and slowing of circulation when oxygen tension is increased.

   h. Many sickle cell patients are healthy, seldom have pain, lead normal lives, and live near-normal life spans.

4. List the essential topics that need to be included in the teaching plan for patients with newly diagnosed sickle cell disease.

5. Compare the three complications of sickle cell disease: (1) thrombotic crisis, (2) aplastic crisis, and (3) splenic sequestration.

6. **Case Study:** The nurse caring for a patient in sickle cell crisis performed a thorough physical assessment, assessed the patient's knowledge level about his condition, attended to the patient's comfort needs, encouraged fluid intake to enhance hydration, monitored the patient for complications, and provided teaching regarding treatment and follow-up care. What other patient needs still need to be addressed, if any?

7. A patient is diagnosed with iron-deficiency anemia.
   a. What physical assessments need to be made?

   b. The patient is started on oral iron supplements. What teaching needs to be done regarding this medication?

8. An older man suspected of having vitamin B_{12} deficiency presents with general signs and symptoms of anemia, including fatigue, pallor, and shortness of breath. What patient findings may help differentiate B_{12} deficiency from other types of anemia?

187

9. A prothrombin time and a partial thromboplastin time test have been ordered for a patient. Why may both of these tests be necessary since they both assess clotting? What do they measure?

10. One patient is to receive platelets and another is to receive whole blood. How do the procedures for administering these products and accompanying nursing care differ?

11. A patient has a platelet count of 100,000 but no evidence of petechiae, bruising, or gingival bleeding. His urine is negative for blood. Is this enough information to detect bleeding in this patient?

12. Identify the hematologic problem or problems for which these nursing activities are most appropriate.

_____ a. Protect patient from potential sources of infection.

_____ b. Monitor for signs and symptoms of abnormal bleeding.

_____ c. Teach patient and family regarding the possibility of hemorrhage after dental extraction, injury, or surgery.

_____ d. Monitor for prolonged prothrombin time and partial thromboplastin time as well as low levels of factors V, VIII, and fibrinogen.

_____ e. Teach patient to avoid the use of drugs such as salicylates, quinine, barbiturates, and coumarin derivatives.

_____ f. Administer granulocyte infusion according to prescribed orders and institution policy.

188

_____ g. Teach patient and family regarding self-administration of cryoprecipitate, if ordered.

13. How do each of these factors contribute to the development of disseminated intravascular coagulation?
    a. Sepsis

    b. Trauma

    c. Burns

    d. Snake venom

14. Explain the paradox that seems to occur with disseminated intravascular coagulation: clotting followed by hemorrhage.

15. **Case Study:** A patient with primary polycythemia vera is being discharged after phlebotomy to reduce his hemoglobin and hematocrit levels. He has received teaching about the nature of the disorder, the importance of continued follow-up care, medications that have been prescribed, and signs of extremity thrombosis that should be reported. What is the nurse's responsibility at this time, or is patient teaching adequate?

16. **Case Study:** A young man is being treated with DDAVP for hemophilia. The young man appears anxious and states that he does not want to die. On further questioning, the nurse learns that he is fearful that he will contract the AIDS virus.
    a. How should the nurse respond?

b. If the patient was receiving antihemophilic factor instead of DDAVP, would the response be different? If so, in what way?

17. What conclusions can be drawn about forms of leukemia based on the following factors?
    a. Age

    b. Symptoms produced

    c. White blood cell levels

18. What conclusions can be drawn about the usefulness of chemotherapy for leukemia as a whole?

19. Give examples of nursing activities that apply to all patients receiving chemotherapy for leukemia, regardless of type.

20. A patient with chronic myelocytic leukemia has been taught about her disease and its effects, how to prevent infections, the names and side effects of prescribed drugs, the scheduling of chemotherapy, the laboratory monitoring needed, symptoms that need to be reported, and follow-up care. What important information has been omitted from the patient's teaching?

21. One patient has Hodgkin's disease and another has non-Hodgkin's disease. How is care for these patients different? Similar?

22. **Case Study:** A patient has recently been diagnosed with Hodgkin's disease. The physician has informed him that he is in stage II. The patient understands that his disease may involve two or more lymph nodes. He tells the nurse that he knows he has a terminal disease process. How should the nurse respond?

23. A 16-year-old is being treated for acute mononucleosis. What is the most important information that can be provided to the patient to reduce her anxiety and indirectly enhance her comfort level?

34 Assessment of the Renal System

1. Match the descriptors with the correct terms.

_____ a. Responds to changes in arterial pressure

_____ b. Composes the outer layer of the kidney

_____ c. Performs both excretory and regulatory functions

_____ d. Consists of the glomerulus and Bowman's capsule

_____ e. Alters the volume and composition of the ultrafiltrate to form urine

_____ f. Basic functioning unit of the kidney

_____ g. Assists in concentration and dilution of urine

A. Nephron
B. Renal cortex
C. Renal medulla
D. Renal tubule
E. Cortical nephron
F. Afferent arteriole
G. Renal corpuscle

2. Correct any false statements pertaining to renal physiology.
   a. The proximal and distal tubules are primarily responsible for maintaining normal electrolyte balance.

   b. Ultrafiltrate contains constituents similar to those of plasma.

   c. The cortical hormone angiotensinogen causes increased sodium reabsorption, thereby resulting in water conservation.

   d. Glucose and calcium are the only urinary constituents that are filtered and 100% reabsorbed.

193

e. Between 85% and 90% of the water filtered by the kidneys is reabsorbed in the proximal tubule.

f. The kidneys achieve acid-base balance most efficiently by actively secreting hydrogen ions in the proximal and distal tubules.

3. Briefly describe the process by which the kidneys maintain homeostasis of the body's internal environment.

4. Explain how the kidneys respond to each of the following conditions.
   a. Hypotension

   b. Hyperkalemia

   c. Blood loss anemia

5. Give examples of questions that may be asked to solicit information from patients about the following.
   a. Urinary incontinence

b. Urinary frequency

c. Nocturia

d. Hesitancy

6. Patient A is a 23-year-old man and patient B is an 80-year-old man. How does their renal status differ on the basis of normal renal physiology?

7. Suspecting that a patient has a urinary infection, the nurse practitioner requests a clean catch specimen and urine culture. To ensure accurate results, what instructions need to be given to the patient?

8. Both a creatinine clearance test and a serum creatinine test may be obtained on the same patient. How do these tests differ?

9. A patient being treated for malabsorption syndrome has a normal serum creatinine level of 1.2 mg/dl and an elevated blood urea nitrogen level of 25 mg/dl. Interpret these findings.

10. Explain the following diagnostic tests to a patient in lay terms.
    a. Renal ultrasound

    b. Abdominal KUB

11. **Case Study:** When assessing a patient after renal biopsy at 4:00 PM, the nurse notes that the patient is lying flat on her back with a sandbag to her right side. The patient denies pain but states that her back is hurting from lying in the same position. The biopsy was performed at 9:00 AM. How should the nurse respond?

12. Describe the similarities and differences among the following diagnostic tests.
    Test A: intravenous pyelogram

    Test B: renal angiogram

    Test C: renography

    Test D: computed tomographic scan

35 Kidney and Urinary Tract Problems

1. Identify the commonality that exists among these individuals regarding their renal status.
   a. A nurse on a busy nursing unit does not take time to empty her bladder even though she feels the need to void.

   b. A 78-year-old woman has an indwelling urinary catheter.

   c. A 67-year-old man has prostatic hypertrophy.

2. A young woman is about to leave the clinic after treatment for a mild urinary tract infection. The nurse teaches her the need for returning in 1 week for another urinalysis; reporting increases in frequency, urgency, or burning on urination; calling the clinic immediately if she has fever or chills; and completing all the prescribed medication as ordered. Evaluate the nurse's teaching.

3. **Case Study:** A patient with acute pyelonephritis has had dysuria for 2 days accompanied by frequency, urgency, and nocturia. She states that she is nauseated and very tired. Her urine is cloudy and has a foul odor.
   a. What further data are needed?

   b. The patient wants to know if her kidneys are going to be permanently damaged. How should the nurse respond?

4. A 50-year-old patient is taking the drug gentamicin for a severe respiratory tract infection. Identify laboratory tests that must be monitored and explain why.

5. Correct any false statements about acute glomerulonephritis.
   a. It is an acute infection of the kidney that occurs as a complication of post-streptococcal pharyngitis.

   b. Glomerular inflammation and swelling result in proteinuria and hematuria.

   c. It causes hypertension from fluid retention and stimulation of the renin-angiotensin system.

   d. Decreased urine specific gravity, increased serum creatinine, and decreased urine output are clinical manifestations of acute glomerulonephritis.

6. If acute glomerulonephritis is an inflammatory condition rather than an infection, explain why patients are placed on antibiotic therapy.

7. Identify at least two nursing or collaborative actions that address the following patient problems associated with acute glomerulonephritis.
   a. Fluid overload

b. Hypertension

c. Knowledge deficiency

8. A patient has significantly reduced renal function from chronic glomerulonephritis. The patient voices surprise when told of his condition, stating that he hasn't had any kidney problems in the past and only recently noticed puffiness around his eyes and ankles. How can the nurse best address the patient's surprise and concern?

9. Diagram the pathologic changes occurring with nephrotic syndrome that lead to generalized edema.

10. A 17-year-old girl has acute glomerulonephritis related to a poststreptococcal throat infection. A 14-year-old girl has nephrotic syndrome from an unknown cause.
    a. Identify the similarities and differences between these two patients.

    b. Which nursing diagnoses are appropriate for both of these patients?

11. Identify the renal vascular disorder described in each statement.

_____ a. Medical emergency that requires immediate intervention to prevent permanent renal damage.

_____ b. A leading cause of end-stage renal disease.

_____ c. Vigorous therapy is required to control the associated hypertension.

_____ d. Glomerular damage results in proteinuria, although signs and symptoms are generally mild.

12. A patient has a urinary obstruction from an unknown cause. An identified nursing diagnosis is impaired urinary elimination: obstruction. Nursing activities include monitoring fluid intake and urine output at least every 8 hours; maintaining patency of the urinary drainage system; maintaining sterility of the urinary drainage system; monitoring for hematuria, proteinuria, and the color and odor of urine; and maintaining activity level as tolerated. Which important nursing activities have been omitted, if any?

13. **Case Study:** After outpatient surgery a patient states that he needs to urinate. The nurse provides privacy and gives him a urinal. He voids approximately 50 ml of urine. An hour later, he again reports the need to urinate and voids only 30 ml of urine.
a. What should the nurse suspect?

b. What actions, if any, need to be taken?

c. Which serious complication can result from urinary retention?

14. Which type of catheter will most likely be used for each patient?

_____ a. A patient with prostatic hypertrophy is unable to void.

_____ b. A patient with renal calculi has a blocked ureter.

_____ c. A patient who gave birth this morning has postpartum urinary retention.

_____ d. A trauma patient has blood in her urine.

15. A patient is unable to urinate. What can the nurse do to help him void rather than perform a catheterization?

16. A patient has recently passed a kidney stone and is seeking your advice about preventing future stone formation. He states that the pain was excruciating and that he is willing to do whatever is necessary to avoid having another one. His stone was classified as a uric acid stone. What advice can you give him?

17. Explain the differences between the procedures percutaneous lithotripsy, extracorporeal shock wave lithotripsy, and candela laser therapy.

18. Patient A had a nephrolithectomy. How will her care be similar to that of another patient who underwent surgical removal of a bladder tumor?

19. A patient confides that she has noticed blood in her urine over the past few months. She denies pain, urgency, frequency, or other symptoms. What advice should the nurse give to the patient? Why?

20. A patient has just returned to his room after urologic surgery. On assessing him, the nurse notes that he is cool, clammy, and restless. His blood pressure is 104/86 mm Hg, pulse is 120 beats/min, and respirations are 30/min. What further data are needed?

21. A patient is scheduled for a conduit urostomy after removal of her cancerous urinary bladder. She has been taught about the surgical procedure, including preoperative and postoperative expectations, and provided with information about the stoma. What other nursing activities may be helpful at this time?

22. Identify each patient's urinary diversion.
    a. The patient's ureters have been moved from the bladder and attached to a segment of ileum that has been resected. A stoma is present, and urine is eliminated by the segmented ileum into a plastic pouch.

    b. The patient has an internal reservoir that has been constructed to store urine. The stoma must be catheterized to drain urine from the reservoir.

23. A patient with a urinary diversion reports that she is having difficulty wearing her pouch for the prescribed 5 days because it leaks. How can the nurse help the patient address this problem?

24. Identify the type of incontinence being experienced by these individuals based on their symptoms.

    _____ a. "I leak urine frequently while performing exercises in my stretching class."

    _____ b. "I had a stroke a few months back. I dribble urine if I cannot get assistance to the toilet on a regular basis."

    _____ c. "I feel the need to void, but I urinate before I can get to the bathroom."

25. A 35-year-old married woman with three children has no difficulty with voiding or urinary incontinence. Why, then, has her health care practitioner suggested that she perform perineal (Kegel) exercises on a regular basis?

26. A young woman has been recently diagnosed with polycystic kidney disease. Her primary concern is that she will develop renal failure. Are her fears justified? Why or why not?

36 Kidney Failure

1. Identify the primary similarities and differences between acute and chronic kidney failure.

2. A 29-year-old man who is an exterminator is admitted to the hospital for persistent flank pain. He denies urinary frequency, urgency, or pain. He denies recent illnesses or injuries except for a sore throat 3 weeks ago that subsided without treatment. His family history is positive for hypertension and diabetes. He is taking no medications. Identify this patient's risk factors for developing kidney failure.

3. **Case Study:** A 42-year-old patient is being treated for acute renal failure secondary to hemorrhagic shock.
   a. What type of acute renal failure does she have? Why?

   b. The patient is in the oliguric phase of acute renal failure. Which findings need to be reported to the health care provider?
      Urine output of 30 to 45 ml/hr
      Serum creatinine of 2.6 mg/dl
      Blood pressure of 140/90 mm Hg
      Serum potassium of 5.6 mEq/L

205

c. What could happen if this information is not reported promptly?

d. The patient's condition deteriorates and she becomes severely uremic. What complications may occur if treatment is not initiated?

4. **Case Study:** A 67-year-old woman was admitted to the cardiac care unit 2 days ago for acute coronary syndrome. She continues to have chest pain, which requires narcotic analgesia. Her extremities are cool but free from peripheral edema; she is oliguric and her blood pressure is 110/84 mm Hg. She is receiving beta-blockers and is wearing a nitroglycerin patch. Her medical history includes an 8-year history of hypertension controlled by diet and medication. She takes acetaminophen for occasional headaches and has had no recent illnesses, surgery, or trauma. Her laboratory data indicates a serum creatinine level of 2.4 mg/dl, blood urea nitrogen level of 68 mg/dl, and a cardiac enzyme profile supportive of acute coronary syndrome.

a. What conclusions can be drawn on the basis of the patient's data?

b. What ongoing assessments need to be made on this patient?

c. The patient develops acute renal failure secondary to acute coronary syndrome and progresses to the oliguric phase. Identify clinical manifestations expected during this stage of acute renal failure.

d. The patient is treated with slow, continuous ultrafiltration. Why is this procedure more suitable for this patient than other forms of dialysis?

e. Explain the rationale for placing the patient on a high-carbohydrate, moderate-fat diet.

f. The patient's renal status improves with treatment, and discharge plans are underway. What patient teaching is necessary before discharge?

g. What other problem warrants attention before the patient's discharge? Why?

5. Correct any false statements about acute renal failure.
   a. Any nephrotoxic injury may precipitate acute renal failure.

   b. A sudden, severe decrease in the glomerular filtration rate is one of the first pathophysiologic changes that occur with acute renal failure.

   c. During acute renal failure Na^+ reabsorption from the proximal tubules is increased.

   d. Nausea, vomiting, and diarrhea can occur from either metabolic acidosis or hyperkalemia.

   e. Lethargy and confusion occurring during the oliguric phase of acute renal failure are caused by hypovolemia.

6. Match the clinical manifestations and characteristics with the correct stage of chronic renal failure.

_____ a. Nocturia is common

A. Decreased renal reserve
B. Renal insufficiency
C. Uremia (renal failure)
D. End-stage renal failure

_____ b. Glomerular filtration rate is 10% to 20% of normal

_____ c. Oliguria is common

_____ d. Patient may be asymptomatic

_____ e. Glomerular filtration rate is 20% to 40% of normal

_____ f. Severe azotemia

_____ g. Fixed urine specific gravity of 1.010

_____ h. Serum creatinine begins to elevate

_____ i. Patient may develop anemia

_____ j. Blood urea nitrogen and serum creatinine levels are normal

_____ k. Associated with mild azotemia

_____ l. Glomerular filtration rate is 40% to 50% of normal

_____ m. Urine specific gravity is low

7. **Case Study:** A 57-year-old woman has had lupus erythematosus (an autoimmune disease) for 10 years. She has been treated intermittently with prednisone to control symptoms. Her disease has been slowly progressive but has not interfered with her ability to work. She is married and has two grown daughters. She is 5 feet 4 inches tall and normally weighs 132 pounds. During the past week the patient has felt unusually tired, but she attributes her fatigue to her disease and her need to get up once or twice each night to urinate. In an attempt to get more rest she has decreased her daily fluid intake.

a. What risk factors does the patient have for kidney failure?

b. What is likely happening to the patient?

c. What is the relation between nocturia and renal insufficiency?

d. How will the patient's glomerular filtration rate be altered if she has renal insufficiency?

e. Within what range will the patient's serum creatinine and blood urea nitrogen be during this time?

8. **Case Study:** A patient is admitted with reports of excessive fatigue, mild nausea, headache, and shortness of breath. His blood pressure is 200/118 mm Hg, temperature is 99.2° F orally, heart rate is 108 beats/min, and respirations are 36/min. He states he has gained 20 pounds over the past month. He has crackles in both lung bases, and 1+ pitting edema of both lower extremities. A vein is accessed and an indwelling urinary catheter is placed. The patient is diagnosed with chronic kidney failure.

   a. Which patient finding supports the presence of kidney failure?

   b. List at least four laboratory values that are altered by kidney failure.

   c. What is the best choice of treatment for the patient's kidney failure? Why?

   d. While receiving hemodialysis the patient reports dizziness and nausea. He is mildly hypotensive, diaphoretic, and has a pulse rate of 112 beats/min. What is happening, and how will the nurse respond?

   e. The patient has an arteriovenous fistula constructed in his left arm as a permanent access site. Before discharge, he is taught to avoid blood pressure measurements and venipunctures in his left arm, avoid wearing constrictive clothing, and recognize signs and symptoms that indicate infection. What other teaching needs to be done, if any?

9. Identify the process that occurs during dialysis.

   _____ a. Movement across membrane as a result of artificially created pressure gradient

_____ b. Movement of particles from an area of high concentration to low concentration

_____ c. Movement of fluid from an area of high concentration to low concentration

10. Match the process that clears each substance during dialysis.

_____ a. Creatinine   A. Osmosis
                            B. Diffusion
                            C. Ultrafiltration

_____ b. Urea

_____ c. Water

_____ d. Uric acid

_____ e. Phosphate

_____ f. Waste products

11. Explain the cause of each complication to hemodialysis or peritoneal dialysis. Identify an appropriate nursing response to each.
    a. Hemodialysis
       1. Hypotension

       2. Vomiting

       3. Headache

       4. Blood loss

b. Peritoneal dialysis
   1. Peritonitis

   2. Hyperglycemia

   3. Low back pain

12. A 68-year-old woman has been on dialysis for 14 years. Her quality of life has slowly deteriorated, and she has chosen to discontinue treatment. What are the most appropriate nursing actions to assist and support the patient at this time?

13. Which type of organ rejection is being experienced by each of these patients?
    a. A patient who underwent kidney transplantation 4 months ago notes a decrease in urine output, dull flank pain, ankle swelling, and a 10-pound weight gain.

    b. Immediately after anastomosis of arterial vessels, cytotoxic antibodies infiltrate a patient's newly transplanted kidney. Kidney infarction occurs.

14. Identify the major potential complications of renal transplantation and the clinical manifestations of rejection.

15. Identify at least two nursing responsibilities or actions for patients after kidney transplantation.

16. Explain why this statement is false: A major advantage of using organ transplantation as a treatment modality is the current availability of donor organs.

17. Explain the difference between a non–heart beating donor and a deceased donor.

18. If the ideal drug could be designed to prevent organ rejection, what characteristics would it have to possess?

19. Correct any false statements about kidney transplantation.
    a. The transplanted kidney is placed extraperitoneally, in the iliac fossa.

    b. Efficient revascularization of the transplanted kidney is essential to prevent ischemic injury.

c. The postoperative care of a live donor differs significantly from patients having other types of kidney surgery.

d. Dehydration must be avoided after kidney transplantation to prevent renal hyperperfusion and possible tubular damage.

e. A blood clot in the indwelling catheter is a common cause of early postoperative obstruction after renal transplantation.

f. The first priority for discharge preparation after kidney transplantation is dietary teaching.

37 Assessment of the Endocrine System

1. Reflecting on the endocrine feedback loop, create an analogy to illustrate how the mechanism works.

2. Compare the feedback mechanisms for antidiuretic hormone and thyroid hormone. What are their similarities and differences?

3. Explain the concept of intrinsic rhythmicity as it relates to acetylcholine levels.

4. How do factors such as stress and infection affect acetylcholine levels?

5. Identify the clinical consequence of each of these endocrine alterations.
   a. Increased antidiuretic hormone secretion

b. Decreased cortisol secretion

c. Decreased aldosterone secretion

d. Decreased insulin secretion

e. Decreased T4 secretion and plasma T3 levels

f. Decreased vitamin D and estrogen

6. Identify the priority assessments that need to be made on patients with any type of endocrine disorder.

7. The nurse has collected data from a patient suspected of having an endocrine disorder. Are any of the findings significant? Explain.
a. Weight loss

b. Family history of diabetes mellitus

c. Blood pressure, 148/80 mm Hg lying, 142/76 mm Hg sitting, 140/74 mm Hg standing

d. Decreased libido

e. Nervousness, irritability

8. Compare the water-deprivation and vasopressin tests as tools for differentiating diabetes insipidus (caused by absence of antidiuretic hormone) from nephrogenic diabetes insipidus (inability of the kidney to respond to antidiuretic hormone).

9. Explain the differences between the exocrine and endocrine function(s) of the pancreas.

10. Correct any false statements about the endocrine system.
    a. Estrogen in men and testosterone in women are under feedback control.

    b. Extrinsic factors such as stress and pain can prevail over the normal feedback mechanisms and increase hormone secretion.

    c. The hypothalamus has control over the entire endocrine system because it controls the anterior pituitary.

    d. Iodine is necessary for the production of growth hormone.

    e. The adrenal cortex produces epinephrine and norepinephrine.

    f. An elevated serum calcium level causes decreased release of calcitonin by the thyroid with a subsequent increase in parathyroid hormone.

11. Differentiate between factors and conditions that stimulate (S) and inhibit (I) the secretion or release of antidiuretic hormone. In other words, which individuals are likely to have an increase in urine output (decreased antidiuretic hormone) versus a decrease in urine output (increased antidiuretic hormone)?

_____ a. A 42-year-old postoperative patient receiving morphine

_____ b. Patient receiving hypertonic intravenous fluids

_____ c. A 56-year-old patient in fluid overload

_____ d. An 86-year-old confused patient admitted for dehydration

_____ e. A 36-year-old patient with psychogenic polydipsia

_____ f. Postoperative patient with internal hemorrhage

12. A 48-year-old man is suspected of having an adrenal tumor (pheochromocytoma), which secretes an excess of catecholamines. Knowing the functions of the adrenal medulla in relation to epinephrine and norepinephrine, indicate the expected (E) and the unexpected (U) findings.

_____ a. Increased blood pressure

_____ b. Tachycardia

_____ c. Fatigue

_____ d. Diaphoresis, pallor

_____ e. Hypotension

_____ f. Signs and symptoms of hypoglycemia

_____ g. Nervousness, excitation

_____ h. Tachypnea

13. Analyze the clinical situations for both of these patients. Discuss the significance of the clinical manifestations based on the patients' ages.

Patient A: A 72-year-old patient reports fatigue, decreased activity level, and chronic constipation. She states that she feels mentally sluggish but attributes these findings to retirement and her change in lifestyle. Her husband states that she is becoming more forgetful.

Patient B: A 34-year-old legal secretary reports fatigue and lethargy for 4 months. She has gained 10 pounds and takes a laxative three times weekly for constipation.

14. A 40-year-old man visits his family physician with symptoms of thinning hair, feeling depressed, and diminished sexual drive. On physical examination the physician notes no abnormal findings. The patient's wife thinks he is going through a midlife crisis and is imagining these problems. Discuss the significance of the patient's symptoms.

Chapter **37** **Assessment of the Endocrine System**

38 Pituitary, Thyroid, Parathyroid, and Adrenal Gland Problems

1. Describe how the hormone prolactin acts differently in men than in women.

2. How does postoperative teaching for patients undergoing an adenectomy differ from that for patients undergoing hypophysectomy?

3. Compare the pathophysiology of syndrome of inappropriate secretion of antidiuretic hormone (SIADH) with that of diabetes insipidus.

4. On the basis of the above differences, explain the fluid requirements for persons with SIADH versus those with diabetes insipidus.

5. Explain why the thiazide diuretics are the best choice for treating diabetes insipidus.

6. **Case Study:** A 50-year-old man has just returned from surgery after a transsphenoidal adenectomy for a pituitary tumor. The nurse places the nursing diagnosis of *risk for deficient fluid volume* on his plan of care as a priority nursing diagnosis.
   a. Why is this problem being addressed as a priority nursing diagnosis?

   b. Twelve hours postoperatively, the nurse notes that the patient's blood pressure is 142/88 mm Hg, heart rate is 86 beats/min, respiratory rate is 16/min, and urine output within the last 4 hours is 1000 ml. The patient's urine specific gravity is 1.003. On the basis of these findings, what may be happening to the patient? What additional information would be useful?

   c. On the patient's second postoperative day, despite teaching, the patient strains to have a bowel movement. The nurse notes increased drainage on the patient's gauze nasal dressing. What action should the nurse take and why?

   d. During an outpatient follow-up visit, the patient reports lack of appetite, weight gain, weakness, and fatigue. On assessment the nurse notes that the patient's serum glucose level is decreased and his oral temperature is 96.8° F. Offer an explanation for these findings.

7. **Case Study:** A 47-year-old patient being treated for oat cell carcinoma begins to report nausea and unusual fatigue (malaise). The nurse notes that he has gained 4 pounds within the last day but had urine output of 300 ml within the past 4 hours. He has no peripheral edema.

   a. The nurse would be correct to expect the presence of which problem in this patient?

   b. Serum laboratory values confirm the presence of SIADH secondary to lung neoplasm (cancer) secreting antidiuretic hormone. The patient's serum Na$^+$ levels have dropped from 120 to 115 mEq/L. What effect will this change have on the patient's status? Explain.

   c. Explain why edema does not occur with SIADH.

   d. A 3% sodium chloride solution is administered to the patient intravenously along with 40 mg of IV Lasix (furosemide). Explain the purpose of these medications when treating SIADH.

8. **Case Study:** A 36-year-old woman with a history of bronchial asthma presents to her health care provider with reports of nervousness, difficulty sleeping, missed menstrual periods, weight loss, diarrhea, and heart palpitations. Symptoms have been present for more than 3 months, but she thought it was stress related to the death of her father.

   a. What additional information is needed to determine the cause of the patient's symptoms?

   b. Physical exam shows no evidence of exophthalmos. On the basis of this finding, should Graves disease be ruled out?

   c. Diagnostic testing reveals that the patient has a low thyroid-stimulating hormone level. Explain the relation between decreased thyroid-stimulating hormone levels and hyperthyroidism.

Chapter **38** **Pituitary, Thyroid, Parathyroid, and Adrenal Gland Problems**

d. The patient is ultimately admitted to the hospital with fever of 102° F orally, heart rate of 120 beats/min, and blood pressure of 168/94 mm Hg. She is restless and apprehensive. Treatment includes the administration of 2 mg IV dexamethasone q6h. Why was this drug administered?

e. The nurse administers a tepid bath, places a cooling blanket over the patient, and phones the health care provider to obtain an order for aspirin suppositories. Evaluate the actions of the nurse.

9. Match the classification of drug that would be given in each patient situation.

_____ a. A patient needs immediate reduction of thyroid hormone stores.

    A. Antithyroid drug
    B. Iodides
    C. Adrenergic blocking agent

_____ b. A 45-year-old with hyperthyroidism develops a respiratory tract infection.

_____ c. A 50-year-old with hyperthyroidism has chest pain and a heart rate of 120 beats/min.

_____ d. A 58-year-old with a history of congestive heart failure is being prepared for a subtotal thyroidectomy.

_____ e. A 36-year-old will undergo a total thyroidectomy in 2 days.

_____ f. A 61-year-old with Graves disease is in atrial fibrillation.

_____ g. A 44-year-old has iodine-induced hyperthyroidism.

10. **Case Study:** A 50-year-old patient with Graves disease is hospitalized for radioactive iodine therapy. She is given one oral dose of ^{131}I and placed on radiation precautions. Which patient statements indicate that she has an adequate understanding of radiation therapy?

    a. "I'm glad I only have to take one dose of this medication."

    b. "I should be able to see improvement of my symptoms by tomorrow."

    c. "I didn't realize I'd be radioactive for several weeks."

    d. "I'm glad this radiation solution comes out of my body rather quickly."

    e. "It's rather strange to think that I might have to take thyroid medication after all this is over."

    f. "It's a relief to know that this radiation will eliminate all my thyroid problems!"

11. Compare the etiology, clinical manifestations, and nursing care priorities for patients with the following conditions.

    a. Thyroid storm

    b. Myxedema coma

12. Explain how goiter formation, if present, is indicative of primary hypothyroidism as opposed to secondary hypothyroidism.

13. A patient is being treated for hypothyroidism with L-thyroxine. Identify assessment findings that indicate effective response to this treatment.

14. The nurse is planning to teach a 65-year-old patient with hypothyroidism about his hormone replacement therapy. Identify special considerations, if any, that the nurse should focus on because of the patient's age.

Chapter **38** **Pituitary, Thyroid, Parathyroid, and Adrenal Gland Problems**

15. What are the possible consequences to the parathyroid glands if injured during thyroidectomy?

16. After thyroidectomy, a patient reports respiratory distress. What should the nurse suspect and what actions need to be taken?

17. List nursing diagnoses appropriate for patients with hypersecretion or hyposecretion of endocrine hormones as a whole.

18. Compare the dietary needs for patients with hypersecretion of thyroid, adrenal, and pituitary hormones with those who have hyposecretion of these glands.

19. What conclusions, if any, can be drawn about endocrine disorders and their subsequent effects on other endocrine glands?

20. List at least two desired outcomes for patients who have endocrine disorders.

21. A 47-year-old patient with hypoparathyroidism secondary to thyroidectomy is hospitalized for low serum calcium levels. The patient is quite anxious and hyperventilating. Why is addressing both problems important in this patient? What action(s) should the nurse take?

22. Identify at least two nursing diagnoses and corresponding nursing actions for patients with cortisol excess.

23. Explain the meaning of iatrogenic Cushing's syndrome.

24. A 45-year-old patient is suspected of having pheochromocytoma. Which assessment findings, if present, will help substantiate the diagnosis?

227

39 Diabetes Mellitus and Hypoglycemia

1. Patient A has an autoimmune disease. Patient B is 90 pounds overweight and sedentary but is otherwise healthy. How are these patients similar regarding their risk for developing diabetes mellitus?

2. Match the hormones involved in glucose metabolism with their correct function.

_____ a. Controls blood glucose levels during stress

_____ b. Increases lipolysis

_____ c. Boosts gluconeogenesis

_____ d. Increases the breakdown of fats

_____ e. Prevents fat breakdown

_____ f. Slows cellular uptake and use of glucose

_____ g. Influences cortisol secretion

_____ h. Inhibits the release of insulin

A. Cortisol
B. Acetylcholine
C. Glucagon
D. Insulin
E. Growth hormone
F. Epinephrine

3. Explain how relative and absolute insulin deficiency differ. Identify the final result of both conditions.

4. List at least two consequences of relative or absolute insulin deficiency on the following.
   a. Liver

   b. Skeletal muscle

   c. Adipose tissue

5. **Case Study:** A 68-year-old patient with type 2 diabetes is being treated for pneumonia. The nurse notes that the patient is unusually lethargic. When questioned, the patient reports that she has a headache and is nauseated. Her heart rate is 118 beats/min and regular, blood pressure is 104/72 mm Hg, and respirations are 30/min. She is flushed and feels warm and dry. Her urine output for the morning exceeds 800 ml, and her serum glucose level is 310 mg/dl.
   a. What may be happening to this patient?

   b. What data support the problem that may be occurring?

   c. What laboratory tests will confirm the presence of the problem?

d. What are the priority nursing interventions for the patient at this time?

e. How does hyperglycemic hyperosmolar nonketotic coma (HHNC) differ from what this patient is experiencing?

f. How will assessment findings for the patient with HHNC differ from this patient?

g. Identify nursing actions that are the same for this patient and patients with HHNC.

6. A patient with type 1 diabetes is reporting a headache, fatigue, and inability to focus when reading. Assessment reveals pale skin, diaphoresis, and tachycardia. What may be happening to the patient? How should the nurse respond?

7. What is the impact of each of these conditions or situations on the patient who has diabetes mellitus?
   a. Smoking two packs of cigarettes each day

   b. Increasing loss of vision over several months

   c. Uncontrolled hypertension

d. Abnormal monofilament test

8. Explain the importance of preventing diabetic foot in any patient with diabetes mellitus.

9. Patient A received 15 U regular insulin and patient B received 15 U Lente insulin at 0730 (7:30 AM) today. If both patients eat all of their prescribed meals, how will their insulin needs differ at 1730 (5:30 PM)?

10. A patient who works rotating shifts reports that her blood glucose level is difficult to control because she is unable to eat at consistent time intervals. Suggest an insulin regimen that may help her deal with this problem.

11. A patient with diabetes mellitus confides to the nurse that her blood glucose level is steadily increasing even though she maintains her diet and takes her usual dose of daily insulin. How should the nurse respond?

232

12. Explain hemoglobin A1c to a patient with newly diagnosed diabetes mellitus in a manner he can understand.

13. Explain why intensive insulin therapies are superior to once a day, day and night, or mixed insulin treatment regimens.

14. Match the antidiabetic drug with its correct action.

_____ a. Decreases insulin resistance

_____ b. interferes with absorption of carbohydrates

_____ c. Augments insulin secretion

_____ d. increases insulin sensitization

_____ e. Augments action of insulin

_____ f. Provides exogenous insulin

_____ g. Inhibits digestion of carbohydrates

A. Metformin HCL
B. Alpha-glucosidase inhibitor
C. Insulin
D. Sulfonylurea

15. Plan a 1-day menu for a person with diabetes mellitus who is on a 1200-calorie exchange diet.

16. The nurse has assessed the physical, emotional, psychosocial support, and financial status of a patient with diabetes mellitus. What other important assessment(s) need to be made?

17. Correct any false statements about diabetes mellitus.
    a. Patients with diabetes mellitus have glycosylated hemoglobin levels that are approximately half the level of those without diabetes.

    b. When patients express their feelings about having diabetes, their fears are likely to diminish.

    c. Patients with diabetes mellitus are at increased risk for dehydration from osmotic diuresis, which is caused by increased blood glucose levels.

    d. When patients' blood glucose levels exceed 100 mg/dl, their urine ketones need to be assessed.

    e. Patients who are able to accurately select foods according to their prescribed diets are meeting their primary dietary goals.

    f. Because patients with diabetes mellitus have similar needs, planning and implementing educational programs to meet their needs equally is easy.

g. When drawing up two different types of insulin, the long-lasting insulin is drawn up first to prevent contamination from the short-acting regular insulin.

h. The patient with diabetes mellitus should be able to verbalize the need for excellent skin care before discharge from the hospital.

18. A patient with type 1 diabetes mellitus has a fever of 101° F, is nauseated, and has diarrhea. She is unable to eat or drink anything for breakfast because of her nausea. Should her insulin be administered? Why or why not?

19. A patient states that she self-administers her insulin in the right thigh repeatedly because it is convenient and less painful for her. Should the nurse intervene? Explain.

20. Explain how injection site complications can interfere with insulin absorption.

21. Identify nursing actions that will benefit each person described, classifying the action according to the type of prevention it represents.
    a. A 48-year-old patient has recently lost 20 pounds but has increased thirst and hunger.

b. A 27-year-old patient has had diabetes mellitus since age 12 years. She has a 3-month-old infant.

c. A 42-year-old man leads a sedentary lifestyle at work and home.

d. A 63-year-old woman resides by herself. She is economically disadvantaged and has no means of grocery shopping on a regular basis.

22. **Case Study:** A patient with diabetes mellitus on insulin therapy has just undergone an abdominal hysterectomy. What precautions need to be taken for this patient that may not be required for patients without diabetes?

23. **Case Study:** A patient who ate lunch approximately 2 hours ago is now reporting headache and feelings of jitteriness. Assessment reveals that the patient is diaphoretic and trembling.
a. What should the nurse suspect?

b. What actions should the nurse take, if any?

24. Think about how you might feel if you were told that you have diabetes mellitus and need to take insulin for the rest of your life. What concerns or fears might you have? What information do you think you would want to receive from your nurse?

40 Assessment of the Gastrointestinal, Biliary, and Exocrine Pancreatic Systems

1. Compare the esophagus and stomach. How are they similar? Different?

2. Person A has just finished a meal high in carbohydrates. Person B has just eaten a meal high in protein. How is the digestive process different for these two individuals?

3. A patient underwent an upper gastrointestinal series 2 days ago and is scheduled for a barium enema today. What assessment data does the nurse need to obtain before sending the patient to radiology?

4. After colon surgery for cancer, a patient's carcinoembryonic antigen level drops from 12 to 6 ng/ml. Six months after being started on chemotherapy, his carcinoembryonic antigen value is 10 ng/ml. Discuss the significance of this finding.

5. Interpret the meaning of the following diagnostic findings.
   a. Serum albumin level of 2.5 mg/dl

   b. Serum calcium level of 7.2 mg/dl

   c. Urine bilirubin level of 3.7 mg/dl

   d. Lipase level of 200 U/L

   e. Alkaline phosphatase level of 100 U/dl

6. Two patients in the same room are having endoscopic procedures. One is having an esophagogastroduodenoscopy, the other an endoscopic retrograde cholangio-pancreatography. The patients ask the nurse how these tests are different. How would you explain the difference? How will nursing care be different or similar after these procedures?

7. Correct any false statements regarding aging and the gastrointestinal system.
   a. As persons age, saliva increases, which increases the person's susceptibility to infection.

   b. Decreased esophageal motility occurs with aging but has a minimal effect in the healthy individual.

   c. Chronic gastritis commonly occurs in older adults and is usually the result of achlorhydria.

   d. Chronic constipation occurs in older adults because of reduced contractions of the large intestine.

e. Decreases in the production of immunoglobulin A can lead to more frequent and severe infections.

8. **Case Study:** A 67-year-old man is admitted to the hospital for weight loss and fatigue. He has a 15-year history of diverticulitis, which has primarily been treated by diet. In addition to the data collected below, what other information is needed, if any, to assess this patient's condition adequately?
   a. Nutritional status: loss of appetite for 2 weeks, unable to tolerate raw fruits or vegetables, drinks 2 to 4 cups of coffee per day, uses no tobacco, has full dentures

   b. Abdominal pain: pain is a cramping sensation occurring within 1 hour of eating, occasionally associated with nausea, no vomiting

   c. Energy level: no report of fatigue or weakness

   d. Elimination pattern: occasional constipation, no blood noted in stools, stools normally brown in color

9. Regarding the patient in question 8, which objective findings are significant and should be reported to the physician? Discuss the significance of each finding.
   Weight of 178 pounds
   Full dentures
   Abdomen firm with tenderness noted over the left lower quadrant
   Bowel sounds present and hyperactive throughout
   Reddened, visible hemorrhoids
   Small white patches on tongue that cannot be removed with tongue blade

Chapter **40** **Assessment of the Gastrointestinal, Biliary, and Exocrine Pancreatic Systems**

41 Mouth and Esophagus Problems

1. Identify at least two independent nursing activities that may benefit patients with each of these mouth disorders.
   a. Gingivitis

   b. Candidiasis

   c. Parotitis

   d. Herpes simplex

2. Compare hiatal hernia with gastroesophageal reflux regarding clinical manifestations, nursing care, and treatment.

3. Consider each person's risk of developing cancer of the mouth and/or esophagus. On a scale of 1 to 3 (1 = low risk, 3 = high risk), rank each person's risk.

   _____ a. A 60-year-old man with chronic gastroesophageal reflux

   _____ b. An 18-year-old African-American who chews smokeless tobacco

   _____ c. A 35-year-old Asian who is chronically malnourished

   _____ d. A 65-year-old African-American with a 45-year history of smoking and recently diagnosed alcoholism

_____ e. A 58-year-old Asian man with poor oral hygiene, who drinks socially, and dislikes fruits and vegetables

_____ f. A sexually active teen who smokes one pack of cigarettes per day and drinks beer daily

_____ g. A 75-year-old woman who smoked briefly in her teens, never uses alcohol, and eats at the senior center

_____ h. A 40-year-old man with dysphagia and a 20-year history of smoking and alcohol consumption

4. **Case Study:** A patient with esophageal reflux voices concern about the expense of taking omeprazole (Prilosec) indefinitely. She is frustrated because her insurance company insists on physician validation of the need for this medication each time a prescription needs to be refilled. What additional information does the nurse need to collect to help problem-solve in this situation?

5. **Case Study:** The nurse is reviewing the documentation of a 56-year-old patient newly admitted to the medical unit. The patient has a history of multiple sclerosis, asthma, and diverticulitis. His chief complaint is difficulty swallowing over the past 6 months, a 10-pound weight loss, and foul breath.
   a. Are additional data required to plan the care for this patient? If so, what other information needs to be collected?

   b. What data suggest that the patient may be suffering from achalasia?

c. What suggestions can the nurse make to help improve the patient's swallowing and nutritional intake?

6. **Case Study:** A 62-year-old man is being cared for by a nursing student during the immediate postoperative period after esophagectomy. He has a chest tube, nasogastric tube, and an intravenous infusion of D5 0.45% sodium chloride running at 125 ml/hr. The patient is upset and withdrawn because he knows that the tumor growth was extensive. As part of the plan of care, the student has identified four nursing diagnoses with rationales. Do you agree with the nursing diagnoses and rationales? Explain.

1. Anticipatory grieving related to loss of ability to eat
   Rationale: Because the patient has a poor prognosis, the focus of care should be on the patient's psychosocial needs.
2. Imbalanced nutrition: less than body requirements related to NPO status
   Rationale: Promotion of adequate nutrition should include maintaining NPO status and irrigating the nasogastric tube every 2 hours with normal saline. If the patient continues to lose weight and albumin level decreases, the physician should be notified for possible tube feedings.
3. Risk for aspiration related to loss of lower esophageal sphincter function
   Rationale: The patient should be kept in high Fowler's position to prevent regurgitation and possible aspiration.
4. Potential complication: anastomotic leakage and pulmonary compromise
   Rationale: Promoting coughing and deep breathing and assessing lung parameters should occur at least once per shift. Increased drainage in the chest tube may indicate leakage of the anastomosis.

42 Stomach and Duodenum Problems

1. Match the stomach condition or problem with its correct descriptor.

_____ a. Characterized by acid oversecretion

_____ b. Can be caused by salmonella or staphylococci

_____ c. Characterized by exacerbations and remissions

_____ d. Often related to ingestion of irritating or corrosive agents

_____ e. Nonsteroidal antiinflammatory drugs impair mucosal defenses and bicarbonate secretion

_____ f. *Helicobacter pylori* damages mucosa and impairs bicarbonate secretion

_____ g. Generally self-limiting disorder

_____ h. Common after radiation or chemotherapy

_____ i. Antibodies attack parietal cells

_____ j. Buffering of gastric acid is impaired because of increased rate of gastric emptying

_____ k. Symptom rather than a disease

A. Acute gastritis
B. Chronic gastritis
C. Duodenal ulcer
D. Gastric ulcer
E. Dyspepsia

2. A patient presents with bloating, a feeling of fullness, and burning epigastric pain occurring approximately 2 hours after meals that is sometimes relieved with antacids. Is the patient's medical history helpful in differentiating between a gastric and duodenal ulcer? What other information will help differentiate these two conditions?

3. Identify the advantages and disadvantages of each of these drugs as treatment for duodenal ulcer.
   a. Maalox

   b. Cimetidine

   c. Carafate

   d. Omeprazole

4. Evaluate the teaching plan for a patient with a duodenal ulcer. Correct any incorrect nursing actions or rationales.
   a. Action: Instruct the patient to eat six small meals each day and include a snack before Bedtime. Rationale: Research supports the ability of a full stomach to decrease acid production and mucosal irritation.

   b. Action: Teach patient to use ibuprofen for minor pain or headaches. Rationale: Ibuprofen is the least irritating of the antiinflammatory agents.

   c. Action: Discuss implications of smoking on ulcer development. Rationale: Smoking may exacerbate disease process.

   d. Action: Encourage use of relaxation and stress reduction techniques. Rationale: Stress reduction measures may decrease acid secretion and subsequently reduce pain.

e. Action: Teach patient how to take prescribed *H. pylori* medications and the need for completing the recommended treatment. Rationale: Many patients are unaware of the role of *H. pylori* in ulcer development and may not complete the recommended treatment, which can lead to relapse.

5. A patient states that he does not understand the surgery he is scheduled to undergo. Which explanation best answers the patient's questions regarding the scheduled vagotomy and pyloroplasty?
   a. "The surgery will decrease acid production in your stomach, but you will remain at risk for ulcer recurrence."
   b. "The vagus nerve will be severed, which will decrease acid production. The bottom of your stomach will be widened to improve drainage."
   c. "Your surgeon will be removing 50% of your stomach to reduce acid secretion. You may have intermittent diarrhea after the surgery."
   d. "Your surgeon will remove 75% of your stomach and reconnect the remaining portion to the small intestine."

6. **Case Study:** A 55-year-old man is hospitalized for gastrointestinal bleeding secondary to peptic ulcer disease. Throughout the day he has had abdominal cramping, tarry stools, and coffee ground emesis. He calls the nurse to his room, and she notes that he is vomiting bright red emesis. On further assessment the patient is noted to be tachycardic, restless, and apprehensive. His blood pressure is 96/76 mm Hg.
   a. What should the nurse do first? Why?

   b. What additional nursing actions need to be taken?

   c. Why is iced saline contraindicated for gastric lavage in this patient?

   d. Discuss the advantages and disadvantages of thermal coagulation, injection therapy, and surgery as a means of controlling gastric bleeding.

7. **Case Study:** A patient has an ileus after an automobile crash in which she and other members of her family were seriously injured. The patient has a nasogastric tube in place and attached to low suction.
   a. What findings, if noted, need to be reported immediately?

   b. Why is this patient at increased risk for a stress ulcer?

8. A healthy young woman with a family history of stomach cancer asks the nurse's advice about staying healthy. What advice can the nurse give the woman?

9. A patient with stomach cancer states that she does not understand the meaning of stage II cancer. What is the best way to describe staging to this patient?

10. A patient is recovering from gastric surgery. After eating approximately 50% of lunch, the patient reports nausea. The nurse advises the patient to not eat any more food. The nurse then lowers the head of the patient's bed, pulls the curtains, and closes the door so the patient can rest. Approximately 20 minutes later the patient reports severe nausea and requires medication. Evaluate the nurse's actions.

250

11. Describe at least three nursing activities that may decrease or control dumping syndrome after gastric surgery.

12. A patient is nauseated after extensive abdominal surgery. Both cyclizine and metoclopramide are prescribed for the patient. Which drug may be most effective for controlling the patient's nausea? Explain.

13. Explain the differences between malabsorption and protein-calorie malnutrition and their treatments.

14. Correct any false statements regarding enteral feedings and total parenteral nutrition.
    a. High-density enteral feeding formulas tend to be less hypertonic and may contribute to diarrhea.

    b. Residual volumes are checked before each intermittent feeding and at specified intervals between.

    c. Bulking agents, slow delivery rates, and formula dilution are methods used to prevent diarrhea in patients receiving enteral feedings.

    d. Peripheral parenteral solutions contain glucose content that does not generally exceed 20%.

e. Blood glucose levels are checked daily when total parenteral nutrition is initiated to determine if endogenous insulin adjustments have occurred.

f. Catheter problems, infection, and metabolic imbalances are primary complications associated with total parenteral nutrition therapy.

43 Intestinal Problems

1. Identify at least two independent nursing actions that may be helpful for persons with the following conditions.
   a. Constipation

   b. Diarrhea

2. A patient with fecal incontinence has been started on a bowel training program. Identify several nursing actions that address fecal incontinence other than the actual toileting procedure itself.

3. A patient suspected of having acute appendicitis has been placed on NPO status and bed rest. When assessing the patient the nurse notices that he has a heating pad placed over his lower abdomen. The patient states that a family member brought it from home hoping it would alleviate his pain. What should the nurse do or say?

4. A 63-year-old patient is preparing for discharge after treatment for acute diverticulitis. She has been taught about her illness and its treatment. Which patient statement indicates the need for further teaching? Why?
   a. "I should increase my intake of dietary fiber."
   b. "If I develop pain in the left lower part of my abdomen, I should notify my doctor."
   c. "I will no longer be able to eat foods such as popcorn, nuts, or strawberries."
   d. "Changes in my bowel pattern may mean that one of the pouches is becoming inflamed."

5. A patient has acute pain from peritonitis caused by a ruptured diverticulum. The patient tells the nurse that she does not understand why she is so sick and wants to know what can be done to relieve or eliminate the problem. What explanation can the nurse offer the patient about peritonitis and its treatment?

6. Patient A has ulcerative colitis. Patient B has Crohn's disease.
   a. How are these disorders similar? Different?

   b. How is nursing care for these disorders similar? Different?

7. Identify at least two nursing activities for patients with inflammatory bowel disease that address the following factors.
   a. Pain and discomfort

   b. Maintenance of fluid and nutritional status

   c. Emotional well-being

8. A patient has just returned to his room after bowel surgery for inflammatory bowel disease. Assessment reveals the absence of bowel sounds. What should the nurse do?

9. A patient has an ileoanal reservoir after surgery for ulcerative colitis.
   a. Identify the advantages and disadvantages of this procedure over other surgical treatments for ulcerative colitis.

   b. Why would this procedure be contraindicated if the patient was 55 years or older?

10. **Case Study:** A patient had a perineal resection and colostomy for rectal cancer 2 days previously.
    a. What is the most significant factor influencing the patient's ability to manage the ostomy independently and maintain a good pouch seal?

    b. The patient voices concern about the appearance of the stoma, which is red, swollen, and draining serosanguineous drainage. How can the nurse best address the patient's concern?

    c. The patient calls the nurse to the room and reports burning and discomfort around the stoma. The nurse notices papular lesions and redness. What approaches may be used to manage the patient's skin, pouch selection, and reapplication of the stomal pouch to prevent further stomal irritation?

    d. The patient confides to the nurse that he is fearful of impotence and intimacy. How can the nurse address the patient's fears?

11. A 49-year-old patient presents to the emergency department with sudden-onset mid-abdominal cramping that he describes as "continuous." He is vomiting intermittently. Abdominal assessment indicates high-pitched intermittent bowel sounds. His serum electrolyte levels are Na$^+$, 132 mEq/L and K$^+$, 3.1 mEq/L. Identify data that support the presence of small bowel versus large bowel obstruction in this patient.

12. Compare the pathophysiology, clinical manifestation, and risk of bowel obstruction for these two patients.
    a. A 70-year-old man has a sliding abdominal hernia. He reports nausea and vomiting and his abdomen is slightly distended.

    b. A 69-year-old man has adenocarcinoma of the distal sigmoid colon, stage B. Occult blood is present in his stool, and he reports constipation with pencil-shaped stools and vague abdominal discomfort.

13. Certain nursing actions are common to patients with any type of intestinal obstruction, regardless of the cause. Identify at least five nursing actions that are appropriate for patients with intestinal obstruction regardless of cause.

14. Correct any false statements about intestinal disorders.
    a. Surgery is definitive therapy for colorectal cancer.

    b. Preparation of the bowel before surgery cleanses the colon and prevents post-operative bacterial infections.

c. Incisional pain is typically severe after abdominal surgery but rarely interferes with lung expansion.

d. The incidence of colon cancer is heavily skewed toward the older population.

e. Patients who undergo extensive lymph node dissection in the pelvic region can be reassured that sexual dysfunction rarely occurs postoperatively.

f. Conditions commonly associated with hemorrhoid development include pregnancy, obesity, congestive heart failure, and chronic renal disease.

g. The blood loss from hemorrhoids can be large enough to cause significant iron depletion causing anemia.

h. Anal fissures most often occur from the obstruction of gland ducts in the anorectal region by feces.

44 Gallbladder and Exocrine Pancreatic Problems

1. Explain the differences and relations among cholelithiasis, cholecystitis, and choledocholithiasis.

2. Outline your understanding of the formation of gallstones.

3. Identify each of the following surgical procedures.
   a. Anastomosis of the gallbladder to the stomach

   b. Incision into the common bile duct

   c. Removal of the gallbladder

   d. Anastomosis of the common bile duct with the duodenum

   e. Creation of an opening into the gallbladder for drainage

   f. Anastomosis of the common bile duct with the jejunum

   g. Incision into the common bile duct to remove a stone

4. **Case Study:** A 47-year-old woman presents to the emergency department with nausea, chills, and severe right shoulder pain. She is diaphoretic, tachycardic, restless, and has a fever.

   a. If gallbladder disease is suspected, why does the patient not have pain in her right upper quadrant?

   b. Which assessment findings support both cholelithiasis and cholecystitis?

   c. How does preoperative care for patients having open cholecystectomy differ from that of patients having laparoscopic cholecystectomy?

   d. When is an abdominal incision considered more appropriate than a laparoscopic procedure for cholecystectomy?

5. Patient A is returning from postanesthesia recovery after a laparoscopic cholecystectomy. Patient B is returning after a cholecystectomy by an abdominal incision. Compare their postoperative care on the basis of the following factors.

   a. Postoperative pain

   b. Nutritional needs

c. Teaching

d. Postoperative restrictions

6. **Case Study:** A patient with a long history of inflammatory bowel disease is admitted to the hospital with symptoms of fatigue, fever, abdominal pain, pruritus, and weight loss occurring over the past several months. Assessment data include jaundice and elevated liver enzymes, serum bilirubin, and alkaline phosphatase. On the basis of these findings, which disorder should the nurse suspect? What treatments are available for this disorder, if any? What teaching will the nurse need to do if the patient's diagnosis is confirmed?

7. A 53-year-old woman is hospitalized for evaluation of weight loss, jaundice, and vomiting. While completing her admission history, the nurse learns that the patient has had intermittent upper abdominal pain, anorexia, and nausea for at least 6 months. Her abdomen is tender and mildly distended. Which finding strongly suggests that the patient may have biliary cancer as opposed to cholecystitis?

8. A 57-year-old man is being treated for acute hemorrhagic pancreatitis. Another is being treated for acute interstitial pancreatitis. How do these diseases differ in pathophysiology and prognosis?

9. **Case Study:** Nursing assessment of a patient with non–alcohol-induced acute pancreatitis reveals a temperature of 100.6° F orally; pulse of 98 beats/min; respirations of 28/min; blood pressure of 130/78 mm Hg; tender, rigid abdomen; decreased bowel sounds; negative Cullen's sign; poor skin turgor with a yellow cast; dry mucous membranes; and urine output of 30 to 45 ml/hr.

   a. What important item of data is missing?

   b. What alterations are expected in these diagnostic studies within 24 to 48 hours of the onset of the patient's illness?
      1. Serum amylase
      2. Serum lipase
      3. Urinary amylase
      4. Alkaline phosphatase

   c. What conclusions, if any, can be drawn about the patient's pancreatitis on the basis of review of her diagnostic findings?

   d. The patient is scheduled for an ultrasonogram. Offer an explanation for this procedure to the patient.

10. Match the complication of acute pancreatitis with the affected system.

_____ a. Decreased insulin release

_____ b. Acute respiratory distress syndrome

_____ c. Hypoalbuminemia

_____ d. Encephalopathy

_____ e. Varices hemorrhage

_____ f. Disseminated intravascular coagulation

_____ g. Gastritis

_____ h. Increased blood urea nitrogen level

_____ i. Hypovolemic shock

_____ j. Peptic ulcer hemorrhage

_____ k. Increased blood glucose level

_____ l. Atelectasis

_____ m. Oliguria

_____ n. Anemia

A. Cardiovascular
B. Hematologic
C. Respiratory
D. Gastrointestinal
E. Pancreatic/hepatic
F. Renal
G. Metabolic
H. Neurologic

263

11. What is the desired effect for these collaborative interventions implemented for patients with pancreatitis?
   a. Nasogastric suctioning

   b. Insulin administration

   c. Total parenteral nutrition

   d. Monitoring intake and output

12. List at least two nursing activities that address problems experienced by patients with acute pancreatitis.
   a. Pain

   b. Fluid and electrolyte balance

   c. Risk for complications

   d. Risk for imbalanced nutrition

   e. Patient education

13. How do assessment findings for a patient with chronic pancreatitis differ from those for a patient with acute pancreatitis?

14. Identify at least three priority nursing diagnoses for the patient with chronic pancreatitis.

15. Correct any false statements about pancreatic cancer.

a. Cigarette smoking is thought to be an important causative agent of pancreatic cancer.

b. The pain of pancreatic cancer is often described by patients as epigastric in location, intermittent in character, and relentlessly progressive in nature.

c. Diarrhea and steatorrhea commonly occur in patients with pancreatic cancer if bile duct obstruction is severe.

d. Surgical resection is the only curative option available for pancreatic cancer.

e. Most patients are ideal candidates for surgical management of pancreatic cancer because most tumors are still operable at the time of diagnosis.

f. A celiac plexus block may be performed when a patient's pain associated with pancreatic cancer is unrelenting and cannot be effectively managed with medications.

g. Pain management, depression, and fatigue are some of the problems addressed by palliative care specialists with patients who have pancreatic cancer.

45 Assessment of the Hepatic System

1. Identify two diagnostic tests for distinguishing between hemolytic jaundice, hepatocellular jaundice, and obstructive jaundice. Explain why these tests are useful.

2. Think about the major metabolic functions of the liver. What conclusions can be drawn about the nutritional requirements of an individual with liver dysfunction?

3. A 28-year-old woman reports extreme fatigue, loss of appetite, and a 10-pound weight loss. The nurse notes slight yellowing of her sclerae. Identify specific questions the nurse can ask to help rule out a hepatic problem.

4. A patient has just undergone a liver biopsy. Identify possible complications for which monitoring is needed and list priority nursing measures for the patient during the postprocedural period.

5. How is postprocedural care for patients undergoing paracentesis similar to that of patients undergoing liver biopsy?

6. Identify five or six nursing diagnoses appropriate for patients with hepatic dysfunction.

7. Match each of the hepatic-related terms with their correct definitions.

_____ a. Lipogenesis

_____ b. Glycogenolysis

_____ c. Gluconeogenesis

_____ d. Glycogenesis

A. Conversion of simple sugars into glycogen
B. Breakdown of glycogen
C. Conversion of carbohydrates into fat
D. Formation of glucose from amino acids

8. **Case Study:** A 54-year-old man is admitted to the hospital with symptoms of abdominal pain, nausea, anorexia, pruritus, and a 15-pound weight gain. His sclerae are slightly yellow. His medical history includes depression, acute coronary episodes, and chronic leukemia.
   a. What questions can be asked by the nurse to help identify any social, personal, or lifestyle factors that may be significant?

b. Why is obtaining a thorough medication history on this patient important?

c. Offer an explanation for the patient's weight gain given that he is anorexic and nauseated.

d. Analyze the patient's laboratory findings and offer an interpretation. Are all these tests equally effective in supporting the presence of liver dysfunction?
   PT: 18 seconds (control seconds, 12)
   NH3: 70 mcg/dl
   Total bilirubin: 1.5 mg/100 ml
   AST: 25 U/L (slightly elevated)
   ALT: 100 U/L (high elevation)
   LDH: 480 U/L (moderate increase)
   Alkaline phosphatase: 140 U/L (marked increase)

46 Hepatic Problems

1. Clinical manifestations of cirrhosis are directly related to pathophysiology. Match the pathophysiology with its resultant clinical manifestations of cirrhosis.

_____ a. Decreased glycogenolysis and gluconeogenesis

_____ b. Decreased bile and fat metabolism

_____ c. Decreased vitamin K synthesis

_____ d. Increased estrogen in men

_____ e. Increased testosterone in women

_____ f. Increased aldosterone

_____ g. Decreased albumin production

_____ h. Increased ammonia levels

_____ i. Increased total bilirubin

_____ j. Decreased intestinal excretion of bilirubin

_____ k. Increased urobilinogen

_____ l. Decreased phagocytosis

_____ m. Decreased protein synthesis

A. Clay-colored stools
B. Fatigue, low energy, weight loss
C. Facial hair
D. Increased infection potential
E. Gynecomastia
F. Altered healing
G. Tea-colored urine
H. Intolerance to fat, weight loss
I. Ascites, fatigue
J. Jaundice
K. Increased bleeding potential
L. Edema, hypokalemia, orthostatic blood pressure
M. Confusion, decreased coordination

271

2. A nurse is planning a class for teens on alcoholism and alcoholic cirrhosis. Identify aspects of alcohol cirrhosis that the nurse needs to make sure are included in the class.

3. A patient with Laënnec's cirrhosis is receiving discharge instructions after a portal-systemic shunt to control his ascites. He understands that his poor nutritional habits have contributed to his liver disease and ascites, but he is confused about the lifelong restriction of dietary protein that he must adhere to. How can the nurse clarify this important concept?

4. **Case Study:** A patient hospitalized for alcoholic cirrhosis is irritable, has a mild hand tremor, and is having difficulty concentrating on the conversation. She is alert and oriented. She reports abdominal pain, ranking it as 7 on a scale of 0 to 10. What should the nurse suspect based on these assessment findings, and what action needs to be taken?

5. A patient who has ascites from liver cirrhosis has difficulty breathing and taking in adequate food and has output that does not equal input. Give the rationale for each nursing activity implemented for this patient.
   a. Patient placed in high Fowler's position

b. Flotation pad placed on patient's bed

c. Serum potassium levels monitored

d. Bleeding precautions instituted

e. Small, frequent meals served

6. An 8-year-old child has ingested poisonous mushrooms. A 52-year-old woman is receiving high-dose methotrexate for leukemia. Both are exhibiting clinical manifestations of toxic hepatitis. Explain the difference between these two patients based on the effect of each hepatotoxin.

7. Correct any false statements about the various types of hepatitis.
   a. Autoimmune hepatitis is an acute necroinfectious liver disorder associated with circulating autoantibodies.

   b. Corticosteroids are the mainstay for treatment of autoimmune hepatitis.

   c. Viral hepatitis B is the most frequently reported infectious disease in the country.

d. Inflammation, degeneration, and regeneration of the liver occur simultaneously in viral hepatitis.

e. Jaundice, a common manifestation of viral hepatitis, is caused by a disturbance in bile metabolism.

f. Persons requiring hospitalization for hepatitis have serum bilirubin concentrations greater than 25 mg/dl or liver failure.

g. Hepatitis B, A, and C are vaccine-preventable diseases.

h. Patients with viral hepatitis need approximately 2000 ml/day of fluids because of increased fluid needs from vomiting and febrile illness.

i. The major aim of care for the patient with viral hepatitis–related pruritus is prevention of scratching and resultant skin injury.

j. The level of activity allowed for patients with viral hepatitis is determined by their amount of fatigue and severity of their illness.

8. Explain the differences between focal and diffuse hepatocellular disorders. Give examples of each.

9. Prioritize nursing diagnoses for the patient with an acute pyrogenic liver abscess exhibiting signs of shock.
   a. Imbalanced nutrition: less than body requirements related to anorexia, increased metabolic needs

   b. Impaired oral mucous membrane related to dry mouth, fever, fluid loss

c. Deficient fluid volume related to fever and vomiting

d. Acute pain related to liver abscess, febrile illness, and pruritus

10. **Case Study:** A 39-year-old man is brought to the emergency department with possible liver trauma after a severe car crash. Physical assessment reveals pale skin, diaphoresis, blood pressure, 90/64 mm Hg; pulse, 122 beats/min; respirations, 24/min and shallow; absent bowel sounds; abdominal tenderness on palpation; bloody urine; and no penetrating wounds. The patient reports abdominal and chest pain intensified by inspiration and shortness of breath. What has most likely happened to the patient? Speculate about the patient's prognosis.

11. Discuss reasons why primary liver cancers are less common in the United States than in other countries.

12. Explain why patients undergoing liver resection are at increased risk for
    a. Hemorrhage

    b. Infection

    c. Portal hypertension

13. Identify at least two nursing responsibilities or actions for patients after liver transplantation.

Assessment of the Nervous System

1. Fill in the correct word(s) to complete each statement.

   a. The _____ is the basic structural and functional unit of the nervous system.

   b. The _____ is specialized for the transmission of information away from the cell body to adjacent neurons.

   c. In the resting state all neurons possess a potential for action and are said to be _____.

   d. When a neuron is stimulated, membrane permeability to sodium significantly _____.

   e. A strong stimulus _____ give rise to a larger action potential.

   f. The presence of myelin causes nerve fibers to be called _____ fibers.

   g. Large fibers have a _____ conduction velocity than small fibers.

   h. Transmission across a synapse is essentially a(n) _____ process.

   i. Chemicals allowing _____ transmission are acetylcholine, norepinephrine, dopamine, and serotonin.

   j. Nerve endings _____ regenerate.

   k. Passage of substances into the brain is _____ compared with other body organs.

   l. The blood-brain barrier _____ entry of plasma protein.

2. Each patient has a cerebral lesion. Identify the lobe of the cerebrum that is affected based on the data provided. F = frontal, P = parietal, T = temporal, O = occipital

   _____ a. A 55-year-old who cannot comprehend written instructions

   _____ b. A 67-year-old who has difficulty with verbal expression

_____ c. A 76-year-old who cannot remember if he just ate

_____ d. A 58-year-old who cannot differentiate right from left

3. Match each brain structure with its function.

_____ a. Thalamus   A. Postural reflexes

                        B. Maintenance of equilibrium

                        C. Perception of sensory impulses

_____ b. Midbrain   D. Controls rhythmic quality of respirations

                        E. Cardiac, respiration, and vasomotor control

_____ c. Pons

_____ d. Medulla

_____ e. Cerebellum

4. Match the spinal tract with the activity that it controls.

_____ a. Ventral corticospinal   A. Knee-jerk response

                                    B. Balancing on one leg

                                    C. Raising both arms

_____ b. Reticulospinal   D. Walking

                                    E. Winking the right eye

                                    F. Perception of feather touching the cheek

_____ c. Lateral corticospinal   G. Firm thigh muscles

                                    H. Burning sensation in left arm

_____ d. Lateral spinothalamic

_____ e. Ventral spinothalamic

_____ f. Olivospinal

_____ g. Tectospinal

_____ h. Vestibulospinal

5. Identify the term for the disorder each patient has.

_____ a. The patient speaks fluently but the content is not meaningful.

_____ b. The patient has explosive speech with sustained sounds.

_____ c. The patient is unable to maintain balance walking heel to toe.

_____ d. The patient identifies a safety pin as a pair of scissors by touch.

_____ f. The patient has absence of smell.

_____ g. The patient has loss of vision in half of both visual fields.

6. Match each assessment technique with the neurologic parameter it is designed to test.

_____ a. Ability to identify a coin in the hand with eyes closed

_____ b. Passive range of motion

_____ c. Discrimination between sharp and dull

_____ d. Standing, feet together, eyes closed

_____ e. Stroking plantar surface of the foot

A. Crude touch sensation
B. Perception
C. Superficial pain perception
D. Proprioception
E. Muscle strength
F. Muscle tone
G. Reflexes

_____ f.   Assessing ability to feel a cotton swab

_____ g.   Placing a tuning fork on bony prominences

7. Identify which of the 12 cranial nerves (I through XII) is assessed by each technique.

_____ a. Identifying alcohol odor

_____ b. Identifying whispered words

_____ c. Testing pupil equality and reflex

_____ d. Observing the opened mouth for jaw deviation

_____ e. Observing the tongue for deviation

_____ f. Reading fine newspaper print

_____ g. Noting sour versus sweet tastes on side of tongue

_____ h. Testing touch and pain sensation of the face

_____ i. Testing for gag reflex

_____ j. Moving an object into each visual fiel

_____ k. Watching for symmetrical facial movement

_____ l. Identifying taste on posterior third of tongue

_____ m. Assessing ability to shrug the shoulders

_____ n. Observing for ptosis or dropping of upper eyelids

_____ o. Assessing ability to look up, down, and either side

8. On the basis of the information provided, identify the patient who has incurred trauma to Broca's area and which patient has an abnormality in Wernicke's area.

   Patient A: A 56-year-old woman is admitted to the hospital with a diagnosis of acute cerebrovascular accident. She was found on the floor in her bathroom with right-sided weakness. On admission she is trying to speak but is unable to verbalize clearly. She nods appropriately to "yes/no" questions.

   Patient B: A 58-year-old woman is admitted to the hospital also with a diagnosis of acute cerebrovascular accident. She exhibits right-sided weakness but can verbalize fairly clearly. However, she responds inappropriately to simple questions. For example, when asked how old she is, she states that she "needs to go to church this evening."

9. Compare circulatory characteristics of the brain with those of the body in relation to compensatory vasodilation and vasoconstriction.

10. A 68-year-old woman is admitted to the hospital with signs and symptoms of cerebrovascular compromise. She is scheduled for a digital subtraction angiogram. Before the procedure, the patient states, "How is this test different from the cerebral angiogram I had several months ago?" In understandable terms, explain the main differences between these two procedures.

11. **Case Study:** The nurse is performing a neurologic examination on a 22-year-old college student. Evaluate the nurse's findings. Identify abnormal findings and possible cause(s). What additional tests would be useful in establishing the correct diagnosis?

Some resistance noted on passive neck flexion; unable to extend legs completely without pain (rated as 3 on 1 to 5 scale). T, 100.2° F; P, 98; R, 28; BP, 150/60. Reflexes 2+ bilaterally. Complains of headache. Oriented to person and place but not to time. Difficulty interpreting the proverb "a bird in the hand is worth two in the bush" and subtracting 9 from 100 serially. Speech is fluent and articulate; difficulty following simple verbal commands when distracted by other activities in the room. Able to hear whispered words bilaterally. Visual assessment: optic disk 1.5 mm flat and sharply defined. Slight ptosis noted with decreased facial sensation. Able to move eyes up and down symmetrically but had difficulty moving eyes in lateral positions. Pupillary reaction equal but sluggish. Grip and dorsiflexion strength equal bilaterally; steady gait. Hyperreacts to light touch stimulation.

12. A 47-year-old patient with symptoms of severe back pain of 2 months' duration is scheduled for a lumbar myelogram with an oil-based dye. A 45-year-old patient also reporting chronic back pain is scheduled for a lumbar myelogram with a water-based dye. Explain the differences in these procedures and differences in the care and preparation of each patient.

48 Traumatic and Neoplastic Problems of the Brain

1. Identify the patient's state of awareness based on the nurse's documentation. Use the categories of
   A = alert
   B = confused
   C = obtunded (semiconscious)
   D = stupor (semicomatose)
   E = comatose

   _____ a. "Unarousable and unresponsive to all stimuli."

   _____ b. "Patient states he is at his son's home but shortly thereafter states he is in the hospital. Responds to his name. Asks questions of the nurse repeatedly."

   _____ c. "Grimaces when noxious stimulus applied to fingernail. Unresponsive to verbal stimulation."

   _____ d. "Alert and oriented to persons, place, and time. Able to follow verbal commands."

   _____ e. "Patient easily arousable and responds appropriately to simple questions that often need repeating. Extremely lethargic when not being stimulated."

   _____ f. "Very lethargic with blank, gazing facial expression. Verbally unresponsive and arouses only with vigorous stimulation."

2. Consider each patient situation and label the patient's behavior as an illusion (I), delusion (D), or hallucination (H).

   _____ a. Patient tells the staff that the devil has invaded his body.

   _____ b. Patient calls out at 0100 and is observed sitting up in bed, stating a man is in the room stealing her purse. Respiratory therapist at bedside of other patient in room.

_____ c. Patient quietly lying in bed, picking at the air, stating that she is trying to get the spider webs down from the ceiling.

3. Label the documented behaviors according to the correct seizure category:
   T = tonic-clonic (grand mal)
   A = absence (petit mal)
   M = myoclonic
   CP = complex partial (psychomotor)
   S = simple partial (focal)

_____ a. A 30-year-old patient suddenly begins to stagger around the room, picks up items, and throws them on the floor. He is talking as if in response to someone conversing with him. After 45 seconds, he urinates on the floor, lays down on the couch, and goes to sleep.

_____ b. A 42-year-old patient reports lightheadedness and smelling burning wood. Ten seconds later she falls to the floor in an unconscious state. She begins to have jerking-relaxing movements for approximately 30 seconds.

_____ c. A 28-year-old patient suddenly has a strong, rapid, involuntary contraction of the left arm and thigh.

_____ d. A 56-year-old woman tells her husband that the right side of her face and hand feel numb. Shortly thereafter, she begins smacking her lips and salivating heavily, after which she begins having muscular jerking of her hand.

_____ e. A 16-year-old boy is observed by his teacher to be vacantly staring at the blackboard with eyes focused straight ahead, unresponsive to verbal stimuli.

4. Patient responses have been documented by two different nurses. Discuss how the terms used by both nurses might be misleading to other nurses or health care personnel.

   Nurse A: Patient not oriented to time, place, or person. Obtunded with no verbal response to painful stimuli.
   Nurse B: Patient appears to be in a stupor. Very drowsy with a short attention span. Responds appropriately to painful stimuli by withdrawing extremity.

5. Using the Glasgow Coma Scale, rate the patient's response based on the nurse's documentation.

   "Patient reacts specifically but inconsistently to stimuli. Generally pulls arm away when painful stimulus initiated. Arouses and opens eyes when name called several times. Verbalizes but does not communicate in complete or comprehensible sentences."

   _____ Eye response   _____ Verbal response   _____ Motor response

6. Discuss the potential positive and negative consequences of using or not using restraints for patients with altered levels of consciousness.

7. Critique the following documentation, evaluating content for clarity and thoroughness in describing a grand mal seizure. Was any necessary information missed or omitted?

   "Patient c/o seeing unusual things before his eyes. Cried out loudly and fell back on the bed from a sitting position. Noted flexion of arms and extension of legs. Vital signs: P, 64; BP, 118/60; no spontaneous respirations. Shortly after contractions stopped, patient unable to recall seizure activity or aura; patient c/o headache."

8. A young high school student is discharged after 24 hours of observation after a minor head injury. The nurse will teach the parents to call the physician or emergency department immediately if their child develops which conditions?

9. **Case Study:** A 69-year-old man admitted to the hospital with confusion has a longstanding history of congestive heart failure. He takes Lasix 80 mg daily. His wife states he is not eating. Laboratory data reveal hemoglobin, 8.9 g/dl; hematocrit, 29%; potassium, 3.6 mEq/L; sodium, 133 mEq/L; and albumin, 2.2 g/dl. Analyze the data and determine what additional assessment data are needed to help identify the cause of this patient's altered level of consciousness.

10. **Case Study:** A 52-year-old auto mechanic who works the 1500 to 2300 shift is admitted to the hospital with a report of headaches that have escalated over the past 2 to 3 months. The patient attributes his headaches to the usual noise and loud music in his work environment. His wife states that he has become increasingly hostile and moody. Neurologic examination and computed tomography scan confirm the diagnosis of brain tumor. Three days after craniotomy, he is transferred to the oncology unit from the intensive care unit. As the shift begins, the nurse notes that the patient's verbal and motor performance have changed as indicated by Glasgow Coma Scale ratings (verbal was 4, now 2; motor was 5, now 3). Vital signs are blood pressure, 140/68 mm Hg, pulse, 90 beats/min; respirations, 32/min; temperature, 101.4° F. Indwelling urinary catheter is patent. The patient is incontinent of stool. During morning care, the patient is unable to assist with bathing and grooming activities because of diminished cognition and motor responses. The physician is notified of the new findings, and the patient is returned to the intensive care unit with increasing intracranial pressure. Analyze this patient situation and write five or six nursing diagnoses that address the patient's primary problems.

11. **Case Study:** Analyze the following patient's diary for key factors that may be triggering her headaches.

"Oct. 21. No headache today. Nonstressful day at work. Did yard work despite the heat. Had cereal, milk, and toast for breakfast; ham sandwich and carrot sticks for lunch; grilled chicken, baked potato, and tossed salad for dinner."

"Oct. 22. Slept well. Was asked to do extra work assignment. Felt I should accept, although I am falling behind on the new building project. Had lunch with several co-workers at a new bar and grill. Ate peanuts before lunch and had a chef's salad. Had pizza with the family for dinner and enjoyed several beers after mowing the lawn. Went to bed at midnight after working on new project. No headaches today. Felt great! P.S. Ate five chocolate chip cookies before bed!"

"Oct. 23. Awoke with intense headache on the right side of my head. Felt mildly nauseated throughout the day. Could not concentrate at work. Went home 1 hour early."

12. **Case Study:** A patient underwent a craniotomy for a brain tumor 48 hours ago. Nursing assessment reveals a Glasgow Coma Scale score of 15, urine specific gravity of 1.029, very dilute urine, and serum sodium 150 mEq/L. What is the patient most likely experiencing based on the data? Write an appropriate nursing diagnosis for this patient and discuss collaborative care expectations in this situation.

49 Vascular and Degenerative Problems of the Brain

1. Correct any false statements about stroke.
   a. A stroke is a disease that causes decreased cerebral blood flow and sudden focal neurologic deficits.

   b. Nonmodifiable risk factors for stroke are age, sex, race, diabetes mellitus status, and hypertension.

   c. Brain ischemia causes an influx of fluid-activated white blood cells and coagulation factors that clog the microcirculation.

   d. The overall effect of cerebral edema from stroke may peak by 48 hours after infarction and remain present for up to 1 week.

   e. Urinary frequency, urgency, and incontinence are common problems in the initial days after stroke.

   f. Visual defects are uncommon after stroke unless the visual pathways have been involved.

   g. Depression after stroke is often compounded by frustration over losses in functional abilities and communication.

2. Identify each brain condition based on the descriptions.

   _____ a. Occurs suddenly during waking activities and produces severe defects at the time of event.

   _____ b. Defect usually reverses within 48 hours but may extend up to 3 weeks.

   _____ c. Stable syndrome of neurologic defects occurring within 1 hour; comprises 60% of all strokes.

289

_____ d. Related to ruptured vessel caused by hypertension; generally occurs during waking hours; carries a high mortality rate.

_____ e. Relatively brief episode of neurologic deficit that resolves without residual effects.

_____ e. Neurologic defect occurs in stepwise progression; can progress up to 72 hours.

3. How do comprehension and expression aphasia differ? Identify nursing interventions for each.

4. A patient is diagnosed with a right cerebral hemisphere stroke. Discuss how the nurse assesses for the presence of sensory-perceptual deficits such as hemianopia, unilateral neglect, or agnosia.

5. **Case Study:** A 70-year-old man is admitted to the emergency department with neurologic deficits. After an emergency computed tomography scan, a diagnosis of embolic stroke is made. The patient's blood pressure is 180/96 mm Hg, pulse is 100 beats/min, and respirations are 18/min. The physician orders intravenous 0.9% NaCl and a heparin drip. Antihypertensive medications are not ordered. Discuss the rationale for administering intravenous saline and withholding antihypertensive medication in this situation.

290

6. The nursing staff at a rehabilitation facility is preparing a standard protocol for addressing *imbalanced nutrition: less than body requirements*. Identify specific nursing interventions and related activities that should be included in the protocol to help the majority of patients who have had either a vascular or degenerative neurologic disorder.

7. Explain whether the type of stroke (thrombotic, embolic, hemorrhagic) is an important consideration when planning nursing care.

8. Fill in the blanks to complete the sentences about cerebral aneurysm and arterio-venous malformation.

   a. A cerebral aneurysm is a thin-walled _____ or

      _____ of a(n) _____ in the brain.

   b. Between _____ and _____ of persons

      having _____ of a cerebral aneurysm die at the time of

      _____.

   c. When a cerebral aneurysm ruptures, blood at _____ pressure is

      forced out into the _____, usually into the

      _____ space.

   d. The classic symptom of _____ from either an aneurysm or

      arteriovenous malformation is the _____

      _____ of a violent _____.

   e. The focus of nursing care for patients with aneurysm or arteriovenous

      malformation is careful patient _____ and implementation of

      aneurysm _____ precautions.

9. Correct any false statements about the degenerative disease multiple sclerosis.

a. Multiple sclerosis is an acute, degenerative, autoimmune disorder characterized by infection, demyelination, and scarring of the myelin sheath.

b. A total of 70% to 75% of cases of multiple sclerosis are diagnosed in women, with the average age of onset being 30 years.

c. The most common form of multiple sclerosis is relapsing/remitting, which involves periods of disease exacerbations and remissions.

d. Research evidence suggests that a latent bacterial infection initiates the autoimmune response occurring in multiple sclerosis.

e. Acute inflammation increases the thickness of the myelin sheath surrounding the axons and nerve fibers, which slows or blocks the conduction of nerve impulses.

f. The basic goal of drug therapy for multiple sclerosis is to decrease the inflammation and destruction of the myelin sheath.

g. Multiple sclerosis is a debilitating rather than a fatal disease process that requires patients and families to cope with disease challenges for many years.

h. Urinary tract infection is a common cause of death in patients with multiple sclerosis and cannot always be prevented.

10. **Case Study:** An older adult man was recently diagnosed with Parkinson's disease. Family members ask the nurse how they can help when the patient begins propelling forward or freezes while walking. Provide several strategies that the family can use to promote the patient's safety.

11. **Case Study:** A patient is admitted for acute exacerbation of myasthenia gravis. The nurse administers a dose of Mestinon at 0730 before breakfast. At 0930 the patient reports a significant increase in weakness, nausea, and difficulty swallowing saliva. The nurse realizes that the patient could be in one of two types of crises associated with myasthenia gravis (myasthenic or cholinergic). Offer a conclusion and support your choice.

12. Explain how the use of Tensilon can differentiate between myasthenic crisis and cholinergic crisis.

13. Write at least two nursing diagnoses that are relevant for a patient with amyotrophic lateral sclerosis as well as the patient with Guillain-Barré syndrome.

50 Spinal Cord and Peripheral Nerve Problems

1. Identify the terms related to mechanisms and types of spinal cord injury.

_____ a. Extreme lateral flexion or twisting of the head and neck resulting in highly unstable spine.

_____ b. Decreased perfusion and ischemia of the spinal cord from damaged blood vessels.

_____ c. Extreme vertical force causing the vertebra to shatter or burst.

_____ d. The cord is compressed and bleeding into the cord results in bruising and edema.

_____ e. Injury causes significant damage from pronounced downward and backward arc of the head's movement.

_____ f. Complete or incomplete severing of the spinal cord with loss of neurologic function below the level of injury.

_____ g. The head and neck are forcibly hyperflexed and may be snapped backward into forced hyperextension.

_____ h. Cord is severely jarred or squeezed but without identifiable pathologic changes.

_____ i. Permanent injury occurs from an actual tear in the cord.

_____ j. Injury caused by an object in direct contact with the spinal cord.

2. Use an analogy that explains or demonstrates the relation between upper and lower motor neurons.

3. Predict the muscle function that will remain after the following injuries:
   a. A 29-year-old man with a transection of the cord at C3

   b. A 34-year-old woman with an injury at C6

   c. An 18-year-old man with a transection of the cord at T10

   d. A 22-year-old woman with an injury at L2

4. Correct any false statements about the pathophysiology and complications of spinal cord injury.
   a. After spinal injury, a cascade of biochemical and cellular changes occurs, resulting in secondary damage to the spinal cord.

   b. The process of secondary injury begins within hours of the original spinal insult.

   c. Neurogenic shock occurs primarily in patients with injuries to the lumbar and sacral spine.

   d. Spinal shock refers to the hemodynamic instability caused by the loss of innervation from the brain to the parasympathetic nervous system.

   e. Spinal cord injury is considered complete when a total loss of sensory and voluntary motor function is present below the level of injury.

   f. Central cord compression refers to loss of strength, pain, and temperature sensation below the level of the injury.

g. The syndrome caused by cone-shaped termination of the spinal cord at the L1-2 level is known as cauda equina syndrome.

h. Paraplegia indicates a lesion in the thoracic, lumbar, or sacral segments of the spinal cord.

i. Patients with spinal cord injury between the levels of C1 and C4 can initiate breaths normally but may have hypoventilation from the loss of intercostal and accessory muscle strength.

j. The effects of spinal cord injury on bowel, bladder, and sexual function vary based on whether upper or lower motor neurons have been damaged.

k. Hypoventilation, ineffective breathing patterns, pooling of secretions, and difficulty clearing the airway are ongoing concerns throughout the life of patients with spinal cord injury.

l. The use of pharmacologic interventions and pneumatic compression devices has not significantly reduced the incidence of deep vein thrombosis in patients with spinal cord injury, although they do provide comfort.

m. Neuropathic pain is difficult to control and more responsive to antidepressants and anticonvulsants than traditional analgesics.

n. Stretching exercises and hot pack therapy are the two primary interventions for managing spasticity in patients with spinal cord injury.

o. An overdistended bladder is the most common cause of autonomic hyperreflexia.

p. Spinal cord injury is a significant risk factor for development of gastric ulcers, which is further increased by use of high-dose steroids.

5. **Case Study:** A young man is being evaluated in the emergency department after a motorcycle accident. Physical findings include flaccid paralysis and loss of sensation below C6, blood pressure of 92/58 mm Hg, pulse of 56 beats/min, respirations of 16/min and shallow, and temperature of 94° F. His skin is warm/dry, pedal pulses are diminished, bowel sounds are absent, and he is incontinent of bowel and bladder shortly after the accident. Urinary output over the past 2 hours equals 60 ml of concentrated urine. Analyze the assessment findings. Determine which data, if any, support spinal neurogenic shock. Is any evidence of hypovolemia present? If so, note indicators.

6. Match the correct use for each medication used in the care of patients with spinal cord injury.

_____ a. Muscle relaxant   A. Enoxaparin

                                 B. Dibucaine

                                 C. Bisacodyl

_____ b. Anticonvulsant   D. Gabapentin

                                 E. Baclofen

                                 F. Tizanidine hydrochloride

_____ c. Anticoagulant   G. Dantrolene sodium

_____ d. Antispasmodic

_____ e. Topical anesthetic

_____ f. Stimulant suppository

7. **Case Study:** Three weeks ago, a 16-year-old boy incurred a complete spinal cord injury at the level of T2 during football practice. His mother overhears him talking with his high school friends as they make plans for the upcoming football season. The conversation leaves her with the impression that her son has not accepted his paralysis. She conveys her concerns to the nurse. How should the nurse respond? What actions, if any, should the nurse take?

8. Patient A sustained a spinal cord injury during an automobile accident. He exhibits hyperreflexia and spastic paralysis of the lower extremities, and he is able to trigger his bladder to empty by tapping over the bladder. Patient B injured L5 and S1 in a fall. He exhibits flaccid paralysis of the lower extremities, absent reflexes, and muscle atrophy and requires urinary catheterization every 4 to 6 hours.
   a. Which patient has an upper motor neuron lesion, and which patient has a lower motor neuron lesion? Identify the data that support your conclusion.

   b. What aspects of care will be similar or different for these two patients?

9. **Case Study:** A 28-year-old man is 6 months into a rehabilitation program after a complete spinal cord injury at C6. The patient has a spastic bladder and has been able to trigger bladder emptying. During range-of-motion exercises the nurse notes that the leg she is exercising appears pale and feels cool, and the patient's face is flushed. Discuss questions the nurse should ask the patient. What other assessments are necessary? Prioritize a plan of action based on assessment findings.

10. Complete each of the statements regarding nursing care of the patient with spinal cord injury by selecting the appropriate word or words within the parentheses.
    a. Individuals with a spinal cord injury at the level of C4 (will/will not) be able to breathe without ventilator support.

    b. Loss of the intercostal muscles interferes with expansion of the (rib cage/diaphragm), decreasing alveolar ventilation.

    c. The accessory muscles are innervated from the spinal cord at the level of (C2-8/T1-7).

    d. Studies show that continuous turning is (effective/ineffective) in preventing pooling of secretions in patients with spinal cord injury.

e. Suctioning in the patient with spinal cord injury can result in profound (bradycardia/tachycardia).

11. Care of the patient with a spinal cord tumor is most like care of the patient with which type of spinal cord injury? Explain.

12. **Case Study:** A patient is noted to be avoiding brushing her teeth and eating any solid foods. When questioned, she barely opens her mouth, stating that the pain is too severe. What should the nurse suspect? What other triggers could stimulate the patient's pain? If the patient elects to undergo stereotactic radiosurgery, how long will it be before she obtains pain relief?

13. Write two or three nursing diagnoses that address common problems patients experience from Bell's palsy.

51 Assessment of the Musculoskeletal System

1. Identify the similarities and differences between cortical and cancellous bone.

2. List the five major functions of bone and give an example of a condition or situation in which each of the functions is compromised.

3. **Case Study:** A 22-year-old man with type 1 diabetes mellitus was involved in a motorcycle accident in which he incurred a fracture to his right femur, rib contusions, and several lacerations. His fracture was surgically reduced and immobilized with a cast. A rib splint was applied and his lacerations were sutured. Six weeks later radiographs demonstrated a nonunion of his fracture. Identify factors that placed the patient at risk for a nonunion.

4. Identify each type of muscle contraction based on the definitions.

   _____ a. Involuntary contraction caused by stimulation

   _____ b. Stronger twitch contractions in response to regularly repeated, constant, strength stimuli

_____ c. Jerky reaction to a single stimulus

_____ d. Continual partial contraction vital in maintenance of posture

_____ e. Synchronous contraction of individual fibers

_____ f. Tension within the muscle increases but the muscle does not shorten

_____ g. Contraction in which the muscle changes length but the tension within the muscle is unchanged

_____ h. Sustained contraction produced by a series of stimuli in rapid succession

5. What are the major differences between cartilage and ligament?

6. **Case Study:** A 63-year-old woman with a musculoskeletal disorder requires the use of a cane and is unable to stand up straight. Her history reveals no known allergies; the intake of 200 mg ibuprofen twice daily; nonsmoker status; consumption of one glass of wine per week; ability to perform all activities of daily living without assistance; and no changes in weight. Her height has decreased by 1.5 inches over the past 5 years. She works 2 days per week at a floral shop that requires long periods of standing, eats well-balanced meals, but tends to skip breakfast. She drives her own car and does not rely on community services, family, or friends.
a. What further data are needed, if any?

b. How should the nurse respond if any of these problems are noted during assessment? Why?
  1. Redness over finger and wrist joints
  2. Cool, pale lower extremities
  3. Small areas of alopecia
  4. Joint tenderness of several joints
  5. Subcutaneous nodules

7. A patient's documentation reads, "Ulnar drift is present bilaterally, kyphosis is notable, and lower extremities are mildly atrophic." Explain this description.

8. Interpret the following assessment findings and explain the significance of each.
  a. 1+ deep tendon reflexes

  b. Crunching sound on joint movement

  c. Joint subluxation

  d. Flaccid muscle

9. Suggest an appropriate nursing response to each of the following situations.
   a. A patient has been admitted for suspected rheumatoid arthritis. A serum complement level has been ordered. The patient wants to know about the test.

   b. The patient is concerned about her elevated antinuclear antibodies. She states, "I thought I had an autoimmune disease, but now I know I have cancer."

   c. While being prepared for a myelogram, the patient confides that he is not afraid to have the procedure but is really dreading the headache that will follow.

   d. A patient is apprehensive about a scheduled double-contrast arthrogram.

   e. A patient asks why a computed tomography scan is not as effective as a magnetic resonance imaging scan for diagnosing his musculoskeletal problem.

   f. A patient scheduled for an electromyogram states he is relieved that the procedure is painless.

52 Trauma to the Musculoskeletal System

1. Explain the major differences between the following:
   a. Avulsion and comminuted fracture

   b. Malunion and pseudoarthrosis

   c. Stress and bowing fractures

   d. Spiral and impacted fractures

2. A plastic cast has just been applied to a patient's fractured arm. She understands that showering is okay because water will not alter the effectiveness of the cast. What additional information does the patient need to understand about her cast?

3. What problems are common to all patients with traction regardless of the type of traction used?

4. Correct any false statements about traction.
   a. The Ilizarov external fixator corrects deformities by applying gentle traction to the fracture, stimulating bone growth, and lengthening the bone.

305

b. Bone can be harvested from the iliac crest and used as an allograft for nonhealing fractures.

c. Neurocirculatory checks must be completed every 2 hours for 12 hours, then every 4 hours after internal fixation of a fracture.

d. Patients with hip fractures need four assessments: motor or sensory function, edema, color and temperature of the foot on the affected side, and vital signs.

e. The nurse can be confident that patients undergoing open reduction of hip fractures are free of infection as long as their dressing remains clean and dry.

5. Identify at least two independent nursing actions for each of the following fracture-related patient problems.
   a. Deficient knowledge

   b. Risk for infection

   c. Self-care deficit

   d. Risk for impaired mobility

   e. Pain

6. **Case Study:** A patient is experiencing pain from a lower leg fracture in spite of adequate pain medication. A heel pad has been placed and sheets beneath his leg are free of wrinkles. The nurse is becoming frustrated, and the patient continues to complain. What else can the nurse do, if anything?

7. What aspects of care for the patient with fractures can be generalized to other patient populations?

8. List several nursing actions to help prevent or reduce fracture complications.

9. **Case Study:** A 45-year-old woman who underwent an open reduction and casting for a severely fractured right humerus is reporting intense pain. On assessment, the nurse notes that the patient's right hand and fingers are moderately cool but pink.
   a. Interpret the assessment findings. What should the nurse do?

   b. What should the nurse suspect if the patient's hand was cool and blanched, with diminished or absent pulses?

   c. What collaborative management goals are appropriate for this patient, and how can they be achieved?

   d. Why is monitoring the appearance of the patient's urine important?

10. **Case Study:** A patient who has just returned to his room after knee arthroplasty states that something is "wrong." He is restless and has fine petechiae over his chest and neck. His oral temperature is 101° F.

a. What should the nurse suspect?

b. How should the nurse respond if the suspected problem is occurring?

c. Explain why the patient is at increased risk for this complication.

11. **Case Study:** A 73-year-old patient has undergone open reduction and internal fixation for a left intracapsular hip fracture. Before his fall and subsequent surgery, the patient was essentially healthy, lived alone, and was able to adequately care for himself.

a. What factors will affect, either positively or negatively, the patient's ability to return to his normal lifestyle?

b. How does an intracapsular fracture differ from an extracapsular fracture?

c. What limitations are required during the patient's recovery?

d. Identify several achievements that can be expected of patients recovering from hip fracture surgery by their fourth postoperative day?

e. Considering his limitations, what support systems will be necessary for the patient to return home?

12. **Case Study:** A patient is being discharged home after surgical treatment for a fractured hip. She is ambulatory with the assistance of a tripod cane. She lives by herself, but her son checks on her daily. Her apartment is small and has tile floors. Her bedroom is adjacent to the bathroom. She has a small dog. What home assessments need to be made before she returns home?

13. **Case Study:** A 39-year-old man had a spinal fracture during a work-related accident. Surgical stabilization of the fracture was accomplished and he is 1 day postoperative.
   a. Identify aspects of care for hip fracture patients that apply to the care of this patient.

   b. What aspects of care are different?

14. Identify the soft tissue condition described by each of the following statements.

   _____ a. Assessment reveals joint deformity, instability, and hemarthrosis.

309

_____ b. Administration of nonsteroidal antiinflammatory drugs and immobilization are often adequate treatment.

_____ c. An audible "pop" or "snap" may be heard when stress occurs during hyperextension and external rotation.

_____ d. This condition is accompanied by swelling and often referred to as "joint locking."

_____ e. Surgical reconstruction may be indicated, which involves grafting and extensive rehabilitation.

_____ f. Surgical intervention is commonly required when complete rupture occurs.

_____ g. A splint or cast may be beneficial, but surgical arthrotomy may be necessary.

_____ h. This is a common baseball injury.

_____ i. The injury is associated with deceleration and changes in direction.

53 Degenerative Disorders

1. A 24-hour urine collection for uric acid is ordered for a patient with reports of right toe pain and swelling. Why is this test indicated in view of the patient's symptom? Explain how the drug allopurinol (Zyloprim) may be useful in improving the patient's condition.

2. Compare gout and bacterial arthritis.

3. **Case Study:** An anxious patient calls the emergency department stating that he has a tick on his leg. He does not know how to remove the tick and is concerned about contracting Lyme disease.
   a. What additional information is needed from the patient?

   b. What advice can the nurse give the patient about removing the tick?

   c. Is the patient at risk for contracting Lyme disease? Explain.

4. **Case Study:** A 35-year-old woman with a 4-year history of systemic lupus erythematosus is hospitalized for an acute exacerbation. She has a fever, joint inflammation, and persistent proteinuria. The woman is fatigued and obviously does not feel well. She states that her aunt had arthritis that left her with unsightly deformities. She is concerned that the same thing will happen to her. She further states "I don't understand why this happened. I've done everything possible to prevent my lupus from coming back."

a. What is an appropriate response to the patient's statement?

b. What information can be provided to reassure the patient about her lupus-associated arthritis?

c. The patient has 4+ proteinuria. How should the nurse respond in light of this finding?

d. The patient is hypertensive and requires medication to reduce her blood pressure. Her practitioner suspects central nervous system involvement. What actions should the nurse take in response to this information?

5. Correct any false statements about lupus erythematosus, ankylosing spondylitis polymyositis, and dermatomyositis.

a. Each episode of acute inflammation of the spine results in greater deformity in patients with ankylosing spondylitis.

b. Antiinflammatory medications may help retard the disease process and relieve pain in patients with ankylosing spondylitis.

c. Rest is discouraged in patients with ankylosing spondylitis unless a fracture is present.

d. Polymyositis is an inflammatory disease of striated muscle, whereas lupus is an inflammatory connective tissue disease.

e. Polymyositis generally affects the distal muscles first, producing symmetrical weakness.

f. Polymyositis may produce dysphagia, cardiomyopathy, and Raynaud's phenomenon, whereas dermatopolymyositis generally results in calcinosis, rash, and fatigue.

g. Nursing actions for comfort promotion in the patient with polymyositis are similar to those for the patient with ankylosing spondylitis.

6. **Case Study:** A patient with osteomyelitis of the right femur has been placed on bed rest, given an analgesic, and started on intravenous antibiotics.
   a. Why is osteomyelitis more difficult to eradicate with antibiotics than other types of localized or systemic infections?

   b. What aspect of nursing care for this patient is different from that of patients with other types of bone disorders?

7. A 29-year-old truck driver who is a heavy smoker is required to load and unload his own vehicle. He has no history of serious injuries or illnesses. He presents with complaints of low back pain. If the patient must continue in his present line of work, how can he reduce his risk for further injury or disability?

8. One patient has a herniated intervertebral disk. Another is being treated for degenerative joint disease. Differentiate between these two disorders.

9. A patient has just returned from the postanesthesia care unit after lumbar spinal fusion with grafting. He is flat and a turning sheet is beneath him. The nurse has checked his drain for suction and output, inspected his surgical incision for drainage or hematoma, and inspected his donor sites. What has the nurse failed to assess, and why is it important?

10. Identify several topics that need to be discussed with the patient who is scheduled to undergo surgical correction of scoliosis.

11. A patient has bilateral Dupuytren's contractures with mild deformity. What techniques may help him maintain maximal hand mobility?

12. Try to imagine how you might feel if you had to make the decision for yourself or a family member about amputation or limb salvage surgery for bone sarcoma.
    a. Which surgery do you think you would select?

    b. What feelings are invoked when considering such a decision?

314

13. Identify several psychosocial problems that individuals with musculoskeletal disorders have in common regardless of specific type of disorder.

14. In what ways may educating people with musculoskeletal disorders help them cope with the psychosocial problems you listed for question 13?

54 Osteoarthritis and Rheumatoid Arthritis

1. Correct any false statements about osteoarthritis.
   a. By age 75 years, more than 80% of the population have clinical manifestations of osteoarthritis.

   b. Obesity is a serious modifiable risk factor for osteoarthritis.

   c. Regular moderate exercise has been shown to increase existing degenerative joint disease in most patients.

   d. Pain is the primary feature of osteoarthritis and is usually described as deep, aching joint pain.

   e. Leukocyte counts in excess of 2000 to 3000 μL indicate inflammation and subsequent osteoarthritis.

   f. Acetaminophen has been shown to be superior to nonsteroidal antiinflammatory drugs in improving knee and hip pain in persons with osteoarthritis.

   g. Nonsteroidal antiinflammatory drugs may cause serious gastrointestinal side effects that are potentially fatal.

   h. Studies have shown that nonsteroidal antiinflammatory drugs increase blood pressure by 5 mm Hg in normotensive and hypertensive persons.

   i. Intraarticular injection of steroids is effective in controlling pain and improving function in patients with osteoarthritis.

2. Identify at least three priority nursing interventions for patients with osteoarthritis during the postoperative phase after total joint replacement.

3. Complete the blanks regarding surgical management of osteoarthritis.

a. Surgical management of the patient with osteoarthritis is indicated to relieve

_____, improve _____, or correct

_____.

b. Surgical procedures for osteoarthritis include those that preserve or restore

_____ _____ and those that

_____, _____, or _____

joints.

c. Procedures to restore or preserve cartilage include joint _____,

abrasion _____, and replacement of _____

cartilage with _____.

d. Materials for prosthetic implants include _____, high-density

_____, _____, and other synthetics.

e. A particular risk associated with total joint arthroplasty is _____,

which usually necessitates _____ of the prosthesis.

f. Persons having knee or hip joint replacement are at risk for development of

_____ _____ _____ and

_____ or _____ embolism.

g. Without prophylactic _____, the frequency of

_____ _____ _____ in

persons undergoing hip replacement may be as high as _____ %.

h. Erythropoietin-alpha administered _____ joint replacement surgery

is effective in stimulating _____ and reducing the need for

_____ _____ by _____ %.

318

i. The venous foot pump is an alternative method of _____

_____ _____ and reducing the risk for

_____ _____ _____ after

joint surgery.

j. _____ management is an important aspect of

_____ care for patients after joint replacement.

4. Correct any false statements about rheumatoid arthritis.
   a. Rheumatoid arthritis is thought to be an autoimmune process in which immunoglobulin A interacts with rheumatoid factor.

   b. The proliferation of the synovial membrane along with erosion of articular cartilage and subchondral bone are the primary pathologic features of rheumatoid arthritis.

   c. Cartilage degeneration causes the pain experienced by patients with rheumatoid arthritis.

   d. Patients with rheumatoid arthritis differ from those with osteoarthritis because they have morning stiffness from synovitis.

   e. Rheumatoid arthritis can affect other body systems, with rheumatoid nodules developing in the heart, lungs and spleen.

   f. Complications associated with rheumatoid arthritis are localized and rarely cause systemic manifestations.

   g. The erythrocyte sedimentation rate is generally decreased in patients with rheumatoid arthritis.

   h. The purposes of pharmacologic therapy for rheumatoid arthritis are pain relief, control of inflammation, and reversal of bone erosion.

   i. Nonsteroidal antiinflammatory drugs should not be used as monotherapy for rheumatoid arthritis but used in combination with disease-modifying antirheumatic drugs and steroids.

j. Disease-modifying antirheumatic drugs have shown to better decrease functional disability, pain, joint tenderness and swelling than nonsteroidal antiinflammatory drugs.

k. Disadvantages of disease-modifying antirheumatic drug therapy for rheumatoid arthritis includes high cost, toxic effects, and short onset of action.

l. Human tumor necrosis factor has shown promise in treatment of rheumatoid arthritis because it retards radiographic progression of disease.

5. Identify the type of surgical procedure for either osteoarthritis or rheumatoid arthritis based on the descriptions.

_____ a. Removal of part or all of the synovial membrane

_____ b. Moving a tendon from its usual position

_____ c. The opening of a joint

_____ d. Replacement of part of a joint with a prosthesis

_____ e. Removing articular hyaline cartilage for bones to grow together

_____ f. Reconstruction of a joint

_____ g. Cutting a bone to change its alignment

_____ h. Replacement of both sides of a joint with a prosthesis

6. **Case Study:** A 71-year-old woman with degenerative joint disease (osteoarthritis) has joint enlargement of her hands and knees, morning stiffness, and pain with weight bearing. A 46-year-old woman with rheumatoid arthritis has joint tenderness, symmetrical joint swelling of her wrists and knees, and subcutaneous nodules.

   a. What aspects of care are similar for these women?

   b. What aspects of care are different?

7. Identify the benefit of each activity for patients with either osteoarthritis or rheumatoid arthritis.

   a. Balancing exercise with rest

   b. Applying heat or cold to affected joints

   c. Verbalizing one's feelings

   d. Wearing shoes when ambulating

8. Explain why each nursing diagnosis is appropriate for patients with rheumatoid arthritis.

   a. Impaired mobility

   b. Chronic pain

   c. Fatigue

   d. Situational low self-esteem

55 Assessment of the Reproductive System

1. Discuss how the ovaries and testes parallel one another in function.

2. A 65-year-old woman sees her physician for a routine physical that includes a pelvic examination. The physician notes ovarian enlargement on the right side. Discuss the significance of this finding.

3. How would you explain to a male patient that an elevated prostatic specific antigen test does not necessarily mean cancer?

4. Explain how the nurse can help diminish the anxiety of a young woman who is being prepared for her first Pap smear.

5. A patient is discharged home after a hysterosalpingogram. Several hours later the patient calls the nurse. The patient is quite anxious, stating that she sees dark stains on her vaginal pad. What is the most appropriate response from the nurse?

6. A young woman tells the nurse about having a thin, gray vaginal discharge. The nurse performs a pelvic examination and wet mount. Microscopic findings show clue cells and bacteria. The whiff test is positive. Offer an interpretation of these findings.

7. A woman performs a pregnancy test at home and the results are positive. During a visit to her gynecologist, a serum human chorionic gonadotropin level reveals a value of 512 mIU/ml. What conclusion, if any, can be drawn about gestation?

8. Match each characteristic with the appropriate sexually transmitted disease. Answers may be used more than once.
   S = syphilis, C = chlamydia, G = gonorrhea, H = herpes simplex

   _____ a. The most common sexually transmitted disease in the United States

   _____ b. Multiple painful genital blisters

   _____ c. Caused by *Treponema pallidum* organism

   _____ d. Urethral or vaginal discharge

_____ e. DNA probe test used for screening

_____ f. Painless chancre at site of exposure

_____ g. May be accompanied by flulike symptoms

_____ h. First-voided urine sample can be used for screening

_____ i. Chronic disease can trigger reactivity in serologic tests

9. Complete each sentence by selecting the correct word within the parentheses.
   a. The female external genitalia are collectively called the (vulva/vestibule).

   b. (Bartholin's/Skene's) glands secrete a mucus that provides lubrication during intercourse.

   c. After puberty, the vaginal pH changes from a neutral pH 7.0 environment to a more (acidic/alkaline) pH.

   d. The (myometrium/endometrium) is the layer of the uterus that responds to the cyclic changes in estrogen and progesterone levels.

   e. Production of testosterone by the testes is stimulated by (luteinizing hormone/follicle stimulating hormone).

   f. The majority of sperm are stored in the (epididymis/vas deferens).

   g. During the proliferative phase of menstruation, larger amounts of estrogen cause the endometrium to become (thinner/thicker) and (decreases/increases) cervical mucus.

   h. The removal of the uterus (does/does not) result in menopause.

i. Persistent elevations in prostatic acid phosphatase (always/often/never) indicate the presence of prostate cancer and metastasis.

10. **Case Study:** A 54-year-old man reporting urinary frequency, nocturia, lower abdominal and back discomfort, and fatigue is hospitalized with pneumonia. His physician notes an enlarged prostate gland on rectal examination. Preliminary laboratory reports indicate an increased acid phosphatase level, mildly elevated white blood cell count, and normal hemoglobin level.
    a. How reliable is the elevated acid phosphatase level as a diagnostic indicator of prostatic cancer? Explain.

    b. Prostatic biopsy confirms the presence of prostatic cancer. In view of the definitive diagnosis, discuss the significance of the increased alkaline phosphatase level.

11. **Case Study:** A 32-year-old woman reports vaginal bleeding between her menstrual periods. From the questions listed below select those that are essential to ask the patient regarding her symptom. In addition to these, what other questions are also important to ask?
    a. When did you first start menstruating?
    b. How many pads or tampons do you typically use?
    c. Do you perform breast self-exams regularly?
    d. Have you ever had a miscarriage?
    e. What did you eat for lunch?
    f. Have you ever been physically abused by your partner?
    g. How long do you usually flow during your menstrual period?
    h. What kind of contraception do you use?
    i. Are your parents living?
    j. Are you taking any medication?
    k. When was your last mammogram?
    l. How many days after menstruation do you begin bleeding?
    m. What do you do for fun?

56 Female Reproductive Problems

1. Based on the information provided in your text, consider the risk factors for each patient described and decide if the woman's risk for vaginal infection is low (L), medium (M), or high (H).

_____ a. A 68-year-old postmenopausal woman

_____ b. A 22-year-old monogamous woman using the rhythm method of contraception

_____ c. A 30-year-old pregnant woman

_____ d. A 45-year-old married woman with diabetes taking ampicillin for a leg ulcer

_____ e. A teenage girl with multiple sexual partners and taking oral contraceptives

_____ f. A 28-year-old sexually abstinent, healthy woman

_____ g. A 48-year-old premenopausal woman who uses vaginal suppositories for birth control

2. A 49-year-old woman is being treated with metronidazole (Flagyl) for 7 days and sitz baths for vaginitis caused by *Trichomonas*. Which statements made by the patient indicate the need for further teaching? What does the patient need to know to correct misinformation?
a. "I realize this medication will turn my urine reddish brown."

b. "I'm glad I don't have to give up my daily cocktail while I'm on the medication."

c. "So if I continue to have drainage, I can purchase some Monistat cream without a prescription?"

d. "My husband won't be happy about being abstinent for a while."

e. "I can keep douching three times a week with a dilute vinegar solution."

f. "I should choose vaginal suppositories and foams for contraception during this infection."

3. Develop two or three nursing diagnoses that are consistent with problems common to women with vaginal infections, regardless of cause.

4. The school nurse is planning a teaching session for teenage girls about toxic shock syndrome. Outline prevention information that should be included in the teaching session.

5. A 27-year-old long-distance runner has not menstruated for more than 1 year. She has 15% body fat and is dedicated to running. Discuss the nurse's role in the health care of this woman.

6. Correct any false statements about women's reproductive problems and their collaborative management.
   a. Symptoms occurring in the 9 days preceding menses for four consecutive cycles confirms the diagnosis of premenstrual syndrome.

b. When dysfunctional uterine bleeding cannot be controlled with hormones, endometrial ablation or hysterectomy may be necessary.

c. Hormonal treatment with agents such as danazol, medroxyprogesterone, or oral contraceptives has been effective in reducing the pain of endometriosis.

d. Uterine prolapse represents a relatively minor uterine problem in which the uterus descends through the pelvic floor aperture or genital hiatus.

e. Women with rectoceles may report intermittent diarrhea and develop hemorrhoids.

f. Procedures designed to tighten the vaginal wall are referred to as anterior and posterior colporrhaphy.

g. Fistulas can develop between the vagina and the rectum, bladder, or urethra.

h. When being conservatively managed, nursing interventions for fistulas focus on prevention of constipation and douching to remove fecal matter from the vagina.

i. Ectocervical polyps are usually reddish purple to cherry red, smooth, soft growths that vary in size.

j. Preinvasive cancerous cervical lesions seem to occur in some populations at a very early age and may be related to the sexual practices of teenagers.

k. Cervical cancer produces vaginal drainage and is very painful during the early stages.

l. Chemotherapy has played a significant role in the management of squamous cell cervical cancers.

m. Radical hysterectomy involves removal of the uterus, supporting tissues, distal vagina, and pelvic lymph nodes.

n. The woman receiving intracavitary radiation for cervical cancer often feels alienated and depressed.

7. **Case Study:** A 60-year-old woman consults her gynecologist with reports of vague pelvic discomfort, loss of appetite, and mild urinary frequency. On examination an ovarian mass is palpated. A CT scan of the abdomen confirms the presence of an ovarian tumor. She and her husband run a dairy farm and they have two children, ages 20 and 22 years. She began menopause at age 57 years, and there is no familial history of ovarian cancer.

   a. The patient's CA-125 (ovarian carcinoma antigen) level is elevated, and she is scheduled for a laparotomy for definitive diagnosis. Explain why the physician is not relying on the CA-125 for diagnostic validation.

   b. Identify factors that may have contributed to this woman's development of ovarian cancer.

   c. The patient is diagnosed with stage III ovarian cancer. She is anxious and upset, wondering why she did not realize something was wrong earlier. How can the nurse help diminish her feelings of self-blame?

8. Outline the dos and dont's that should be conveyed to the woman after either an anterior/posterior colporrhaphy or hysterectomy.

9. A young mentally challenged woman is scheduled for sterilization. Discuss the ethical considerations involved in using federal criteria and guidelines for informed consent.

10. Discuss the psychosocial implications of infertility and the process of fertility testing for a young childless couple.

57 Male Reproductive Problems

1. Answer the following questions about epididymitis, orchitis, and prostatitis.
   a. What generalizations can be made about the collaborative care of men with the infectious disorders of epididymitis, orchitis, and prostatitis?

   b. Identify one major difference in caring for patients with these disorders.

   c. Differentiate between the clinical manifestations of these.

2. Compare medical treatment measures for seminomatous and nonseminomatous neoplasms of the testes.

3. A nurse is planning a teaching session for a men's group on disease prevention. Suggest priority topics because time is a limiting factor.

4. Patient A is a sexually active 16-year-old who began to notice tenderness and swelling and pain of his left testis and groin and a urethral discharge beginning approximately 2 weeks ago. The pain diminishes when his scrotum is elevated and increases when he is walking. He has a low-grade fever.

   Patient B, a sexually active 18-year-old, awoke with an acute episode of pain in his right testis and lower abdomen. He is afebrile and reports nausea; his right testis is swollen, red, tender, and appears to be slightly raised. The pain is unrelieved by scrotal positioning.
   a. Based on the data, which patient is exhibiting signs of testicular torsion? Validate your conclusion.

b. Why is accurately distinguishing these conditions in a timely manner imperative?

c. How can a definitive diagnosis be reached?

d. Compare collaborative care management for these two conditions.

5. Correct any false statements about benign prostatic hypertrophy and its management.
   a. Prostate cell growth is stimulated by decreases in androgen and increases in estrogen and dihydrotestosterone.

   b. Prolonged exposure to high bladder pressure can adversely affect the upper urinary tract, causing hydronephrosis and kidney enlargement.

   c. Prostate specific antigen testing is often performed on men age 50 years and older to estimate the volume of the prostate.

   d. Medications used to treat benign prostatic hypertrophy are aimed at either reducing the size of the prostate gland or relaxing the neck of the bladder.

   e. Tamsulosin (Flomax) is the most selective alpha-blocker for the urinary bladder.

   f. Laser surgery for benign prostatic hypertrophy causes greater blood loss and increased recovery time than transurethral resection of the prostate.

   g. Constant bladder irrigation is used after transurethral resection of the prostate to prevent excessive clotting or clot retention.

h. Fertility is not affected after transurethral resection of the prostate even though the man make have retrograde ejaculation.

i. Belladonna and opium suppositories are often prescribed for bladder spasms after prostate surgery.

j. Surgical procedures used to treat benign prostatic hypertrophy carry a high risk of altering a man's ability to have an erection.

6. **Case Study:** A 59-year-old man is admitted to the hospital for difficulty with urination. A routine urinalysis, complete blood count, and chemistry profile are ordered.
   a. During assessment, what questions should the nurse ask to help determine the cause of the patient's symptoms?

   b. Which tests and laboratory findings need to be assessed? Why?

   c. The patient is diagnosed with benign prostatic hypertrophy. Identify at least two major dos and dont's for this patient.

   d. Discuss the potential for noncompliance with prescribed medications such as androgen antagonists.

7. **Case Study:** A 62-year-old man presents to his physician with reports of dysuria, hematuria, and back pain. His prostatic specific antigen and serum acid phosphatase levels are elevated. Prostatic biopsy confirms the diagnosis of prostate cancer. The surgeon recommends radical perineal prostatectomy.

   a. Explain why a prothrombin time and partial thromboplastin time are ordered preoperatively.

   b. The patient is reluctant to have radical surgery. Discuss possible alternative treatment approaches, citing an advantage and disadvantage or potential consequences of each.

   c. The patient was initially thought have stage C prostate cancer, but his surgery confirmed that he is in stage D. What is staging? Interpret the patient's finding.

8. Compare nursing measures for perineal and retropubic approaches to prostatectomy.

9. A nurse in a public health clinic is counseling a couple regarding vasectomy. Both patients are age 37. They have three children ages 11 months, 2 years, and 7 years. Outline important issues to discuss with this couple.

10. A 42-year-old man has been receiving care for a duodenal ulcer. Over the past few months he has felt fatigued, had headaches, and had difficulty achieving an erection. He attributes these problems to his high-stress job, although he is concerned that something more serious is occurring. History includes hypertension controlled by Aldomet and reserpine. The nurse notes that his blood pressure is 197/92. Of what significance is the blood pressure in relation to the patient's report of impotence?

58 Problems of the Breast

1. Identify the degree of risk for breast cancer in each situation. I = increased risk;
   L = lower risk; N = no clear link; C = controversial.

   _____ a. Menarche starting at age 9 years

   _____ b. Sister is a breast cancer survivor

   _____ c. Moderate consumption of alcohol

   _____ d. First child before the age of 30 years

   _____ e. Fibrocystic breast disease

   _____ f. Long-term oral contraceptive use

   _____ g. Radiation treatments for acne

   _____ h. Nulliparity

   _____ i. Total fat daily intake of 40%

2. Any patient newly diagnosed with cancer undergoes a series of emotional reactions,
   including fear, anxiety, and grief. Nurses must be aware of how they communicate
   with these patients. Mark with a 1 the phrases that are therapeutic in talking with
   patients. Mark with a zero 0 those that should not be used.

   _____ a. "You look rather upset."

   _____ b. "I understand how afraid you must be."

339

_____ c. "It must be difficult to face a diagnosis of cancer."

_____ d. "You just relax and leave the worrying to us."

_____ e. "I'm sure you'll feel better in a few days."

_____ f. "I can't imagine how tough it is accepting breast cancer."

_____ g. "I'm sure your husband will be very supportive."

_____ h. "Your doctor is the best surgeon; you needn't worry."

_____ i. "Maybe a humorous movie will cheer you up."

_____ j. "Oh. . . , I see . . . please go on."

3. A 40-year-old woman seeks consultation with the nurse practitioner when she notices a small lump in her left breast. The lump is hard, firm, fixed, and difficult to define. There is "dimpling" of the skin. Discuss the data in terms of malignant versus benign characteristics.

4. Mammography is able to detect 1-cm lesions. The value of breast self-examination in detecting cancer at an early stage is unclear. Provide a convincing argument why women should perform regular breast self-examinations and receive mammogram screening versus mammography alone.

5. A 35-year-old woman diagnosed with stage II ductal carcinoma of the right breast is unsure about which type of breast reconstruction to undergo. Outline the advantages and disadvantages of silicone implants versus autogenous tissue flaps. Be sure to use terminology that will ensure the patient understands the differences.

6. A 45-year-old woman visits the public health clinic and tells the nurse she felt several lumps in her breast. Outline questions the nurse should ask the patient during the interview. Discuss the physical parameters that the nurse should be assessing during the physical examination.

7. A woman is breastfeeding her new infant and reports tender nipples and a discharge. The physician diagnoses acute mastitis. She really wants to breastfeed but is worried about how the infection will affect the baby. The following morning while feeding her infant, the mother is crying, stating that she has decided to stop breastfeeding because of the discomfort. Discuss how the nurse should respond.

8. After a breast biopsy, the patient asks the nurse about possible alternative treatments for the malignancy. She states that she would appreciate the nurse's advice. Discuss the role of the nurse in this situation.

9. Discuss ways in which nurses can advocate for women who either have no health care insurance or otherwise do not use or have access to screening mammography.

10. Mammography results show a 2-cm lesion. The most appropriate conclusion is that
    a. the tumor is malignant.
    b. a tissue biopsy should be performed.
    c. the woman missed the lump on self-exam.
    d. the results could be false because mammograms are unreliable.

11. While waiting for a surgical breast biopsy, the patient asks the nurse about treatment options. The nurse's role in this situation is to
    a. provide information about possible therapies.
    b. acknowledge fears and address options after biopsy results.
    c. encourage the patient to think positively and defer the discussion.
    d. address anxiety and plan to be present when the physician discusses options.

12. A mainstay of treatment for advanced breast cancer is
    a. bone marrow transplantation.
    b. hormonal therapy.
    c. wedge resection.
    d. radiation.

13. Which statement by a patient preparing to go home after a radical mastectomy transverse rectus abdominis muscle flap (TRAM) procedure indicates more teaching is required?
    a. "It's going to be hard keeping my arm immobile until I see the surgeon again."
    b. "I understand I may experience tingling or numbness in my arm."
    c. "I can expect some fluid leakage from around the drain site."
    d. "I'm really looking forward to getting in the bathtub."

14. The primary cause of gynecomastia in elderly men is
    a. poor drug clearance by the liver.
    b. reduced testosterone level.
    c. Klinefelter's syndrome.
    d. decreased body fat.

59 Sexually Transmitted Diseases

1. Identify the sexually transmitted diseases, in descending order, that are most frequently encountered by nurses working in public health or sexually transmitted disease clinics.

2. A 16-year-old confides in the nurse that he has been sexually active and fears he has a sexually transmitted disease. He does not want his parents to know. Can the nurse help the patient without violating his confidence? Explain.

3. You have been invited to join a committee on sex education at a local high school. The topic of concern is the increased incidence of sexually transmitted diseases among freshman students. Offer some suggestions for dealing with this problem.

4. As a nurse, what is your responsibility in controlling the spread of sexually transmitted diseases, if any?

5. Identify at least two independent nursing actions that address each problem related to patients with sexually transmitted diseases.

   a. Promoting self-care

   b. Providing emotional support

   c. Promoting a healthy sexual attitude

6. Identify the likely problem in each patient situation. How should the nurse respond in each case?

   a. A 27-year-old man presents with reports of purulent discharge from his penis and burning on urination, especially the first time he urinates in the morning.

   b. A young woman reports vaginal itching and a thick white discharge. She states that she thinks she has syphilis and wants a penicillin injection.

   c. A patient's VDRL test result is positive.

   d. A patient reports headache and flulike symptoms lasting for several days. Physical assessment reveals a painful, weeping rash on her labia.

   e. A woman presents with reports of foul-smelling, yellowish vaginal discharge, spotting after intercourse, and vague lower abdominal pain. She is concerned because she is 3 months pregnant.

7. Explain how syphilis and genital herpes lesions differ.

8. Identify the sexually transmitted disease that best fits each description.

_____ a. The most prevalent of the sexually transmitted disease in the United States.

_____ b. During the latent period, no clinical signs of this disease are present.

_____ c. Doxycycline is the drug of choice except during pregnancy.

_____ d. Urinary tract infections are common in both men and women as a complication.

_____ e. The patient remains contagious for approximately 2 years if not treated.

_____ f. Lesions can cause severe pain, requiring hospitalization and parenteral analgesia.

_____ g. The pathogenic organism is a spirochete that must be identified by darkfield microscopy.

_____ h. Chronic pelvic inflammatory disease and infertility are complications.

_____ i. A lifelong disease that can produce intense and recurring discomfort.

345

_____ j. A leading cause of pneumonia in newborn infants.

_____ k. Ceftriaxone is the treatment of choice except for strains that are antibiotic resistant.

_____ l. Persons of lower socioeconomic status are at increased risk for development of this disease.

9. **Case Study:** A 24-year-old single patient reports occasional blood in her stools. She recently returned from a trip to Mexico and has been experiencing recurrent cramping and diarrhea. She admits to having more than one sexual partner during the past week. Her oral temperature is 99.9° F, but all other vital signs are within normal limits.
   a. What should the nurse suspect?

   b. What additional information is needed?

   c. What data support the need for further intervention?

   d. Which medications will most likely be prescribed for the woman?

10. What aspects of care for persons with lymphogranuloma venereum and chancroid are similar?

11. **Case Study:** A 37-year-old woman has chronic trichomoniasis. Her practitioner has explained to her that she will need frequent cervical smears to detect cervical cancer if it occurs.

 a. Why is the woman at increased risk for cervical cancer?

 b. What clinical manifestations is the woman likely experiencing?

 c. What treatment is most effective for this disease?

60 Assessment of the Visual System

1. Fill in the blanks to complete the sentences on anatomy and physiology of the eye.

   a. The purpose of aqueous humor is to _____ the lens and

      cornea.

   b. The shape of the eyeball is maintained by a liquid known as

      _____ _____.

   c. Cones are concentrated in the _____ near the center of the

      retina.

   d. The rods contained in the retina are receptors for _____ vision.

   e. Visual information is transmitted to the brain by the _____

      _____.

   f. The _____ provides fine focus for light transmitted to the retina.

   g. The _____ receives images from the lens and is the instrument

      of vision.

   h. The ability of the lens to adjust between far and near objects is known as

      _____.

   i. Pupils _____ when in bright light.

   j. The _____ _____ muscles of the eyeball

      help turn the eye inward.

   k. During near vision, the lens is _____ to accommodate near

      objects.

   l. The _____ provides the main refractive changes for light

      entering the eye.

   m. The _____ regulates entrance of light by contracting or

      dilating the pupil.

   n. Involuntary muscles within the eye that control the shape of the lens and

      pupillary size are known as _____ _____.

o. Nutrients and antibodies are provided to the cornea by the

_____.

p. Tears drain from the lacrimal sac into the _____

_____.

q. A problem with the right optic nerve is manifest by a problem with the

_____ eye.

2. Match the assessment with the function that it tests.

_____ a. Peripheral vision   A. Response to direct light

                                       B. Observe for jaundice, redness

                                       C. Assess for clarity, transparency

_____ b. Pupillary reflex   D. Assess ability to read Snellen chart

                                       E. Observe shape, color, size

                                       F. Ability to identify objects in left visual field

_____ c. Sclera

_____ d. Iris and pupil

_____ e. Lens

_____ f. Visual acuity

3. A nurse is planning a workshop/seminar on the eye and visual changes encountered with aging. The audience is composed primarily of older adults. Identify visual alterations that the nurse should include when teaching this group about normal age-related eye and vision changes.

4. During an eye exam, a person is found to have visual acuity of 20/60. Interpret this finding.

5. Suggest possible causes for each assessment finding. What additional information does the nurse need to collect regarding each condition?
   a. Ptosis

   b. Ectropion

   c. Entropion

   d. Opaque lens

   e. Decreased pupillary reflex

6. Identify the appropriate refractory condition, and explain the physiologic process occurring in each situation.
   a. A 9-year-old child reports inability to read the blackboard at school.

   b. A 28-year-old person notices decreasing ability to read fine print.

   c. A 76-year-old woman tells her husband that objects close to her appear blurred.

7. A 45-year-old woman with diabetes mellitus has decreased visual acuity related to diabetic retinopathy. She is scheduled for a fluorescein angiography. What assessments need to be made before the procedure, and what patient teaching needs to be done?

61 Problems of the Eye

1. Match the drug with the correct classification and action. Answers may be used more than once.

_____ a. Miotic

_____ b. Mydriatic

_____ c. Bactericidal action

_____ d. Osmotic agent

_____ e. Paralyzes ciliary muscles to rest the eye

_____ f. Increases outflow of aqueous humor

_____ g. Controls inflammation

_____ h. Antibiotic

_____ i. Moves fluid from intraocular structures

_____ j. Steroid

A. Cyclopentolate (Cyclogyl)
B. Phenylephrine
C. Cycloplegic
D. Atropine sulfate
E. Pilocarpine (Isopto Carpine)
F. Triamcinolone (Aristocort)
G. Bacitracin
H. Mannitol (Osmitrol)

2. A 52-year-old man reports decreasing visual acuity and difficulty seeing at night. External eye examination reveals redness of the sclera and lid margins. What additional data does the nurse need to further assess the patient's problem?

3. A 10-year-old girl is brought to the emergency department after falling and piercing her right eye with a pencil. The pencil remains embedded. Critique the nurse's actions: lifted the upper right eyelid and irrigated the eye with cold water; removed the pencil and applied direct pressure to the eyeball; covered the other eye with a patch to prevent excessive movement of the injured eye; applied cool compresses to both eyes.

4. Identify several generalizations about the care of persons with any type of eye inflammation.

5. A 78-year-old patient just underwent cataract removal from his left eye. His daughter is with him in the day surgery recovery room. What discharge teaching needs to be completed?

6. Compare open-angle and narrow-angle (angle closure) glaucoma.

7. A 68-year-old patient has newly diagnosed glaucoma. The nurse has just completed a series of instructions regarding the disease and eye care. Evaluate each patient statement and draw conclusions about the patient's understanding of home eye care.
   a. "I think I'll obtain several bottles of my medications pilocarpine and Timoptic so I can keep one with me, one at home, and one at my daughter's house."

   b. "I'm sure hopeful that my iris surgery will help me see again."

   c. "I guess I won't be able to read or sew, since that would cause too much strain on my eyes."

   d. "If my eyes feel tired, or if they look bloodshot, I should report this to my ophthalmologist immediately."

   e. "I've checked with my pharmacist, and he assures me that he can supply my eye medication at any time, day or night, or on holidays."

   f. "I'll sure be glad when I can stop taking the eye medications, but I understand that won't be for a year or two."

8. **Case Study:** A 51-year-old man with bilateral glaucoma is progressively deteriorating. His wife is a nurse and works full time at a local hospital. The patient is an administrator of a large metropolitan business, travels extensively, and has always been independent. The couple has been married for 10 years and are enjoying remodeling their home.
   a. Identify factors that may hinder the patient's adjustment to visual impairment.

b. Identify factors that may help facilitate his adjustment.

9. **Case Study:** A 67-year-old patient with a 20-year history of type 2 diabetes mellitus takes NPH and regular insulin daily. Recently she began "seeing spots in front of my eyes" and having difficulty focusing on reading. On ophthalmic examination the vessels appear tortuous. The patient is extremely anxious and verbalizes her fear of going blind. She is scheduled for a photocoagulation procedure.
   a. Write three or four priority nursing diagnoses based on the patient's assessment data and concerns.

   b. Develop realistic expected patient outcomes for each nursing diagnosis.

10. Correct any false statements about eye disorders.
   a. Symptoms of retinal detachment include showers of floating spots, flashes of light, and progressive loss of vision throughout the visual field.

   b. Pneumatic retinopexy may be used to repair a detached retina when small holes are found in the superior portion of the retina.

   c. The exact location and severity of the detachment governs the patient's specific activity restrictions after retinal surgery.

   d. Reading is permitted after scleral buckle but may be uncomfortable because of ocular tissue swelling.

   e. Adults with new-onset strabismus are generally able to compensate for their double vision.

356

f. Botulinum neurotoxin A (Botox) has not proven successful in the treatment for strabismus.

g. Corneal transplant can restore vision in an eye as long as the iris remains intact.

h. After corneal transplant, activities are restricted to prevent stress on sutures from increased ocular pressure.

i. Small iris tumors may be successfully treated with surgical iridectomy, which sometimes includes a portion of the ciliary body.

j. When enucleation is undertaken as treatment for malignancy, cosmetics and ocular movement can be achieved by wrapping implants in either fascia lata or cadaver sclera.

62 Assessment of the Auditory System

1. Correct any false statements about the structure, function, or assessment of the ear.
   a. The angle of attachment of the ear is greater than 15 degrees when the top of the pinna falls above the eye-occipital line.

   b. Each of the temporal bones can be divided into three parts: the mastoid, petrous, and squamous.

   c. The normal eardrum is slightly conical and appears smooth, shiny, and pearly gray in color.

   d. The pinna is pulled up, back, and out to straighten the ear canal for ease of inspection.

   e. The tympanic membrane conducts sound vibrations and serves as protection for the middle ear.

   f. When examining the ear canal, the presence of ear wax, drainage, swelling, narrowing of the canal, or tophi is considered abnormal.

   g. Presbycusis generally begins in about the seventh decade of a person's life and results in low-pitched hearing loss.

2. A patient is admitted to the emergency department after an automobile accident in which he received numerous facial injuries, including a severed external ear. Explain why the patient will eventually need to have the external ear reconstructed.

359

3. Identify the primary function of each component of the middle ear.
   a. Ossicle

   b. Oval window

   c. Round window

   d. Eustachian tube

4. Compare bone conduction and air conduction.

5. **Case Study:** A 68-year-old man reports a persistent earache over the past 5 days. The onset was sudden, with pain radiating to his jaw. He rates his pain between 4 and 5 on a scale of 1 to 5. He has noticed no drainage but states he is having difficulty hearing. He denies tinnitus or vertigo. He has never had this type of problem in the past.
   a. What additional information is needed?

   b. The nurse performs a whisper test. How is this test performed, and what constitutes a normal test result?

   c. During a Rinne test, the patient states that the tone behind his ear is louder. What is the correct interpretation of this finding?

d. If the patient had vertigo, what conclusion may been drawn about his hearing condition?

e. Will blood tests or ear cultures be useful? Why or why not?

f. The patient is scheduled for a magnetic resonance imaging scan. What explanation can be given to the patient about the purpose of this test?

63 Problems of the Ear

1. Identify the hearing loss described in each statement.

_____ a. Loss of hearing for which no organic lesion can be found

_____ b. Originates in the cochlea and involves the hair cells and nerve endings

_____ c. Loss of hearing through the inner ear

_____ d. Loss of hearing through the external and middle ears

_____ e. Originates in the nerve or brain stem

_____ f. Results from damage to the brain's auditory pathways or auditory center

_____ g. Involves the cochlea and hearing nerve

2. The nurse tells a patient with a hearing loss that "You will have difficulty differentiating between words, hearing surrounding sounds, and responding accurately to oral communication. Consequently, you may find that you need frequent clarification. Don't worry, this really won't affect your life significantly except that you may find it annoying. Do you have any questions?" Critique the nurse's teaching.

3. Older adults generally have some degree of hearing loss. How are older adult patients approached to enhance communications without treating them as if they are deaf, especially when their hearing ability is unknown?

4. The nurse observes a patient attempting to clean his ear with a cotton-tipped applicator inserted into his ear as far as it will go. How should the nurse respond, if at all?

5. A patient who has an external ear infection with moderate drainage is being treated with oral and otic antibiotics. What are the potential consequences if the nurse fails to meticulously clean the patient's ear before administering the eardrops?

6. A nurse selects the correct medication, takes it to the patient's room, washes his hands, verifies the patient's identity, obtains good visualization of the patient's ear canal, pulls up and back gently on the pinna, and instills the prescribed medication. Critique the nurse's procedure for instilling eardrops.

7. The nurse is preparing to irrigate a patient's ear to remove impacted wax. What information will the nurse obtain before performing the actual procedure? Why?

8. What does each sign indicate when noted during assessment of a patient's tympanic membrane?
   a. Dullness

   b. Redness

   c. Bulging

   d. Retraction

9. Patient A has acute otitis media. Patient B has an acute exacerbation of chronic mastoiditis. How will assessments of these patients be similar? Different?

10. Match the diagnostic test with its purpose. Answers may be used more than once.

_____ a. Detects systemic infection

_____ b. Identifies specific microbe(s)

_____ c. Assesses for labyrinth damage

_____ d. Minor surgery

_____ e. Diagnoses fluid osteitis

_____ f. Rules out malignancy

_____ g. Assesses prognosis for paralysis

_____ h. Diagnoses hearing loss

_____ i. Used to visualize tympanic membrane

A. Otoscopic examination
B. Ear culture
C. Biopsy
D. Audiometric testing
E. Imaging
F. Complete blood count
G. Facial nerve testing
H. Electronystagmography

11. Three patients have undergone various surgical procedures for different ear conditions.
    a. Identify the primary concern for the patients as a group, regardless of the surgery performed?

    b. How can the nurse intervene to decrease the patients' concerns?

12. A patient states that the ringing in her ears is so uncomfortable that she cannot sleep. What can be done to increase the patient's comfort?

13. A patient is admitted for evaluation of vertigo. The patient has fallen twice, is unable to perform chores such as sweeping, is unaware of conditions that may have precipitated her vertigo, and is concerned that she has a serious problem, such as a brain tumor. What other information needs to be obtained?

14. Think of an occasion on which you had dizziness (vertigo). How did you feel about the experience? What were your greatest concerns?

64 Assessment of the Skin

1. Complete the sentences related to the structure or function of the skin by filling in the blanks.

   a. The outermost layer of the skin is the _____.

   b. The _____ is the second layer of the skin and is also called the corium.

   c. The purpose of the corium is to _____ the epidermis.

   d. The epidermis is composed of a layer of cells called _____, which gives skin its color.

   e. Another common name for the epidermis is the _____

   _____.

   f. The major function of the stratum corneum is to protect the body against _____ invasion.

2. Match the description with the correct lesion.

   _____ a. 3-cm lesion filled with clear fluid (e.g., blister)

   _____ b. Multiple small lesions filled with fluid and pus (e.g., acne)

   _____ c. Firm, edematous lesion of the dermis (e.g., insect bite)

   _____ d. Solid 0.5-cm lesion (small mole)

   _____ e. Round, flat brown spot (freckle)

   _____ f. 0.5-cm lesion filled with clear fluid (chickenpox)

   A. Macule
   B. Vesicle
   C. Bulla
   D. Papule
   E. Wheal
   F. Pustule

3. Make several "if . . . then" statements (deductions) regarding the effect of impaired skin integrity on the overall integrity of the body.

4. A 10-year-old boy has developed crusty lesions over most of his body. His mother reports that he was recently on a camping trip with his father, but neither recalled coming into contact with poison ivy. What additional data does the nurse need to obtain?

5. A nurse is preparing a teaching project for older adults on skin changes associated with aging. Identify changes to the skin, hair, and nails that commonly occur with aging that the nurse should describe. Explain why these changes occur. Use terminology that is familiar to most individuals.

6. Explain why the lips, earlobes, mucous membranes, and nail beds show cyanosis more readily than the skin in general.

370

7. A 56-year-old African-American woman visits the health clinic for her regular physical examination. She informs the nurse that she has a history of hepatitis. How will this information affect the nurse's assessment of the patient's skin?

8. Evaluate the following deductions and inferences about skin assessment. Determine if they are logical; if not, explain.
   a. Inference: because pigmented skin offers more protection from ultraviolet radiation, people who are dark skinned do not have to worry about developing skin cancer.

   b. Inference: vasoconstriction causes less blood flow to the skin, resulting in decreased redness; therefore vasoconstriction in both dark-skinned and light-skinned individuals will cause pallor.

   c. Dry skin and mucous membranes are symptoms of dehydration, and older adults frequently have dry skin. An 88-year-old patient has dry skin. Deduction: the patient is dehydrated.

   d. Sensitivity to cold, dry and inelastic skin, and dry hair and brittle nails are symptoms of hypothyroidism. A 78-year-old woman has these symptoms. Deduction: the woman has hypothyroidism.

65 Problems of the Skin

1. Identify the bacterial skin infections described in each scenario.

_____ a. 40-year old man, painful eruption on left groin; appears swollen, red, core is yellow

_____ b. 72-year old, swollen right side of face, T 102° F, red line of demarcation noted

_____ c. 10-year-old, multiple pustular, crusty lesions over face and abdomen, afebrile

_____ d. 20-year-old, swelling of eyelid; edge crusted; low-grade fever

2. Evaluate patient understanding of the disease psoriasis. Use an *E* for statements that reflect accurate understanding and thus effective teaching. Use an *I* for statements that require further teaching and reflect ineffective teaching. Correct the inaccurate statements.

_____ a. "I'll be glad when this awful rash leaves for good."

_____ b. "I never sunbathe, so that won't be a problem for me."

_____ c. "I'm glad it's winter; the cold will help decrease this terrible itching."

_____ d. "Before I have ultraviolet treatments, I'm supposed to apply tar medicine."

_____ e. "I know I'm not supposed to use over-the-counter medications while I'm receiving this therapy."

3. Correct any false statements about premalignant and malignant skin lesions.
   a. Premalignant lesions will eventually become malignant.

   b. Erythroleukoplakia has a higher potential for malignancy than leukoplakia.

   c. No known direct relation exists between dental conditions and the development of oral leukoplakia.

   d. All persons with pigmented nevi (moles) will likely develop some type of malignancy.

   e. Squamous cell carcinoma of the lip or ear frequently metastasizes to regional lymph nodes.

   f. Unlike malignant melanoma, basal cell carcinomas rarely metastasize.

   g. Early diagnosis of skin cancer is of little value because most are rapidly invasive and spread early.

   h. The pigment in dark skin helps screen out the sun's rays; therefore African Americans are less likely than people with light skin to develop squamous or basal cell carcinomas of the skin.

4. Discuss the similarities and differences between herpes simplex and herpes zoster.

5. Differentiate between the signs and symptoms of phototoxicity and photoallergy.

6. **Case Study:** A 21-year-old woman presents with reports of a generalized vesicular-type rash. During assessment the nurse determines that the patient works in a fast-food restaurant and washes her hands frequently with soap and water. The patient denies recent changes in soaps or lotions. Recent medical history reveals that she had an upper respiratory tract infection approximately 2 weeks ago.

a. Based on the patient's assessment and history, what should the nurse suspect?

b. Identify any important data that have been omitted from this nursing assessment.

c. Describe the characteristic lesions of all types of dermatitis, regardless of etiology.

d. Identify additional information needed to help distinguish between different types of dermatitis.

e. Prepare a teaching outline for three types of dermatitis: contact dermatitis, eczema, and stasis dermatitis.

7. **Case Study:** A 57-year-old patient with a history of diabetes mellitus and hypertension is 10 days postoperative for a malignant glioblastoma. She responds to commands but is unable to voluntarily move her lower extremities. Recent laboratory values indicate albumin, 2.2 g/dl; hemoglobin, 8.2 g/dl; potassium, 3.0 mEq/L; and metabolic alkalosis. She is receiving tube feedings via percutaneous endoscopic gastrostomy. She has generalized 3+ pitting edema and is incontinent of diarrhea. The nurse's notes indicate that a pressure sore has developed on the coccyx measuring 3 cm in depth and 4 cm in diameter. The wound bed is yellow with a gray border and is draining serosanguineous, foul-smelling drainage (soaking a 4 × 4-inch gauze every 4 to 5 hours).

a. Identify both intrinsic and extrinsic factors that have contributed to the development of this patient's pressure sore.

b. Identify the pressure ulcer stage.

c. Write several priority nursing interventions for the patient on the basis of risk factor assessment.

d. What type of dressing is best for this type of pressure sore? Why?

376

66 Burns

1. Why is identifying the causative agent or mechanism of injury important when assessing and treating patients with burns?

2. Correct any false statements about etiology, epidemiology, or pathophysiology of burns.

   a. The amount and duration of chemical exposure determines the depth of injury, which may be partial or full thickness.

   b. Electrical injuries disrupt electrical activities in the body and can cause cardiac asystole and apnea.

   c. Most exposures to radiation produce systemic manifestations such as erythema, blistering, desquamation, or ulceration.

   d. Children who have blistering sunburns early in life are at significantly increased risk for cutaneous melanoma later in life.

   e. A total of 90% of burns occurring in children are contact burns from flames.

   f. Superficial burns, also known as first-degree burns, involve the epidermal and dermal layers of the skin.

   g. Eschar is a leathery burn covering composed of denatured protein that forms from surface blistering.

   h. The depth of a burn injury is evaluated on the basis of appearance, color, and sensation.

i. The zone of stasis contains cells that are viable even though blood vessels have been damaged and perfusion is decreased.

j. Burns stimulate the release of catecholamines such as epinephrine, which increase cardiac output.

k. Fluid loss from burned tissues and the release of vasoactive mediators can result in orthostatic hypotension.

l. Patients with large surface area burns have edema throughout the body, which can impair peripheral circulation by compressing circulatory vessels.

m. Severely burned patients are at increased risk for acute respiratory distress syndrome because of infection, prolonged immobility, decreased immunity, and inadequate pulmonary hygiene.

n. While serious, infections in patients with major burns rarely lead to sepsis.

o. In 70% of patients with severe burns, an initial lucid period is followed within 48 hours by a period of delirium and other mental status changes.

3. A 13-year-old child is brought to the emergency department after a burn from scalding water. He has burns on the face, arms, and hands. The skin is charred and reddish black with no blanching.
   A 69-year-old woman is on the burn unit for burns sustained in a house fire. Ten percent of her total body surface area is burned with blistering. She is in severe pain and has a history of arteriosclerotic heart disease.
   a. Which of these individuals has the greatest potential for healing without grafting? Why?

   b. Which is at greatest risk for lethal complications? Why?

4. **Case Study:** A patient is in the emergent phase after a severe burn over 30% of the body, including the face.
   a. Describe conditions that place this patient at increased risk for initial fluid shift (hypovolemia).

   b. Explain the events leading to hypovolemia during the initial phase after a severe burn.

   c. Identify the major fluid and electrolyte complications that can occur during the first 1 to 2 hours after a burn. Cite the priority nursing actions for these complications.

5. A 27-year-old patient has major burns to his upper body. He is scheduled for split-thickness skin grafting. Discuss how the nurse can prepare the patient emotionally for this procedure.

6. Summarize the major factors contributing to weight loss in the patient with burns.

7. Analyze the nutritional requirements for a 65-year-old man weighing 167 pounds and having a major burn. Specifically, estimate the daily caloric and protein requirements.

8. Match each description with the correct type of burn treatment.

_____ a. Potential for greater heat loss   A. Closed/occlusive
                                                   B. Open/exposure
                                                   C. Semiopen

_____ b. Requires more wound care

_____ c. Impair wound assessment

_____ d. May impair circulation

_____ e. Strict asepsis required

9. **Case Study:** A 47-year-old man is brought to the emergency department with burns from a fire that started in his basement during the night. He reentered his house to rescue his son when he realized that the boy was still in the burning house. He sustained burns to 3% of his face and 20% of his total body surface area. He weighs 170 pounds.
   a. What critical data can be used to determine if an inhalation injury has occurred?

   b. The patient is intubated, has a right triple-lumen central catheter, a nasogastric tube, and an indwelling urinary catheter. Explain the purpose of each of these initial treatment measures.

c. The physician orders lactated Ringer's solution. How much fluid should the patient receive in the first 8 hours?

d. What are the disadvantages of receiving an isotonic solution such as lactated Ringer's?

e. After the first 12 hours, the physician orders albumin 12.5% to be administered. Explain the purpose and action of this colloid solution.

f. The patient's urine output is 28 ml/hr. Vital signs are blood pressure, 98/62; pulse, 126 beats/min, respirations, 28/min; central venous pressure, 4 mm Hg; and pH, 7.32. He is alert and oriented to time, person, and place. Discuss any conclusion(s) that can be drawn regarding the adequacy of fluid replacement.

10. Explain why reintegration is an important aspect of rehabilitation.

11. Identify two or three nursing diagnoses that address the priority needs of patients during each phase of their injury and recovery: emergent, acute, and rehabilitative. Identify those nursing diagnoses that are common to all three phases of a burn injury.

Answer Key

CHAPTER 1

Scope of Medical-Surgical Nursing

1. a. ANCC Certification
   b. Medical-Surgical Certification
   c. AMSN Certification
   d. Academy of Medical-Surgical Nurses
   e. ANCC Certification
   f. Standards of Medical-Surgical Nurses
   g. AMSN Certification

2. Certification recognizes excellence in nursing practice. It is granted by a professional nursing organization, not the government. Licensure is granted by the government and recognizes a minimal level of safe practice.

3. Examples: Increasing population diversity and aging, increased incidence of chronic illnesses, advances in medical science and technology, the emergence of new diseases (e.g., AIDS), inadequate resources to meet health care demands, and an aging and decreasing number of health care workers.

4. a. False. EBP grew out of efforts to improve medical education through a professional development model of problem-based learning.
   b. False. Optimal economic outcomes are also achieved through EBP.
   c. True.
   d. False. The IOM identified the translation of evidence-based knowledge into clinical practice as a key challenge rather than an easy task.
   e. False. EPB has many differences, the primary one being that it integrates clinical expertise and individual patient rights and situations.
   f. True.
   g. False. Revision is not a stage. The final stage in this model is evaluation.
   h. False. The AHRQ refers to evidence summaries as evidence synthesis. The Cochrane Collaboration refers to them as systematic reviews.

5. The goal/mission of NANDA International is to increase the visibility of nursing's contribution to patient care by continuing to develop, refine, and classify phenomena of concern to nurses.

6. Example: Actual deficient fluid volume related to inability to intake oral fluids. Diagnostic label: fluid volume. Descriptor axis: deficient. Health status axis: actual.

7. NIC refers to a comprehensive, research-based, standardized classification of nursing interventions, such as "Electrolyte Management." NOC is a system for describing patient status after nursing interventions have been implemented. An example is "Fluid Balance."

CHAPTER 2

The Aging Population

1. Primary changes, also known as normative changes, normally occur with aging, are universal, and are not associated with disease. Secondary changes are disease related, are not universal, and occur as a result of disease or lifestyle habits.

2. a. Pneumonia, chronic obstructive pulmonary disease, dyspnea, activity intolerance
   b. Arthritis, muscle atrophy, joint immobility, chronic pain
   c. Indigestion, vitamin deficiency, malabsorption
   d. Cerebral vascular compromise (e.g., stroke), cardiac disease, hypertension

3. a. Assess ability to perform self-care and ADLs; implement safety precautions; encourage self-care to the extent possible; teach how to use assistive devices.
   b. Assist with access to spiritual leaders or spiritual support groups.
   c. Assess ability and desire to engage in sex and factors that may interfere with sexual gratification; refer for treatment of sexual problems, such as vaginal dryness, impotence, loss of sexual interest.
   d. Assess degree of family support and cohesiveness of family; refer to community agencies that provide family support, older adult day care, respite care.
   e. Assess adequacy of dietary and fluid intake, ability to obtain and prepare food; refer to community agencies such as Meals on Wheels or nutrition centers.
   f. Assess for changes in cognitive function; assess for factors that may influence cognitive function (dehydration, depression, drugs, fecal impaction).
   g. Assess hearing and vision; speak slowly; repeat information as needed; encourage use of eyeglasses and hearing aids.

4. a. True.
   b. True.
   c. False. Reminiscence and life review need to be encouraged because they help orient the older adult.
   d. False. Older adults may be less confused if they can see outside; however, bright lights or direct sunlight can be uncomfortable for them.
   e. False. Appropriate touch can decrease fear and anxiety in older adults, even if they are confused.

383

Although the person doing the touching may not be recognized, the gesture is recognized, even by the demented.

5. (1) Alcohol, medication, or drug use, abuse, misuse, or addiction can result in a variety of functional deficits that have negative effects on body systems. (2) Alcohol use in young and middle adulthood can result in functional losses and organ damage that manifest as normal aging occurs. (3) Alcohol and drug/medication interactions can be life threatening. (4) Alcohol/drug actions and interactions may be mistakenly diagnosed as dementia in the older adult.

6. a. False. Known risk factors are older age and family history; however, AD is not a normal part of growing old (primary age-related changes).
   b. True.
   c. False. AD is subtle and progressive, but it often goes unnoticed during the early stages of disease.
   d. True.
   e. True.
   f. False. Caregivers may lose familiar and meaningful family interactions and feel isolated from their friends and social activities.

7. Risk for Falls Assessment Score:
   Age = 1 (72 years old)
   Mental status = 0 (alert and oriented)
   Elimination = 5 (occasional urinary incontinence)
   History of falling = 0 (no history of falls)
   Sensory impairment = 0 (uses glasses and hearing aid)
   Activity = 2 (uses assistance of another person or walker)
   Medications = 1 (uses diuretic)
   Total score = 9

8. Further information needed for assessment includes current medications (prescription, over-the-counter, herbal); side effects or drug interactions that may be occurring; the woman's ability to recall words and recent events; her state of orientation before hospitalization and during the day; her ability to follow instructions.

9. Older adults often have preexisting conditions such as hypertension, cardiovascular disease, renal compromise, and so forth that may or may not be diagnosed before surgery, which significantly increases their risk for intraoperative and postoperative complications. In addition, older adults often have nutritional or fluid deficits. They are more prone to confusion, sleepiness, hypothermia, respiratory depression, and other complications caused by changes associated with aging and the presence of chronic illnesses.

10. Examples: (a) Provide a calendar with the time of day and the number of tablets to be taken for that day. (b) Have the patient describe the order in which tablets are taken throughout the day and on what days the tablets are to be taken. (c) Provide plastic or paper medication cups, labeling each with the time and day its contents are to be taken.

CHAPTER 3

Healthy Lifestyles

1. Answers will vary.

2. a. Examples: What is your usual routine before going to bed? Do you awaken early? What is your sleep environment like? What kind of foods and fluids do you consume before retiring?
   b. Establish a bedtime routine. Avoid vigorous activity before retiring and implement a relaxing activity such as reading or listening to music. Avoid heavy meals and caffeine products at least 4 hours before retiring. Try to alleviate anxiety before retiring for the day.

3. a. S, b. P, c. S, d. P, e. T, f. S, g. P, h. T, i. S, j. T

4. a. True.
   b. False. Exercise increases the proportion of high-density (good) lipoproteins.
   c. True.
   d. False. Exercise directly (not indirectly) affects the development of major disease processes such as coronary artery disease and diabetes mellitus.
   e. False. Approximately 64% of adults older than 20 years and 15% of persons younger than 20 years are overweight or obese in the United States.
   f. True.
   g. True.
   h. False. Women, not men, tend to have more serious sexually transmitted diseases because they seek treatment only after serious problems develop.
   i. True.

5. Barriers to changing the family's eating habits include finances (although this may not be an actual barrier because most convenience foods are more expensive), a busy work schedule, fatigue, and a chaotic or disorganized home schedule. Plans for change should be simple and involve the entire family, such as reserving Saturday mornings for grocery shopping, assigning the children days when they will assist with meal preparation, or preparing nutritional casseroles or other meals on a weekend day that can be stored and cooked as needed during the week.

6. Foremost is the need to help the patient reduce fat intake. A more extensive dietary history is warranted to determine the primary sources of her fat intake. Teaching her about the fat content of whole milk and meat products is a good start. Further suggestions

384

Answer Key

may include increasing complex carbohydrate intake (e.g., fruits, vegetables, whole grains, beans, rice) and decreasing protein intake. An emphasis should be placed on a shift in food selection rather than on a total restriction of favorite foods. Food preparation and ways to reduce fat in recipes need to be major focuses of teaching. Depending on the patient's diet history, recommendations for a variety of foods and a reduction of total sugar intake may be indicated.

7. Many factors may be hindering her cessation attempts: she may not perceive the need to quit smoking as essential; the perceived benefits of maintaining her weight may outweigh those associated with smoking cessation; or she may be reluctant to even attempt a smoking cessation program because of the fear of failure and weight gain. She may perceive the risk of cancer as an external factor, one that she has no control over, because her parents quit smoking and were diagnosed with cancer anyway; she may feel that her parents' cancer diagnoses may produce too much stress for her to quit smoking at this time; or she simply may find that quitting an addictive behavior is extremely difficult.

CHAPTER 4

Complementary and Alternative Therapies

1. Nursing has traditionally viewed health and illness from a holistic perspective, one that cares about the whole person: physical, social, relational, emotional, and spiritual. Therefore the move toward "integrative" therapies, which include a wide range of collaborative approaches to patient care, falls in line with the historic holistic philosophy of the nursing profession.

2. Answers will vary. Each person's response is based on his or her specific spiritual journey and belief system.

3. Examples: They enhance well-being, offer a sense of control, and center around the idea of healing the whole person.

4. a. Many therapies (massage, aromatherapy) may have no negative effect on traditional therapies and may enhance the patient's well-being, thus producing a benefit.
   b. Some herbal remedies could be detrimental if they interact with prescribed medications or reduce the effectiveness of traditional therapies.
   c. The most important nursing action is to get the patient to be totally honest about the use of all homeopathic approaches so that interactions or less-than-positive effects can be avoided. The patient should not be made to feel that he or she is doing something wrong or that the non-traditional therapy is of no value. The patient

needs to understand the need for disclosure so that negative effects can be avoided.

5. a. A, b. B, c. D, d. C, e. A, f. D, g. B, h. E, i. B, j. C, k. B, l. D, m. E, n. B

6. a. False. Although pharmacologic intervention is effective for many, much of the evidence supports the effectiveness of cognitive-behavioral approaches to pain management.
   b. False. Part of the statement is true in that the popularity of CAT continues to grow; however, people are reluctant to report use of such therapies to their physicians.
   c. True.
   d. False. The homeopathic philosophy focuses on treating the person rather than the disease. Although this does include a variety of CAT, the homeopathic philosophy does not necessarily espouse self-prescription.
   e. True.
   f. False. This is not exactly true. Although the research on herbal products is based on self-reports instead of clinical trials, patients should be encouraged to study the available literature.
   g. False. Although herbal products come from plant material, being natural does not always guarantee safety. The content and quality of herbal products can vary depending on when harvesting takes place, the condition of the soil, and which part of the plant is used.
   h. True.
   i. True.

CHAPTER 5

Genetics and Disease

1. a. True.
   b. False. Genes and environmental influences are a major source of human variation in health and disease.
   c. False. Autosomal-dominant inheritance occurs when a person receives an affected gene from only one parent for the disease or characteristic that is manifested.
   d. True.
   e. False. Predisposition is testing that provides a person with information about the likelihood of developing a genetic disorder later in life.
   f. False. Chromosomal gene therapy does not exist. Genes are located on chromosomes. Gene therapies may be somatic or germline.
   g. True.

2. Answers will vary. Display should be similar to Figure 5-12.

3. Identification of diseases that have modifiable risk factors. Examples: coronary heart disease, asthma, diabetes, and melanoma.

385

4. Testing positive for a genetic disorder without a cure can be devastating to an individual and family. Nurses can help people consider the possible impact of information and help them to weigh the risks and benefits of genetic knowledge before they seek testing.

5. Helping people (1) understand the genetic aspect of their medical condition, (2) identify their values, (3) recognize the risks and benefits of diagnostic and treatment costs, and (4) maximize adjustment to living with a genetic disorder.

6. Concern that the knowledge about personal risks will be detrimental to the person tested. On the basis of information received, the person could be discriminated against for employment or insurance, labeled, or harmed socially or economically.

7. a. Autosomal dominant
   b. Possible dilemmas: (1) whether she should become pregnant knowing that she is a carrier for the disease, (2) deciding whether to continue the pregnancy if she becomes pregnant, (3) health care worker concerns about her terminating a pregnancy. Others are possible.
   c. Answers will vary.

CHAPTER 6

Infectious Diseases and Bioterrorism

1. a. D, b. F, c. H, d. B, e. C, f. G, g. A, h. E

2. a. Portal of entry or portal of exit
   b. Reservoir
   c. Mode of transmission
   d. Causative agent
   e. Susceptible host
   f. Reservoir
   g. Mode of transmission
   h. Portal of entry or portal of exit

3. a. An <u>incubation</u> period occurs before the appearance of <u>clinical</u> <u>manifestations</u>.
   b. The second period of infection is the <u>prodromal</u> period, characterized by the onset of <u>nonspecific</u> symptoms.
   c. Infections during the acute period may be <u>localized</u> or <u>systemic</u>.
   d. The final phase of infection is <u>convalescence</u>, during which time <u>healing</u> occurs and <u>symptoms</u> disappear.
   e. <u>Aerobic</u> bacteria require <u>oxygen</u> to grow whereas <u>anaerobic</u> bacteria do not.
   f. Once a <u>virion</u> gains entrance into the host cell, it transforms that cell's <u>metabolic</u> <u>machinery</u> into a <u>viral</u>-producing cell.
   g. Localized <u>fungal</u> infections, known as <u>mycoses</u>, typically occur on the <u>hair</u>, <u>skin</u>, or <u>nails</u>.

h. <u>Prions</u> are not likely to be transmitted from person to person, but <u>bloodborne</u> transmission has been reported.
   i. <u>Protozoa</u> and <u>helminths</u>, the primary <u>parasites</u> that infect human beings, invade <u>deep</u> tissues and reside within the <u>host cell</u> until <u>excreted</u>.

4. Answers may include the following: infections cause significant illness, death, and disability; create financial burdens; tax first responders and emergency personnel; contribute to political instability; challenge governmental ability to respond.

5. Answers may vary. Examples:
   a. Risky behaviors (intravenous drug use, unprotected sex), increased use of child care, increased exposure to woodlands and animal vectors.
   b. Overcrowding, poor hygienic conditions, inadequate sanitation, contaminated drinking water, movement of people from urban to rural areas.
   c. Movement of people and businesses into areas that were formerly not inhabited by people.
   d. Easy movement of food, people, animals, insects, and diseases from one part of the world to another.
   e. Potential widespread distribution of contaminated foods.
   f. Increased human lifespan, increased use of invasive procedures and treatments, increased use of immune-suppressive therapies.
   g. Climate changes favor the proliferation of mice and insects.
   h. Adaptation of microbes and microbial resistance to antibiotics.

6. a. False. *Salmonella enteritidis* is transmitted by these methods. Typhoid is acquired by contact with infected animals or people or by ingesting food or water contaminated with fecal matter.
   b. False. *Campylobacter jejuni* is the most common bacterial cause of gastroenteritis in the world. It does produce severe watery diarrhea.
   c. True.
   d. False. West Nile virus does produce fever in 20% of persons who contract the disease. The majority of persons, however, remain asymptomatic. Hanta pulmonary virus produces a deadly febrile disease carrying a 50% mortality rate.
   e. False. *Borrelia burgdorferi* can produce localize or disseminated disease, but it is known as Lyme's disease, not Dengue fever. Dengue fever produces hemorrhagic fever.
   f. True.
   g. False. Vancomycin-resistant enterococcus is the leading cause of these infections. Methicillin-resistant *Staphylococcus aureus* is associated with surgical wound infections, but not as often as vancomycin-resistant enterococcus.

7. a. Immunizations prevent disease with artificially active immunity. If all persons are immunized,

disease incidence and transmission significantly decreases. Passive immunizations provide temporary protection against pathogenic organisms, thus preventing disease.

   b. Hand washing is the single most important measure for preventing the transmission of infections because it decreases transient and resident flora on the hands and deters cross-infection.

   c. Prevents the harboring of microbes, especially gram-negative bacilli and yeast, beneath the artificial nail.

8. Droplets transmit microbes approximately 3 feet when the patient coughs, sneezes, or talks. Wearing a mask within this range of the patient protects the worker. Airborne microbes are smaller than droplets and circulate around the room. Special air handling and HEPA masks and filters are required to protect workers.

9. a. Anthrax, b. ricin, c. tularemia, d. smallpox, e. botulism, f. plague

10. Nerve agents prevent the transmission of nerve impulses by inhibiting cholinesterase and other enzymes that directly effect neuromuscular receptor sites. They can produce manifestations such as seizures or respiratory arrest. Conversely, vesicants are caustic chemicals that produce skin injury and incapacitate but do not generally cause death. Treatment for vesicant exposure involves decontamination by removing clothing and washing the skin as soon as possible after exposure. Nerve agent exposure also requires immediate decontamination by removing clothing and washing skin; however, drug therapy is also required. Atropine is the primary treatment and is administered intravenously or intramuscularly.

11. c, b, a, d

12. a. The nursery nurse is harboring colonized bacteria on her skin or in her nasal passages. Colonized organisms do not produce injury or elicit signs or symptoms of infection. However, the nurse is capable of transmitting the pathogen to others.

   b. In all cases, strict adherence to hand-washing procedures and use of aseptic technique when changing dressings or performing invasive procedures are essential.

13. (1) Be prepared for possible biologic events. (2) Recognize that an increased number of people presenting with similar clinical manifestations is the first indicator of a biologic attack. In this case, smallpox should be suspected. (3) Immediately isolate the patients from other patients and health care workers to prevent further spread of the disease. (4) Notify the facility and public health emergency preparedness and response teams. Other answers are possible.

CHAPTER 7

Rehabilitation and Chronic Illness

1. a. <u>Shorter</u> hospital stays for <u>acute</u> problems and the <u>aging</u> population with its related <u>chronic illnesses</u> have greatly <u>increased</u> the need for <u>rehabilitation</u> programs and facilities.

   b. Rehabilitation can occur in <u>inpatient</u>, <u>acute care</u>, or <u>outpatient</u> settings.

   c. Rehabilitation is focused on supporting the patient's <u>functional</u> <u>abilities</u> through <u>training</u>, <u>retraining</u>, and use of <u>adaptive</u> <u>devices</u>.

   d. Rehabilitation nursing requires a <u>broad</u> knowledge base to tailor care to patients' <u>ages</u> and <u>diagnoses</u>.

   e. Allowing the patient to master a skill a <u>little</u> at a time is a strategy used to build the patient's <u>self-confidence</u>.

   f. The Level of Rehabilitation Scale includes <u>11</u> items that yield a general <u>assessment</u> of the patient's <u>functional</u> ability.

2. Generally, acute illnesses produce clinical manifestations soon after exposure to the cause, are of short duration, and result in full recovery or death. Examples include pneumonia, appendicitis, and measles. Chronic illnesses have an extended course, produce clinical manifestations at variable intervals after exposure to the cause, and only partial recovery is achieved. Examples include rheumatoid arthritis, chronic obstructive pulmonary disease, diabetes mellitus, and cancer.

3. a. Age
   • Higher incidence of chronic illnesses among older adult persons.
   • Reduction in pediatric death rates and successful treatment of many diseases have allowed a greater number of persons to reach the age at which chronic illness is more common.

   b. Race/ethnicity
   • Some chronic illnesses are more common among some races (e.g., hypertension among African-Americans, chemical dependency among American Indians).
   • Genetic linking of some chronic illnesses.

   c. Culture
   • May give less attention to chronic illnesses than to acute illnesses.
   • May view illness as punishment or a destructive force.

   d. Personal costs of disability
   • Personal and emotional losses.
   • Lack of adequate or no health insurance.
   • Escalating medical debt.
   • Increased need for public assistance.

4. (1) The stage of susceptibility is the presence of risk factors without actual disease, for example, a

cigarette smoker who is hypertensive has two risk factors for cardiovascular disease but does not yet have the disease. (2) The stage of presymptomatic disease involves physiologic changes that have not yet produced signs and symptoms, for example, plaque building in the coronary artery is not yet sufficient to produce symptoms of occlusion. (3) The stage of clinical disease occurs when physiologic changes are severe enough to produce signs and symptoms, for example, the person with renal failure has severely altered urinary output and associated symptoms. (4) The stage of disability occurs when a person's activity is reduced because of acute or chronic illness, for example, the person with multiple sclerosis is no longer able to participate in self-care.

5. a. A, b. B, c. B, d. A, e. B, f. B

6. a. Dying phase
   b. Unstable phase
   c. Comeback
   d. Downward phase
   e. Stable phase

7. a. Examples:
   - Maintain physical integrity.
   - Prevent skin breakdown.
   - Prevent joint deformity.
   b. Examples:
   - Display interest and genuine concern.
   - Allow patient to assist with own care as much as possible to maintain independence.
   - Encourage as near normal lifestyle as possible.
   c. Examples:
   - Allow patient to verbalize concerns and fears.
   - Allow patient to center conversation on self.
   - Convey warmth and genuine concern.
   d. Examples:
   - Assist patient in identifying coping skills.
   - Recognize grief and allow the patient and family to grieve.
   - Listen and help the patient explore his or her own feelings.

8. a. True.
   b. False. Goals of care for those with acute illnesses are recovery or cure. Goals for people with chronic illness center around their adapting to limited activity, disability, treatment schedules.
   c. True.
   d. True.
   e. False. The ability of the individual family to pay its own way is determined in part by which member of the family becomes disabled, not the type of illness the member develops.
   f. False. Epidemiology examines the distribution of chronic disease as well as the measurement of health status in the general population.

   g. False. Verbalizing fears and concerns helps patients and families put their situations in perspective and allows the nurse to correct misinformation or teach, all of which help reduce fear and anxiety.
   h. False. Spouses are more concerned about their health than adult children, who are concerned about family, time, and emotional conflicts.

9. The first family may have been more supportive to one another before the event, making it easier to deal with the crisis when the family member became chronically ill; they may have few personal problems of their own to deal with, or they may be financially secure. The second family may feel inadequate or ill prepared to cope with the situation, have personal problems that overshadow the family member's illness, or have severe financial problems that their member's illness will further tax.

10. a. The nurse does not have enough information to draw this conclusion.
    b. The patient may not understand his dietary restrictions in spite of being taught; he may miss his wife and have no incentive to learn new habits or follow a strict dietary plan; or he may feel deviation from his diet is safe while in the acute care facility and plans to start his diet as soon as he gets home.
    c. Assess the patient's understanding and willingness to implement his dietary restrictions. Correct misinformation. Help him plan his diet so that he can include foods that he enjoys. Assess his feelings about having to prepare his own meals and try to identify obstacles that will prevent him from managing his dietary restrictions. If the man indicates that he has no intentions of following the diet because he does not want to, a nursing diagnosis of noncompliance may be justified.

11. All persons with chronic illnesses face similar problems (managing symptoms, coping with the illness, managing financial burdens, understanding the decreased possibility of cure). Strategies or interventions effective for one person may be just as effective (or ineffective) for other people even though their specific disease state is different.

CHAPTER 8

Palliative and End-of-Life Care

1. a. False. Palliative care is whole person care that is interdisciplinary, but it makes use of adjunctive and complementary therapies that support and facilitate the dying person's goals and impending death.
   b. True.
   c. False. It also includes an advance medical care directive and patient-completed values history.

d. False. A verbal statement may serve as an advance directive even if not documented in the patient's record. However, documentation is advised to assure the patient's wishes are communicated.

e. False. Patients who cannot pay for their pain medications are more likely to be hospitalized than those who can afford their pain medications.

2. a. S, b. F, c. F, d. C, e. S, f. S, g. C, h. F, i. C, j. S

3.

Type of Pain	Descriptors	Effective Treatments
Visceral nociceptive	Sharp, aching/squeezing, cramping, pulling, difficult to localize	Opioids Anticholinergics Octreotide
Neuropathic	Burning, tingling, numbness, shooting, stabbing, radiating, electric-like	Opioids Tricyclic antidepressants Anticonvulsants

4. Intractable nausea and vomiting involves more than one emetic pathway and is difficult to control even when triggers are identified and treated. Those most likely to have intractable nausea and vomiting include younger persons with malignancies, those with anxiety over their disease and treatment, and those with autonomic failure.

5. a. Examples: Control symptoms; address conditions that exacerbate loss of appetite.
   b. Examples: Monitor bowel routines, physical activity, and bowel management agents taken; control nausea and vomiting; relieve dehydration.
   c. Examples: Assess for changes in mental status (confusion, agitation); provide a quiet, safe, and supportive environment; relieve dehydration; administer prescribed pharmacologic agents for delirium and agitated restlessness.

6. Differences between palliative sedation and assisted death are found in the intent of the person carrying out the action. In sedation, death is not intended yet may occur. Assisted death, however, has the direct intent of ending the patient's life.

7. a. The underside of the body becomes <u>darker</u> and skin <u>mottles</u> as <u>circulating</u> <u>blood</u> is reserved for <u>vital</u> <u>organs</u> and is decreased to the body's extremities.
   b. <u>Hearing</u> is thought to be the last sense to be <u>lost</u> even though no evidence supports this belief.
   c. <u>Gurgling</u> sounds occur due to the inability of the patient to <u>cough</u> up normal <u>secretions</u>.

d. Breathing becomes <u>irregular</u> and <u>shallow</u> with periods of no breathing, which is known as <u>Cheyne-Stokes</u> breathing.
   e. Throughout the dying process the nurse must be aware of <u>cultural</u> and <u>religious</u> <u>values</u>, <u>practices</u>, and <u>traditions</u> of the patient and family.

8. Spirituality refers to finding one's meaning in life. Religiosity refers to religious rituals and doctrines. Religiosity is instrumental in spiritual support but does not measure the degree to which one finds meaning in life. Many dying people cannot attend church (religiosity) but pray at home or while hospitalized (spirituality).

9. The mnemonic stands for the causes of breathing difficulty in dying persons, which when identified can be addressed. It stands for *b*ronchospasm, *r*ales, *e*ffusions, *a*irway obstruction, *t*hick secretions, *h*emoglobin (low), *a*nxiety, *i*nterpersonal issues, and *r*eligious concerns.

10. Provide peer support, either formal or informal, including encouraging nurses to reflect on the significant contributions they made to the patient's dying experience, and openly discuss any value conflicts they may be experiencing.

11. Active euthanasia refers to intentionally shortening a person's life by an act of commission. Passive euthanasia refers to letting death occur by withdrawing or withholding treatment as an act of omission. Both active and passive euthanasia (and suicide) are intentional choices and, thus, voluntary euthanasia. Involuntary euthanasia refers to letting someone die by not instituting extraordinary measures to keep the person alive or by discontinuing such extraordinary measures.

12. Death is difficult to define because the term reflects values. Values vary widely among individuals, giving rise to numerous views of when a person is actually dead.

CHAPTER 9

Emergency Care

1. a. Serious. Rationale (may vary): Patient is not hemorrhaging but does have a closed fracture and soft tissue injuries.
   b. Minimal. Rationale (may vary): Patient has minor tissue injuries.
   c. Critical. Rationale (may vary): Patient requires immediate treatment; he had a lethal dysrhythmia and is at increased risk for redevelopment of the same dysrhythmia.

2. a. Level I functions: Advanced technological support readily available; high volume maintained to

ensure skill level of providers. Medical specialists are available 24 hours a day.

   b. Level II functions: Treatment and stabilization. Transfer if specialist or equipment is not available. Medical specialists are on call but not present.

   c. Level III functions: Stabilization and transfer of patients to a level I or level II trauma center. Specialists are not available.

3. a. Head injury
   b. Partial airway obstruction
   c. Shock; head injury
   d. Shock
   e. Shock; hypoxia
   f. Lower airway obstruction
   g. Peripheral or central nerve injury

4. The Good Samaritan statute protects the nurse if aid is offered in good faith and without compensation. However, if the nurse is grossly negligent, he can be held liable for his actions.

5. Perform a quick primary assessment; do not leave the child; summon emergency care; do not allow the child to stand or otherwise move until emergency personnel arrive.

6. a. Subjective: General demeanor, emotional state, presence of pain or discomfort. Objective: Head-to-toe assessment, presence of physical trauma, presence of hair under her nails.
   b. Stay with her, listen to her concerns, and attempt to address her fears in a nonjudgmental manner. Assure her that she will be tested for HIV and other sexually transmitted diseases to establish a baseline of data. She will then be monitored and treated appropriately if such diseases develop in the future.
   c. Provide clean clothes; do not send the victim home alone; seek the assistance of a social worker in finding a safe place of residence for the victim; provide information about the availability of follow-up medical services and counseling services.

7. a. The nurse's approach may actually escalate the man's irrational and belligerent behavior rather than subdue him because he is intoxicated.
   b. If possible, avoid holding the man down. Speak in short sentences with a controlled tone and lowered voice. Avoid making judgmental statements. Make achievable requests.

8. Examples of further data needed: possible consequences of the woman's fall (bruising, hemorrhage, fractures) and any behaviors that may provide additional information about her physical and emotional status.

CHAPTER 10

Critical Care

1. Examples: Minimal environmental stressors (lights, noise); maximal space for equipment and personnel; windows to enhance patient orientation; privacy for patients and families; direct visualization of acutely ill patients.

2. Signs of sleep deprivation include irritability, anxiety, physical exhaustion, respiratory distress, altered metabolic functioning, and changes in the patient's usual behavioral or physical patterns.

3. Examples: Allow the patient to rest for uninterrupted periods; decrease visual, auditory, and tactile stimulation; avoid the use of physical restraints; use reality orientation.

4. Examples: Critical care nurses must make frequent shifts in priorities as changes take place in patients who are generally less stable than patients on the medical-surgical unit; they must interpret data supplied by sophisticated technology and take actions based on those interpretations; they must care for patients with changing databases and a greater number of complex, interrelated problems; and they must work within time constraints imposed by changes in patient condition.

5. A quick head-to-toe assessment needs to be performed to identify the priority problems. More time is spent on in-depth assessment of systems that present the greatest actual or potential threat to the patient's life. As the patient stabilizes, other less important areas are assessed. Both the patient and family or significant other should be solicited for information to complete the history.

6. a. Purpose: Waveform represents the fluctuation of the patient's blood pressure. Arterial pressure correlates with external cuff pressure measurements. Nursing responsibilities: (1) Maintain asepsis of the flush system and catheter insertion site; (2) check catheter for patency, accurate waveforms, and pressure readings; (3) monitor for complications such as hemorrhage, air embolism, infiltration, infection, thrombosis, paresthesia, or distal artery obstruction.
   b. Purpose: Measures cardiac output; provides data regarding left and right ventricular failure; provides data useful in evaluating the effectiveness of vasopressor drugs; assists in management of severe cardiac failure and cardiogenic shock. Nursing responsibilities: (1) Maintain asepsis of catheter insertion site; (2) monitor waveforms to detect catheter tip migration; (3) monitor for complications such as infection, dysrhythmias, pulmonary infarction, pulmonary artery rupture,

balloon rupture with air embolism, or thrombophlebitis.

c. Purpose: Allows continuous observation of the patient's response to therapies aimed at lowering intracranial pressure. Nursing responsibilities: (1) Maintain asepsis of catheter or screw insertion site and all connections; (2) obtain accurate pressure measurements; (3) analyze trends; (4) evaluate patient response to therapy; (5) prevent and monitor for complications.

d. Purpose: Allows continuous monitoring of the patient's response to various modes of mechanical ventilation or to mechanical ventilation itself and monitors the patient's response to therapeutic interventions. Nursing responsibilities: (1) Analyze patient waveforms; (2) modify treatment plan based on analysis.

7. a. Provide an atmosphere of openness and acceptance. Talk openly and honestly with the patient and family. Enhance the patient's ability to communicate by board, notepad, and so forth. Recognize cues in patient's behavior that indicate depression or frustration.

b. Provide simple, repetitive explanations of care and equipment. Inform patient and family of changes in patient's status and treatment plan. Minimize the number of personnel providing explanations so that a therapeutic relationship can be established. Involve alert patients in their own care planning when feasible.

c. Continually direct patient's attention to areas of improvement, even when small. Teach the patient and family to interpret the meaning of signs and symptoms, and teach the purpose of equipment to decrease fears and anxiety. Keep the patient and family informed of transfer plans.

8. a. Maintain day/night orientation.
b. Maintain positive tactile stimulation.
c. Maintain personal/social integrity.
d. Maintain time orientation.
e. Decrease auditory stimulation.
f. Maintain future orientation.

9. The needs of the family should take priority in this situation over the needs of the critical care unit if at all possible. If the patient is in an area (or can be moved to an area) where the family can stay with their loved one without interfering with the care of other patients, the family should be allowed to stay with her during her final hours.

CHAPTER 11

Community-Based Care

1. Several answers are possible. Examples: Show patient how to use a compartmentalized medication dispenser indicating the day and time for the prescribed doses; use a timer that can be set to the hours the medications are scheduled; tape envelopes containing medications to a calendar used only for this purpose.

2. Examples: How long has the client been running a fever? Is any redness, swelling, tenderness, or drainage present at the catheter insertion site? If drainage is present, what is the color? How much? Does it have an odor? Are any other signs of infection present, such as other visible skin lesions? Is the client exhibiting any respiratory or gastrointestinal symptoms suggestive of infection, such as a cough, sputum production, or abdominal cramping or pain?

3. Is the client still taking 4 mg/hr of the fentanyl? Is he taking any other analgesics? Did he resume taking the morphine after he returned home? If so, approximately how many doses has he taken? Is he easily aroused? What are his respirations and pulse rate?

4. The scenario does not provide enough information to suggest that the patient can care for his colostomy alone yet. Because the patient's resources are limited, reducing the number of home visits by the registered nurse to once weekly is reasonable unless the excoriated stoma worsens. Because the patient's sons will be visiting weekly, they could provide skin care management. Another alternative is to solicit the assistance of the neighbor in providing skin care if the patient and neighbor are comfortable with that arrangement.

5. a. Because the patient's daughter is a nurse, the teaching needs for the family may be different from the teaching needs of other families. However, just because the daughter is a nurse, teaching should not be minimized or omitted. Discharge planning in this case will be based on limited home health care reimbursement and focus on patient needs, including the availability of community specialty groups that could possibly donate equipment, such as a bedside commode and wheelchair. Because home management encompasses 24-hour-a-day care, social support systems must be arranged for the family. Respite care options should also be explored.

b. Possible nursing diagnoses include decisional conflict and anticipatory grieving.

6. a. Teaching needs: information about how to incorporate the client's nutrition schedule into a late evening or early morning family mealtime to decrease social isolation, central line care, medication administration, and home activities such as lawn care.

b. Examples of teaching needs: Signs and symptoms of central line infection; when to contact the health care provider if infection is suspected; procedures to maintain patency of the central line and intravenous infusions; actions to take should

391

the antibiotic or solutions become contaminated; troubleshooting steps if the infusion pump malfunctions; signs and symptoms of an allergic reaction and treatment measures; resources available for assistance if problems arise or if assistance is needed; potential complications of nutritional therapy; how to assess blood glucose levels and the steps to take if the glucose level is too high or too low.

   c. Examples: Expense of the prescribed medications, total parenteral nutrition, equipment; complications such as infections or equipment malfunction; social isolation; changes in family lifestyle and roles.

   d. Examples: Encourage interdependence among family members; provide follow up caregiver assistance with phone calls; teach caregivers stress management techniques; encourage caregiver participation in support groups; foster the caregivers' social networking; identify sources of respite care; teach caregivers strategies to access community resources.

7. a. Examples: Infected leg ulcer, limited mobility, diabetes mellitus, need for daily care, patient's preference for being cared for in her kitchen.

   b. Although the kitchen environment may not be ideal, consideration of the psychological importance of this environment to the patient is important. Care can be given in any location of the house. Assessment of environmental safety is, however, a priority because her mobility is limited because of her infection. An assistive device such as a walker will help with mobility. An excellent resource may be the client's neighbor. She may be able to learn to check the client's blood sugar, administer insulin, and even change dressings if she is willing and able. Once taught, the neighbor could also monitor the site for worsening of the infection.

   c. Examples: Does she desire around-the-clock assistance? Does she prefer family or friends administer her care? Does she recognize the possible changes in her daily routine? Does her family have different expectations from her own? How would she react to her friend administering part of her care? Does she feel comfortable asking for help from outside sources? How important to her is maintaining her independence?

CHAPTER 12

Long-Term Care

1. a. False. People ages 85 years and older are the most common users of long-term care.

   b. False. Medicaid, not Medicare, provides these services to financially destitute persons.

   c. True.

   d. False. Less than 7% of long-term care facilities are government owned.

   e. True.

   f. False. The MDS is a core of screening, clinical, and functional status elements that comprise a comprehensive assessment for all residents of long-term care facilities certified to participate in Medicare or Medicaid.

   g. False. A complete clinical record contains an accurate chronologic representation of the actual experiences of the resident.

2. Resident assessments, resident rights, nurse aide training, monitoring of psychiatric medications and restraints, and medical direction.

3. (1) Case mix stratified sample, (2) survey of quality of care furnished, (3) an audit of written care plans and resident assessments, and (4) the review of compliance with residents' rights requirements.

4. To ensure that a minimum standard of care is being delivered to long-term care residents and that their rights are being upheld.

5. Too few professional nurses, inadequate training and supervision of nursing assistants, excessive workloads for direct caregivers, and inadequate government oversight of care.

6. Examples: Heavy work loads, physical demands required for caring for older adult residents with multiple problems, the nursing shortage in general, and the increased number of older adults who need care.

7. All licensed nurses must have at least 30 hours continuing education every 2 years in care of the chronically ill and disabled and/or gerontologic nursing. Nursing assistants must have a minimum of 160 hours of training, including appropriate feeding techniques.

8. a. The long-term care <u>board</u> is accountable for conforming with all relevant <u>rules</u> and <u>regulations</u>.

   b. The <u>Nursing Service Department</u> has by far the most employees, making up <u>60</u>% of all nursing home personnel.

   c. The long-term care <u>administrator</u> is responsible for compliance with all <u>local</u>, <u>state</u>, and <u>federal</u> laws and regulations and for keeping the facility ready for <u>inspection</u> at all times.

   d. Nursing services must be sufficient to provide supportive <u>restorative</u> care that allows each resident to attain and maintain the highest practicable <u>physical</u>, <u>mental</u>, and <u>psychosocial</u> well-being.

   e. Long-term care centers must serve <u>breakfast</u> no more than <u>14</u> hours after the <u>evening</u> meal was served.

   f. Federal law requires an <u>activities</u> program to enhance the <u>quality</u> of <u>life</u> for each resident.

g. The three plagues of <u>loneliness</u>, <u>helplessness</u>, and <u>boredom</u> account for most of the suffering in a <u>human</u> community.

h. <u>Nursing</u> services must ensure <u>safe</u> handling of soiled linens to protect <u>laundry</u> workers.

9. a. Examples: Involve family members in the planning and actual care of their loved one, maintain open communication with the family, promote and support active resident and family councils, respect resident rights.

b. Eating, bathing, dressing, toileting, and transferring ability.

c. Within 7 days after completion of the comprehensive assessment.

d. The registered nurse who is responsible for the resident, the physician, the family, staff from other disciplines as appropriate, the resident's legal representative, and the resident to the extent that she is capable of participating.

CHAPTER 13

Preoperative Nursing

1. The PNDS is a specific, standardized nursing vocabulary that addresses the perioperative patient experience. The PNDS provides a framework for standardized documentation, measurement and evaluation of patient care outcomes, a basis for perioperative nursing research, and validation of the contributions of perioperative nursing.

2. a. False. Contemporary perioperative nursing is more patient centered than task oriented.

b. False. The preoperative phase begins when the decision for surgical intervention is made.

c. True.

d. False. General anesthesia may be required, but minor surgeries usually require the use of local anesthetics.

e. True.

f. False. The opposite is true. Patients undergoing open surgeries, which require opening a body cavity or body part, have greater postoperative pain and longer periods of recovery.

g. True.

h. True.

3. a. Lack of time to adjust to the need for surgery, fear of outcome, fear of death.

b. Fear of incurable diagnosis, fear of deforming disease.

c. Fear that surgery will not be as anticipated, fear that outcome will be worse than the before surgery.

d. Fear of the surgery itself, fear that pain will be increased rather than decreased.

e. Fear that surgery will not produce a cure, fear that surgery will result in chronic pain.

4. No. Signing a consent form does not mean that the patient gave informed consent to the surgery. Informed consent means that the physician has provided the patient with information about the surgical procedure and its associated risks, including the risks involved with anesthesia. It further means that the patient has a clear understanding of the information provided. A signed consent form primarily provides evidence that the consent process has occurred and that the patient is aware of the concept of informed consent.

5. a. D, b. H, c. G, d. F, e. B, f. A, g. D, h. C, i. B, H, and I

6. a. Physical assessments: pulmonary, renal, and cardiac systems. Diagnostics: pulmonary function tests, electrocardiogram, complete blood count, and other tests according to facility protocols.

b. Physical assessments: cardiopulmonary status with particular attention to circulation. Diagnostics: electrocardiogram, renal studies, electrolyte studies, complete blood count, chest radiograph, and other studies according to facility protocols.

c. Physical assessments: cardiopulmonary status and history of recent asthma or respiratory infections. Diagnostics: complete blood count, chest radiograph, and other studies according to facility protocols.

7. The 50-year-old woman with type 1 diabetes mellitus complicated by a systemic condition (renal insufficiency). She is classified as P3, which is higher than the other patients.

8. a. Hypoventilation, increased respiratory secretions, atelectasis, pneumonia, incisional hernia, slowed healing, difficulty with ambulation.

b. Dehydration, fluid and electrolyte imbalance, renal failure, paralytic ileus.

c. Decreased lung expansion, atelectasis, pneumonia.

d. Fluid and electrolyte imbalance, decreased wound healing, continued or exacerbated diarrhea, hypovolemia.

9. a. Reduces the number of intestinal bacteria, preventing injury to the colon and allowing for better visualization during surgery, both of which will reduce the risk for postoperative infection.

b. Removes the soil and transient microbes from the skin, reduces the resident microbial count to subpathogenic amounts in a short period, and inhibits rapid rebound growth of microbes.

10. a. Examples: Increase the woman's sense of control by allowing her to participate in decision making; encourage deep breathing, relaxation exercises, music therapy, guided imagery; involve the

393

family in preoperative teaching; dispel myths about pain and pain management.

b. Examples: Teach patient deep breathing and coughing exercises, splinting of abdomen to reduce pain, use of incentive spirometer; teach patient about the need to move about in bed to prevent stasis of secretions.

c. Decisions will be made during the operative and postoperative periods on the basis of data recorded in the patient's record. Lack of sufficient data or inaccurate data could compromise her safety, the surgery itself, and her recovery.

CHAPTER 14

Intraoperative Nursing

1. Directly: Circulating nurse, scrub nurse (or technician), anesthesiologist, surgeon, and surgical assistants. Indirectly: Pathologists, radiologists, perfusionists, environmental services personnel.

2. All hair and facial hair is covered before donning other operating suite attire to prevent the possibility of hair or dandruff falling onto the scrub suit and contaminating it.

3. The supervisor's decision is a good one if the nursing assistant is qualified to work in sterile services and can demonstrate knowledge of the principles of microbiology. If not, the decision should not have been made, in spite of the heavy workload, because improperly trained personnel can unknowingly violate principles of sterilization and place patients at risk for infection.

4. The surgical hand rub may be used in place of the traditional hand scrub. It consists of prewashing and drying of the hands to remove dirt and debris, followed by use of an alcohol-based hand rub or brushless scrubbing. It is thought to be less irritating to the skin than traditional scrubbing and may have a positive effect on promoting skin integrity even after repeated use.

5. a. Moderate
   b. Epidural
   c. Local
   d. Bier block
   e. Minimal sedation
   f. Spinal

6. Balanced anesthesia involves the use of a combination of inhalation anesthetic gases, muscle relaxants, narcotic analgesics, barbiturates, and other neuroleptic agents.

7. a. Emergence
   b. Induction
   c. Emergence
   d. Emergence

e. Induction
f. Maintenance

8. a. B, F; b. B, F; c. A, D, E; d. C, G, H

9. a. Clinical manifestations: Rapid increase in metabolic rate, extreme hyperthermia, muscle rigidity, respiratory and metabolic acidosis, cyanosis, tachycardia, premature ventricular dysrhythmia. Nursing activities: Identify patients at risk, place patient in ice or on cooling mattress, assist with rapid infusion of intravenous dantrolene.

b. Clinical manifestations: Shivering, speech impairment, cyanosis, decreased blood pressure, weak pulse, dilated pupils. Nursing activities: Monitor core body temperature, apply warm blankets, recognize symptoms of hypothermia.

10. Irritant, type I, and type IV hypersensitivity reactions are possible. Irritant reactions are nonallergic and produce flaking skin, inflammation, blisters, or a dry, pruritic rash. Type I reaction involves an immediate, systemic reaction that is the most serious form of allergy, causing wheezing, bronchospasm, and possibly death. Type IV reaction, also known as contact dermatitis, produces a delayed local reaction to latex that causes discomfort but is not life threatening.

11. a. Protects bony prominences from pressure during the surgery, thus preventing the development of pressure ulcers.

b. Reduces the patient's anxiety, and thus metabolic needs, and prevents hypothermia related to a cold environment.

c. Prevents an electrical hazard, prevents the patient from getting burned or electrocuted.

d. Prevents the patient from being burned, prevents drapes from catching on fire.

e. Prevents the retention of a foreign object and possible exposure to another surgery.

f. Prevents postoperative wound infection.

g. Allows drainage of the surgical site, preventing the accumulation of fluid within a body cavity and subsequent infection or abscess formation.

h. Protects the incision, preventing contamination of the incision and potential wound infection.

12. Expected outcomes may include the following: remains free of signs of skin or tissue injury; remains free of electrical, chemical, or physical injury; remains free of postoperative wound infection; remains free of foreign body retention; is at or near normothermia; and maintains adequate fluid volume.

13. Assess vital signs, especially blood pressure. Immediately notify the anesthesiologist or nurse anesthetist for further evaluation. The patient's manifestations my indicate an adverse reaction to the preoperative medications.

394

14. The increased risks for this patient are related to her age and not necessarily to her diagnosis or surgery. The actions of drugs and anesthetic agents are prolonged in older adults because of increased body fat and decreased ability to excrete such agents.

15. a. False. The respiratory system is the system most affected because positioning can restrict lung expansion at the ribs or sternum.
    b. True.
    c. True.
    d. False. They are counted before the surgical procedure, as additional items are added, at initial closure, and finally at skin closure, all of which occur before the patient leaves the operating room.
    e. False. Core body temperature is measured before, after, and throughout the surgical procedure.
    f. True.
    g. True.
    h. False. Eye surgeries are not considered a high risk for potential infection, but all others listed are.

CHAPTER 15

Postoperative Nursing

1. a. phase II, b. phase III, c. phase I, d. phase II, e. phase I, f. phase II, g. phase I

2. A decreased oxygen saturation level may represent impaired gas exchange or hypoventilation. The nurse should arouse the patient and encourage her to take several deep breaths.

3. The report did not include all necessary information. The type of general anesthetic and amount of fentanyl administered, known allergies, and pertinent preoperative physical or psychological problems should have been communicated to the PACU nurse.

4. a. False. Respiratory complications are the leading cause of morbidity and mortality and include airway obstruction, hypoxemia, hypoventilation, aspiration, and laryngospasm.
    b. False. Hypoventilation, not hyperventilation, decreases the exchange of oxygen between the alveoli and atmosphere.
    c. True.
    d. False. Decreased preload occurs secondary to hypovolemia and is the most common cause of hypotension.
    e. True.
    f. True.
    g. True.

5. a. Emergence delirium is an alteration in level of consciousness that most commonly occurs in children, the elderly, and persons with a history of drug dependence or psychiatric disorders.

    b. The most common postoperative respiratory complications are atelectasis, pneumonia, and pulmonary embolus.
    c. Common presenting clinical manifestations of atelectasis are dyspnea and hypoxia, which may be accompanied by fever, crackles, or diminished lung sounds.
    d. Assessment for pulmonary embolus is challenging because symptoms are vague and nonspecific.
    e. Postoperative blood clots often form in the vein of the foot, calf, thigh or pelvis.
    f. Nausea and vomiting prolong recovery time, increase length of stay and hospital costs, and increase postoperative morbidity.
    g. Acute gastric dilation may result in restlessness; rapid, weak, thready pulse; and hypotension, which indicate shock.
    h. Compartment syndrome occurs when increased pressure causes ischemia and compromises the viability of tissues within the space.
    i. Prolonged immobility leading to urinary stasis may contribute to postoperative urinary tract infection.

6. a. An 8-year-old has the advantage of youth and rapid healing because of increased metabolism and good circulation.
    b. Excess glucocorticoids delay healing by inhibiting fibroblast proliferation and decreasing the rate of epithelialization and collagen synthesis.
    c. A contaminated wound carries a higher risk of infection. An infected wound will not heal until the infection has been eliminated.
    d. The patient's intake of vitamins, especially C, A, B, zinc, magnesium, and copper, will be beneficial to the healing process; however, her insufficient intake of protein may impede short-term healing, because protein is essential for the production of collagen, as well as subsequent healing.
    e. The patient's healing will be influenced by his age and chronic illness. Wounds heal more slowly in older adults because of impaired circulation and decreased fibroblastic activity. Patients with circulatory compromise, such as those who are obese, also have delayed healing.

7. a. False. The first action is to cover protruding viscera with a warm, sterile saline dressing. The physician should then be notified for further instructions regarding the patient's care.
    b. False. Malaise should not be ignored because it may be a sign of a systemic reaction to infection.
    c. True.
    d. False. To prevent the development of resistant organisms, antimicrobial therapy is generally terminated during surgery or within 24 hours of surgery.
    e. True.
    f. True.

g. True.

h. False. These interventions will make the patient feel better, but they are also valuable in preventing postoperative complications.

8. a. Prevents cardiac dysrhythmias and other complications related to decreased core temperature. Hypothermia may occur from cool air in the operating suite, cool intravenous solutions, or medications. Hypothermia produces vasoconstriction, tachycardia, increased blood pressure, and increased cardiac workload.

b. Prevents fear and anxiety. Offering reassurance and reorientation to place reduces the patient's fear and anxiety and fosters psychological well-being.

c. Detects major nervous system complications. Hypoxia, hypothermia, metabolic imbalances, hyponatremia, hyperglycemia, or severe hypercapnia, as well as prolonged effects of anesthesia, may be partially detected by abnormal pupillary reaction.

d. Prevents hypoxia, hypotension, and cardiac dysrhythmias. Administration of oxygen by mask, catheter, or cannula is immediate. Oxygen is administered to increase oxygen saturation of circulating blood and ensure adequate perfusion of tissues.

e. Prevents aspiration if vomiting occurs. Until protective reflexes return, the patient receiving anesthesia is at risk for aspiration if vomiting occurs. The side-lying or semiprone position ensures maintenance of a patent airway and allows drainage of blood, mucus, or vomitus.

9. a. Deficient fluid volume and hypokalemia.

b. Fluid shifts into the bowel lumen occurring during bowel surgery.

c. 1977 ml of fluid, calculated by converting her weight in pounds to kilograms (145 × 2.2 [kg] = 65.91 kg) and multiplying her weight in kilograms by 30 ml (65.91 × 30 = 1977 ml).

d. Loss of potassium from nasogastric suction.

e. Deficient fluid and decreased blood pressure.

f. Addiction to narcotic medications is rare when they are used to treat acute pain, such as surgical pain.

CHAPTER 16

Pain

1. Thumb injury → nociceptors in skin → delta fibers → dorsal root → spinal cord → ascending spinal pathways → spinothalmic tract → thalamus → cortex and spinoreticular tract → brainstem → thalamus. Recognition and response will then take place.

2. a. (1) The woman's pain will be in proportion to her fear of bees because the pain is emotional in nature. The person is afraid of bees, therefore the sting will be very painful.

(2) The girl's pain from the bee sting will be minimal because the degree of injury (or in this case the bee sting) is proportional to the pain and the impulse is transmitted directly from the skin to the pain center in the brain. The girl's fear of bee stings will play no part in pain perception.

(3) The pain experience will be a result of both stimulus intensity and pain impulses being sent to the brain. This theory does not account for the psychological aspects of pain. Therefore the intensity of the girl's pain will not be affected by her fear of bees.

b. If the girl stimulated another part of her body, such as with massage, the new sensation would block the perception of pain by closing the gate. Closing the gate refers to interrupting the pain impulse by sending another competitive signal.

3. Possible factors influencing the pain experience of these individuals may include their effective use of distraction techniques, their age, their anxiety level or fear regarding surgery and cancer, a new cancer diagnosis versus recurrence of cancer, their past experiences with pain or cancer, their spiritual beliefs, available support systems, their level of pain tolerance, and effects of analgesia.

4. Patient positioning and teaching the patient how to splint the incision are two noninvasive interventions that are helpful in reducing pain postoperatively. The patient could be taught relaxation breathing techniques and might benefit from therapeutic touch, which could take the form of frequent back rubs.

5. a. C, b. A, c. C, d. A, e. A, f. C, g. A, h. A

6. a. The absence of behavioral indicators of pain is insufficient evidence to conclude that the patient is comfortable. A rating of 3 caused the patient to seek medical attention. The nurse made a personal judgment regarding the level of pain. Finally, pain does not necessarily have to be severe to indicate a serious medical problem.

b. The rating scale is an effective method for assessing pain perception. However, this type of scale does not assess such factors as what provokes the pain; the quality, duration, or frequency of the pain; or the region or sites of radiation. The characteristics mentioned above, including the severity or intensity of pain, would be better assessed using the mnemonic PQRST.

7. a. Repeated doses can cause toxic effects on the central nervous system. The addition of Phenergan increases opioid-related sedation, hypersensitivity, and depression and should not be used for pain relief.

b. May be appropriate, although an around-the-clock schedule would be more effective for chronic pain.

396

c. The antiinflammatory effect is desirable, but use caution related to gastrointestinal disturbances and possibility of ulcer.

d. May enhance pain relief. Use with caution in the elderly, who have decreased peripheral sensation.

e. Although good for antiinflammatory effect, the intramuscular route is not desirable because of the increased risk of bleeding.

f. A good choice because the dosage can be titrated easily to the patient's pain level.

g. An excellent choice in patients with inflammation and bone pain; it may also improve appetite.

8. Based on the assessment data, the nursing diagnosis is incorrect. Data indicate that the patient has acute, not chronic, pain. The expected outcome is unrealistic (pain free second day postoperatively), although no patient should have to experience pain. Stating "the patient reports satisfaction with pain control measures throughout hospitalization" would be better. Second and fourth interventions are appropriate. Corrections and additions follow:

Nursing Intervention	Rationale
Correction: Encourage the patient to report pain before it becomes severe.	Pain is more manageable when treated before it becomes severe.
Addition: Use different pain relief measures such as massage, distraction, and visual imagery.	These techniques augment analgesics by the gate control theory (stimulation of unaffected skin areas and increased sensory input causes the gate to pain transmission to close).
Correction: Administer analgesics on schedule during first postoperative days.	Anticipating acute postoperative pain will help prevent and minimize pain.
Addition: Assess effectiveness of interventions.	To determine, record effectiveness of pain control measures and modify or revise the plan of care accordingly.

CHAPTER 17

Fluid and Electrolyte Imbalance

1. a. A, b. C, c. B, d. D, e. E, f. G, g. F

2. a. False. Water, not plasma, is the largest constituent of the body.
   b. True.
   c. False. The extracellular fluid, not the intracellular fluid, can only tolerate small amounts of potassium.
   d. True.
   e. True.
   f. False. Edema is not the same as overhydration. Edema can occur with or without the patient being overhydrated.
   g. True.
   h. False. Antidiuretic hormone controls water reabsorption and aldosterone controls sodium reabsorption.
   i. False. Renin, not prostaglandin, is secreted in response to decreased fluid volume to raise blood pressure and restore renal perfusion.
   j. True.
   k. False. Vomiting results in loss of sodium. Diarrhea results in loss of bicarbonate.

3. a. SD or WD, b. WE, c. SD, d. SD or WD, e. SE, f. WD, g. SD or WE, h. SD or WD, i. SE, j. WD, k. SE, l. SD, m. SD or WD, n. SD or WD, o. WE, p. SD or WD

4. Age, weight, and underlying condition are all important factors in determining fluid replacement. The size of the patient is important because a smaller adult has less fluid in each fluid compartment. Fluid replacement is often calculated on the basis of trends in weight. Assessment of weight and degree of weight loss, if any, is important. Adults with normal circulatory and renal function are generally given between 2500 and 3000 ml of fluids per day.

5. Patients receiving loop diuretics are at risk for hypokalemia and hypomagnesemia. Both potassium and magnesium are lost in the urine. Both deficits may precipitate life-threatening cardiac dysrhythmias. The patient should be taught to consume foods high in potassium and magnesium, such as fruits and vegetables. If confusion contributed to overdosing by the patient, a plan for ensuring accurate dosing should be instituted (counting out daily pills, taping pills to a calendar, etc.).

6. The patient's malnourished state places him at risk for hypocalcemia. The serum albumin level is important to consider because the concentration of serum calcium can vary with protein levels. The patient may not exhibit symptoms of hypocalcemia because the ionized portion of calcium may still be within normal limits. To further assess the patient's calcium status, knowing the ionized fraction of serum calcium would be helpful. Other assessment parameters include checking for tetany (Trousseau's and Chvostek's signs), cardiac rate and rhythm, and magnesium level (both often occur together).

7. a. Shortness of breath, edema, elevated blood pressure (bounding), increased pulse, low specific gravity.
   b. Congestive heart failure results in decreased cardiac output because of the weakened myocardium. Decreased cardiac output leads to decreased renal blood flow, which triggers Na/H_2O retention (saline retention/isotonic excess).
   c. Increased extracellular volume leads to increased venous pressure and hydrostatic pressure, causing a shift of fluid into interstitial spaces. Because the

397

interstitial fluid space is part of the extracellular space, the transfer of fluid into the tissues explains the weight gain because the fluid is still in the body. However, the fluid has left the intravascular space, therefore leading to manifestations of extracellular deficit. Although the fluid is still in the extracellular compartment, it is no longer available for use.

   d. Decreased chloride and potassium related to diuretics. Serum sodium is normal.

   e. Sodium is a net gain because sodium and water are being retained. However, the gain is not measurable because it is proportionate to the water gain.

8. a. Elevated serum sodium, flushed skin, high specific gravity, concentrated urine, elevated temperature, diaphoresis.

   b. Decreased level of consciousness—confusion related to shrinkage of brain cells, high urine specific gravity, flushed skin.

   c. Tube feedings could lead to greater dehydration related to increased protein and insufficient water intake, which could lead to hypertonicity and continued shift of water out of the cells, compounding the intracellular deficit.

   d. 0.45% NaCl is a hypotonic solution that would hydrate the cells with water and provide some sodium replacement. A solution of 5% dextrose and 0.45% NaCl with 20 mEq of KCl is slightly hypertonic, providing calories, free water, sodium, potassium, and chloride. The nurse should carefully monitor the patient's output to assess hydration status and ensure adequate kidney function for the patient receiving potassium.

   e. Institute safety measures, administer sufficient water with tube feedings, obtain accurate intake and output and weight measurements, assist the patient with water intake, monitor serum sodium levels, assess neurologic status every 4 hours.

9. a. The fact that the patient is taking diuretics and has a history of diarrhea suggests risk for hypokalemia. The report of muscular weakness and lethargy, coupled with the changes in vital signs (namely the pulse), support this suspicion.

   b. Notify the physician immediately because the patient is at risk for life-threatening cardiac dysrhythmias or respiratory paralysis from a dangerously low potassium level.

   c. No; KCl should never be given undiluted because it is caustic to veins, toxic to cells, and could potentially stop the heart. The potassium should be diluted and administered by an infusion pump. The nurse needs to check renal function before giving large doses of KCl in any form.

CHAPTER 18

Acid-Base Imbalance

1. a. B, b. A, c. C, d. D, e. B and D, f. C, g. A, h. B and D, i. A and C, j. C

2. a. Lo, Hi, N, respiratory acidosis, uncompensated
   b. Hi, N, Hi, metabolic alkalosis, uncompensated
   c. Hi, Lo, Lo, respiratory alkalosis, partially compensated
   d. Lo, Lo, Lo, metabolic acidosis, partially compensated
   e. Lo, Hi, Lo, respiratory and metabolic acidosis
   f. Hi, Hi, Hi, metabolic alkalosis, partially compensated

Possible generalizations: When acid-base disturbances are uncompensated, one normal value is present that always indicates that the system is not compensating for the primary imbalance. During metabolic acidosis and alkalosis with partial compensation, all arrows point in the same direction. During respiratory acidosis and alkalosis with partial compensation, the pH value is opposite the other two values ($PaCO_2$ and HCO_3).

3. a. pH, 7.48; $PaCO_2$, 48 mm Hg; HCO_3, 28 mEq/L

Acidic	Normal	Alkaline
$PaCO_2$		pH
		HCO_3
Partially compensated		Metabolic alkalosis

b. pH, 7.22; $PaCO_2$, 50 mm Hg; HCO_3, 30 mEq/L

Acidic	Normal	Alkaline
pH		HCO_3
$PaCO_2$		
Respiratory acidosis		Partially compensated

c. pH, 7.22; $PaCO_2$, 33 mm Hg; HCO_3, 16 mEq/L

Acidic	Normal	Alkaline
pH		$PaCO_2$
HCO_3		

d. pH, 7.46; $PaCO_2$, 38 mm Hg; HCO_3, 32 mEq/L

Acidic	Normal	Alkaline
		pH
	$PaCO_2$	HCO_3
	Uncompensated	Metabolic alkalosis

e. pH, 7.39; PaCO$_2$, 31 mm Hg; HCO$_3$, 20 mEq/L

Acidic	Normal	Alkaline
HCO$_3$		pH
		PaCO$_2$
Partially compensated		Respiratory alkalosis

4. a. Risk for respiratory acidosis associated with alveolar hypoventilation. Teaching plan: focus on ways to improve ventilation and remove secretions, such as encouraging fluids, coughing, deep breathing, and positioning.
   b. Risk for respiratory alkalosis associated with alveolar hyperventilation secondary to pain and anxiety. Teaching plan: measures to enhance coughing; deep breathing; adequate pain relief measures (especially before activity); anxiety reduction techniques such as relaxation; and ways to prevent, recognize, and treat hyperventilation.
   c. Risk for metabolic acidosis associated with ketoacidosis. Teaching plan: focus on ensuring patient understanding of the importance of keeping diabetes under control with prescribed medication and diet, signs and symptoms of ketoacidosis, and how and when to measure blood glucose.
   d. Risk for metabolic alkalosis related to potassium deficit secondary to laxative abuse. Teaching plan: dietary strategies for avoiding constipation, information about the hazards of laxative overuse, and the need for increased potassium consumption in the diet when laxatives are used.

5. a. Respiratory acidosis. Nursing diagnoses: impaired gas exchange related to hypoventilation; risk for injury related to central nervous system depression and altered level of consciousness.
   b. Respiratory alkalosis. Nursing diagnoses: ineffective breathing pattern: hyperventilation related to hypoxia; anxiety; risk for injury related to alteration in level of consciousness.
   c. Metabolic acidosis. Nursing diagnoses: decreased cardiac output related to cardiac arrest; electrolyte imbalance.
   d. Metabolic alkalosis. Nursing diagnoses: risk for injury related to tetany and seizures associated with hypocalcemia; risk for decreased cardiac output related to dysrhythmias secondary to electrolyte imbalances.

6. a. False. Intubation and mechanical ventilation may be required if the PaCO$_2$ is greater than 50 to 60 mm Hg.
   b. True.
   c. False. Rebreathing reverses respiratory alkalosis. It has no effect on metabolic alkalosis.

d. False. Intravenous NaHCO$_3$ is not highly recommended but is a controversial treatment that can cause profound metabolic alkalosis.
e. True.

CHAPTER 19

Shock

1. a. False. The heart, large blood vessels, and microcirculation (not the brain) function together to maintain adequate cardiac output and tissue perfusion.
   b. False. Cardiac output is the amount of blood the heart pumps from vessels in 1 minute.
   c. True.
   d. False. It influences left, not right, ventricular afterload.
   e. True.
   f. True.
   g. False. Oxygen delivery depends on three factors: (1) blood flow, (2) percentage of arterial oxygen hemoglobin saturation, and (3) the amount of hemoglobin available to carry oxygen.
   h. True.

2. a. Hypovolemic. Primary defect: vascular volume reduced by more than 15% by loss of blood, fluid, or fluid shift. Characteristics: decreased blood pressure, pulse pressure, urine output, tissue perfusion; increased heart rate, respiratory rate; pale, cool, clammy skin.
   Cardiogenic. Primary defect: inability of heart to pump sufficient blood to perfuse tissues, related to pump failure secondary to cardiac failure, tamponade, pericarditis, dysrhythmias, pulmonary embolism. Characteristics: decreased blood pressure, diastolic filling time, tissue perfusion; increased heart rate, respiratory rate, oxygen consumption; pale, cool, clammy skin.
   Distributive. Primary defect: profound vasodilatation secondary to neurologic, allergic, or septic insult. Characteristics: decreased pulse pressure, cardiac output, tissue perfusion; increased heart rate, respiratory rate; widened pulse pressure; warm to hot, flushed skin.
   b. Regardless of the cause, the defining characteristics of shock are similar, including decreased blood pressure, increased heart rate, increased respirations, and decreased tissue perfusion. Distributive and cardiogenic shock are not produced by the actual loss of body fluid but are relative hypovolemic states related to vasodilation and pump failure, respectively.

3. Compensatory shock refers to the complex, widespread physiologic changes primarily aimed at maintaining blood pressure within the normal range to adequately perfuse vital organs. Compensatory changes are only able to maintain blood pressure and tissue perfusion briefly; if the underlying cause is

399

not treated, shock will progress to the next stage. Progressive shock refers to the stage of shock during which compensatory mechanisms can no longer compensate and fail to maintain blood pressure to perfuse vital organs adequately. Compensatory mechanisms become ineffective and severe hypoperfusion of organs will lead to multisystem organ failure if the underlying cause of shock is not corrected. Refractory shock is profound shock accompanied by severe cellular destruction that is no longer reversible.

4. a. Significance: severely compromised renal perfusion and possible impending acute renal failure. Stage of shock: progressive. Assessments: cardiac status; presence of peripheral edema, engorged neck veins, or lung crackles; skin turgor.
   b. Significance: fluid escaping form the intracellular and extracellular spaces is caused by loss of cellular permeability. Stage of shock: progressive, and continues to refractory shock. Assessments: all body systems should be assessed.
   c. Significance: indicates that shock is progressing beyond early compensatory stage (pulse pressure widens in septic shock). Stage of shock: begins in compensatory shock and continues during progressive shock. Assessments: all body systems and mental status should be assessed.
   d. Significance: heart rate increases to compensate for decreased blood pressure (pumping faster to circulate less volume). Stage of shock: compensatory shock. Assessments: respiratory rate, lung sounds, urine output, pulse pressure, presence of edema.
   e. Significance: indicates increased pulmonary capillary permeability or cardiac decompensation. Stage of shock: progressive shock. Assessments: neck vein distention, peripheral and dependent edema, decreased urine output.
   f. Significance: indicates neurologic dysfunction associated with decreased tissue perfusion. Stage of shock: begins in compensatory shock and progresses to coma in refractory shock. Assessments: all body systems should be assessed.
   g. Significance: indicates capillary clotting, depletion of clotting factors, and impending diffuse intravascular coagulation. Stage of shock: progressive and refractory. Assessments: all body systems should be assessed.

5. a. Increased perfusion of vital organs and increased myocardial contractility
   b. Vasodilation to reduce afterload
   c. Improved myocardial contractility and cardiac output

6. Administer drug by infusion pump only; monitor vital signs every 5 to 15 minutes; monitor infusion site for signs of infiltration, and discontinue immediately if infiltration occurs to prevent tissue

necrosis; have phentolamine available if intravenous infiltration occurs; monitor urinary output hourly; maintain a mean blood pressure as prescribed or 80 mm Hg.

7. a. Provides temporary circulatory assistance to restore hemodynamic stability for patients in cardiogenic shock.
   b. Temporarily supports the failing ventricle by diverting blood from the failing ventricle back to the aorta.
   c. Raises blood pressure by increasing systemic peripheral resistance and possibly cardiac output.

8. a. B and C, b. F, c. E, d. F, e. C, f. A, g. B, h. D, i. F

9. a. The four primary changes are (1) myocardial depression, (2) massive vasodilatation, (3) maldistribution of intravascular volume, and (4) formation of microemboli.
   b. Warm, hyperdynamic phase.
   c. Profound vasodilatation.
   d. The patient is in a state of relative hypovolemia caused by profound vasodilation and leakage of fluid out of the capillaries. Fluid replacement is necessary to support vascular volume and blood pressure until vascular integrity is reestablished.

10. a. Vasodilation, increased capillary permeability, bronchoconstriction, and coronary capillary permeability.
    b. Shock is a consequence of hypotension secondary to profound vasodilation and low cardiac output.
    c. Anaphylactic shock develops and progresses within minutes to hours, which does not allow time for compensation.

11. a. Assess cardiac status for compromise, become familiar with emergency equipment and drugs to support circulation, monitor for cardiac dysrhythmias.
    b. Encourage deep breathing and coughing, assess respiratory system for compromise, monitor oxygen saturation levels.
    c. Maintain strict asepsis of all invasive lines, monitor for signs of infection, turn frequently to prevent pulmonary stasis.
    d. Eliminate all nonessential activities to promote rest, administer oxygen as ordered, use calm and reassuring manner, explain all procedures, keep skin clean and dry.

CHAPTER 20

Assessment of the Immune System

1. Natural immunity is nonspecific, present at birth, and does not require exposure to an antigen for its development. It is always the same and consists of anatomic and chemical barriers that recognize and respond to foreign or damaged cells. Acquired

immunity begins after birth and results from repeated exposure to antigens. It is quite specific and results in lifelong immunity. Examples of natural immunity include normal flora, intact skin, inflammatory response, and phagocytosis. Examples of acquired immunity include T cells, B cells, and antibodies.

2. a. False. Eosinophils and basophils release vasoactive chemicals, whereas neutrophils and monocytes are phagocytic cells.
   b. False. Neutrophils are the most efficient and responsive.
   c. False. Neutrophils, not eosinophils, are the first cells to migrate when the inflammatory response is initiated.
   d. True.
   e. True.
   f. False. Natural killer cells secrete interferon-γ, which enhances macrophage ability to kill phagocytosed microbes.
   g. False. Complement accentuates or complements the action of immunoglobulin (antibodies).

3. Serum complement initiates or modifies the inflammatory response, lyses cells, and assists with internal protection. Interferon is a protein substance released from virally infected cells that protects nonvirally infected cells.

4. Localized inflammation occurs at the area of injury. Signs of localized inflammation are redness, heat, swelling, pain, and temporary loss of function at site of injury. Systemic inflammation occurs when inflammation spreads to other parts of the body from a localized area, or occurs at differing sites in the body. Signs of systemic inflammation include fever, leukocytosis, and increased erythrocyte sedimentation rate.

5. Example: Cellular immunity is like the Army, and humoral immunity is like the Navy. The Army has soldiers who help the Navy (T-helper cells) bring a halt to actions (T-suppressor cells) and fight the battle (T-killer cells). The Army general will remember the war strategy (T-memory cells). The Navy has a variety of ships (immunoglobulins G, M, A, D, E) made for specific missions. The Navy admiral will remember the war strategy (B-memory cells). The Army and Navy depend on one another to fight the war adequately (cellular and humoral immunity are interdependent).

6. a. Identifies, engulfs, and destroys foreign antigens.
   b. Protein substances, called immunoglobulins, that combine with the antigen that stimulated its production and either destroy the antigen or activate other antigen-damaging processes.
   c. Regulate other T-cell functions and augment production of antibodies by B cells.

d. Prevent or modify the functions of T-helper and T-cytotoxic cells.
   e. Involved in delayed hypersensitivity in fungi and mycobacteria allergic responses.
   f. Destroys foreign antigen on contact.
   g. Remembers contact with antigen and responds immediately on subsequent exposure to the same antigen.

7. Primary response occurs on first exposure of the immune system to each new antigen. There is a time delay between antigenic exposure and production of antibodies. On subsequent exposures to previously recognized antigens, a secondary response occurs, which is more rapid, of greater intensity, and longer lasting than the primary response.

8. Decreased relative proportions of T-helper and T-suppressor cells, increased autoantibody production, decreased rate of T cell proliferation, decreased numbers of T-killer cells, reduced production of interleukin-2, decreased ability to respond to viral antigens.

9. a. History of allergies, asthma, cold; presence of lung crackles, flaring nares, chest retraction.
   b. History of recent injuries or skin or joint problems; presence of swelling, redness, or pallor; deformity of joint; involvement of other joints.
   c. History of allergies or recent illness; presence of wheezing, rash, or edema in other areas.
   d. History of fatigue, recent illness, chronic illness; presence of weakness of extremities; alterations in skin integrity.
   e. History of recent upper respiratory tract infection or other illness; vital signs, especially temperature; lung sounds for rales or wheezing.
   f. History of recent illness, history of occurrence of lymph node tenderness, presence of enlarged or painful lymph nodes, fever, vital signs.

10. a. White blood cell count is within normal range for age and is therefore not significant.
    b. Lymphocytosis is present, which indicates a possible viral infection.
    c. Indicates the possibility of infection, malignancy, or inflammation related to an autoimmune process.
    d. Decreased number of mature neutrophils and increased immature cells, indicates acute bacterial infection.
    e. The CH50 is elevated, indicating the presence of an inflammatory reaction.

11. a. Elevated eosinophil count, elevated IgE levels.
    b. Elevated IgG, IgM, and IgA levels; elevated CH50; elevated erythrocyte sedimentation rate.
    c. Decreased IgG, IgM, and IgA levels; elevated erythrocyte sedimentation rate.

401

d. Elevated IgG and IgA, elevated CH50; elevated white blood cells; elevated lymphocytes, elevated erythrocyte sedimentation rate.
   e. Elevated IgE level.

12. a. IgM antibodies, indicative of rheumatoid arthritis.
    b. Gamma globulins produced against cell nucleus properties.
    c. Serum antibodies produced against red blood cells, indicates person's Rh factor.
    d. Specific antibodies produced against a particular pathogen such as HIV; indicates exposure to the pathogen.
    e. Neutrophils containing large groups of abnormal DNA, may indicate systemic lupus erythematosus.

13. People may respond to the test at different intervals; therefore several readings are taken for accurate interpretation. A positive test does not mean that he has histoplasmosis, only that he is has been previously exposed to the disease and is hypersensitive to the antigen particles in the injection.

14. a. Fever, joint pain, fatigue, loss of appetite, and rash.
    b. Presence and type of recent infections; when her rash was first noticed, how long she has had it; when her fever started, any pattern associated with it, and how high it has been; the presence of lymph node enlargement; sleep pattern; usual ADL; when her fatigue started; the severity of her joint pain and any relief measures; known allergies, type of reaction, and preventive measures or treatments used.

CHAPTER 21

Immunologic Problems

1. a. Both are highly susceptible to infection and treatment failures because of their compromised immune systems. Both require a well-balanced, nutritious diet and need to avoid excessive fatigue. Both need to be taught infection prevention methods.
   b. The first patient is immune suppressed from chemotherapy; consequently, he has a secondary immunodeficiency. His immune system will likely recover when his chemotherapy is completed. The second patient has a primary immunodeficiency. He will require bone marrow transplantation to treat his immunodeficiency problem. He cannot recover from his illness and will require lifelong therapy.

2. a. Destruction of lymphocytes (primarily T cells) to prevent allograft rejection.
   b. Form IgG to block attachment of IgE to mast cells for the purpose of desensitizing the person to specific allergens.
   c. Blocks the inflammatory response decreasing swelling, pain, and other signs of inflammation.

d. Suppression of a specific antigen to prevent rejection of the Rh-positive fetus during pregnancy.

3. Monoclonal gammopathies refer to plasma cell dyscrasias, whereas polyclonal gammopathies refer to diffuse increases in antibody synthesis from inappropriate antigen stimulation. Both result in high susceptibility to infection. Their clinical manifestations and treatments are quite different.

4. a. Hemoglobin and hematocrit (decreased), white blood cell count (leukopenia, possible thrombocytopenia), serum electrolytes (hypercalcemia), serum uric acid (increased), immunoglobulin assays (decreased immunoglobulins), the presence of Bence-Jones protein in both her serum and urine. Her beta 2 microglobulin value will be less than 339 nmol/L.
   b. Orthopedic fixation devices may be used to prevent cord compression.
   c. It is a monoclonal gammopathy or plasma cell dyscrasia. It inhibits the production of normal antibodies because it induces the overproduction of ineffective immunoglobulins, thus altering the immune response.

5. a. A, b. D, c. A, d. C, e. A, f. B and C, g. B, h. D, i. E, j. A, k. C, l. B, m. D, n. E, o. C, p. A

6. The patient was previously sensitized to something that cross-reacted with penicillin (identified as genetically similar), such as molds. Because penicillin is a mold derivative (he resided in a damp climate), his previous sensitization (primary sensitization) left him vulnerable for systemic anaphylaxis from the second (challenging) dose.

7. The patient with atopic allergy may have rhinitis, hay fever, asthma, contact dermatitis, or food allergies. The patient with nonatopic allergies may not have indications of the hypersensitivity until the offending antigen is encountered. At that time the reaction will likely be more severe and may include urticaria, angioedema, or systemic anaphylaxis.

8. a. Stop the intravenous antibiotic immediately to stop the flow of antigens triggering the reaction. Administer 0.3 to 0.5 ml of intramuscular epinephrine. Place him in high Fowler's position, start oxygen, assess his level of consciousness, maintain a patent airway by suctioning if necessary, and prepare for emergency intubation or tracheotomy. Stay with him and have another nurse notify his physician.
   b. The first and second doses served as primary sensitizers. By the time he received the third dose, his immune system was fully primed and ready to react against the allergen.
   c. The data are supportive but further data are needed, such as the presence or absence of wheezing, use

of accessory muscles, cyanosis, nasal flaring, and signs or verbalizations of anxiety.

    d. Avoidance of the allergen. Because the patient's hypersensitivity is to a drug, the drug can be avoided. He needs to wear medical alert identification or carry allergy information and always warn health care providers about his hypersensitivity.

9. No. People with type O blood do not have either A or B antigens (ABO system); therefore they cannot receive another type of blood without having a reaction. Persons with AB blood are universal recipients. People with Rh-negative blood (Rh system) do not have the Rh antigen and will develop jaundice if given Rh-positive blood. People with O blood can receive only O blood, but because they have no A or B antigens they are universal donors.

10. a. She is having either an acute hemolytic reaction or a febrile reaction.

    b. Collect additional data. If she is having a febrile reaction, she will likely report headache and muscle aching. She will appear flushed and anxious. If she is having an acute hemolytic reaction, assessment will demonstrate tachycardia, hypotension, and impending shock.

    c. Febrile reaction: stop the transfusion. Give antipyretics as prescribed. Send the blood back to the laboratory for analysis. The physician may consider giving leukocyte-poor blood products rather than whole blood. Acute hemolytic reaction: stop the transfusion. Treat shock and continue to monitor her closely. Give diuretics as prescribed to prevent renal complications. Monitor for signs and symptoms of diffuse intravascular coagulation.

11. Neither causes immediate reactions; rather, they have delayed responses. Both produce fever.

12. Careful checking of the label against the patient's arm band for accuracy, proper identification of the blood or blood product being infused, making certain the blood date has not expired, obtaining baseline patient data for later comparison, running the infusion slowly for the first 15 minutes, frequently assessing vital signs to compare against baseline, and administering the product through a filter if indicated.

13. The patient has been exposed to the tuberculosis bacillus at some time even though she is unaware of it because she is sensitized. She reacted in a hypersensitive manner to the tuberculin skin test that served as the challenge dose.

14. Example: Autoimmunity refers to a state in which the body produces substances called antibodies against its own cells. Antibodies are usually protective to the body, but occasionally they are directed against the body and injure its own cells. Such injury produces the clinical manifestations that occur from autoimmune disorders.

15. A fatigue diary may help the person identify fatigue triggers, such as ways in which fatigue starts and progresses and how the fatigue generally manifests itself. It may also help the person evaluate the effectiveness of interventions designed to reduce fatigue.

CHAPTER 22

HIV Infection and AIDS

1. HIV infection means the person has contracted and is infected with the human immunodeficiency virus but is not ill from immune deficiency. Persons infected with HIV may have a clinically silent infection, may not know they are infected, have only minor immunologic abnormalities, and have no opportunistic infections. Persons with AIDS may be quite ill, generally know they are infected, have significant loss of immune capability, and may have one or several opportunistic infections.

2. a. No conclusions can be drawn yet. The individual may be in the "window period" of infection, meaning that exposure has taken place but antibodies to HIV have not yet reached detectable levels. It takes between 6 weeks to 3 months to develop detectable levels of antibodies to HIV. Or the patient may not have been infected with the virus.

    b. Follow-up is essential. Another enzyme-linked immunosorbent assay will be performed 4 to 6 months after the first screening. If that test is positive, further testing will be completed.

3. Hand washing is the single most important action for maintaining effective infection control for patients infected with any bloodborne pathogen.

4. *Mycobacterium avium* complex often occurs late in the AIDS disease process and produces many of the same symptoms as severe immunodeficiency disease and other opportunistic infections; therefore it may not be readily recognized. Persistently high fevers (104° F), weight loss, diarrhea, and positive blood cultures support the presence of *Mycobacterium avium* complex.

5. Examples: Risk for complications of drug therapy, activity intolerance, risk for imbalanced nutrition: less than body requirements, risk for injury.

6. These infections can cause disseminated disease; they all produce fever, fatigue, and weight loss; amphotericin B is the drug of choice as primary treatment; the infections can be controlled but not cured.

7. Assessments: serum electrolytes, weight, intake and output, skin turgor, and skin integrity are priority

assessment parameters. She is at very high risk for malabsorption and electrolyte imbalance from frequent, voluminous, watery diarrhea.

8. Cats often harbor *Toxoplasma gondii,* which can result in encephalitis with accompanying seizures and mental status changes. The patient needs to be taught about the need for wearing gloves while changing the cat litter or having someone else dispose of the litter to prevent contraction of the infection. He does not have to give up his pets as long as he avoids the cat litter.

9. Opportunistic infections as a whole are quite serious in people with AIDS and in many cases may lead to death if not recognized and treated. None requires dietary restriction or activity limitations. All are difficult to eradicate. Drugs used to treat the infections can be highly toxic to individuals who are already immunocompromised and physically compromised.

10. The nurse should attempt to explore his concerns. Offering suggestions and explaining the need for informing his parents are appropriate actions; however, he does have a right to confidentiality if he so chooses.

11. Cancer chemotherapies are too toxic to treat the person with AIDS. Kaposi's sarcoma is rarely the cause of death in patients with AIDS. Palliative therapy is the only therapy for Kaposi's sarcoma currently available to patients with AIDS.

12. The incidence of AIDS among older adults is steadily increasing because of current treatments. People with AIDS are living longer, and many are predicted to reach older adulthood. In the future nurses who care for older adults are highly likely to be caring for some individuals who are HIV infected or have AIDS.

13. Examples: Solicit the help of high school students to assist with education of their peers and campaign for sexual abstinence, solicit community financial resources to make condoms available to individuals who are in high-risk categories, volunteer to assist drug treatment facility personnel with identification and treatment of intravenous drug users, volunteer at an HIV free health care clinic.

14. a. A, b. C, c. E, d. B and D, e. A, f. D, g. A, h. E, i. D, j. A, k. C

15. a. Laboratory: category 2 or 3, depending on the actual number of CD4 T cells. Clinical category: category C.
    b. The HIV virus has infected her CD4 T-helper cells and used those cells to replicate. As viral particles are released, T cells eventually die, depleting their numbers, which results in a dramatic loss of immune protection. The con-

sequence of this loss is significantly increased susceptibility to infections.
    c. Monitor for side effects of drug therapy, headache, vomiting, red blood cell anemia, or granulocytopenia. Assess lung status, mental status, skin, mucous membranes, temperature, abdominal status, level of discomfort, level of anxiety or fear, and intake and output.
    d. Impaired skin integrity: perineal excoriation, increased risk for fluid and electrolyte imbalance, imbalanced nutrition: less than body requirements, fatigue, self-care deficit, fear, powerlessness, ineffective individual coping.
    e. She has a caring, supportive sister who is willing to take part in her care. A supportive relative is important because she can assist the patient with identification of fears, provide emotional support, assist with physical comfort, and provide assurance of the patient's worth as a person.
    f. Care of intravenous lines or intravenous medications, nutritional needs, signs and symptoms of recurrent infections, skin care, mucous membrane care, side effects of medications.

16. a. He has progressed to symptomatic HIV infection. He is a candidate for antiretroviral drug therapy.
    b. The Centers for Disease Control and Prevention recommend that all patients with advanced HIV infection, and those with symptomatic HIV infection without AIDS, should be treated with combination drug therapy including protease inhibitors combined with nucleoside and/or nucleotide reverse transcriptase inhibitors, regardless of plasma viral levels.
    c. Advantages: potential reduction of viral load, prevention of progressive immunodeficiency, delayed progression from HIV to AIDS. Disadvantages: numerous side effects and toxic effects, potential development of drug resistance, unknown duration of effectiveness.
    d. Viral suppression and immune recovery.

17. a. Findings are suspicious for oral *Candida* infection. The infection may involve her esophagus because her emesis contains thick white material.
    b. Drug therapy, such as oral nystatin, clotrimazole, or ketoconazole.
    c. Intravenous amphotericin B will be added to the protocol.
    d. She may develop fever and chills, headache, and generalized pain. Comfort will be her primary problem while receiving this drug.

CHAPTER 23

Cancer

1. a. True.
   b. False. The incidence of breast and lung cancer in women continues to increase, but these increases have slowed in recent years.

c. False. Older adults are diagnosed with advanced cancers more frequently because they do not participate in prevention and screening programs as often as do younger adults.

d. False. White women have the highest cancer incidence, but African-American women have the highest cancer mortality rate.

e. False. Genetic differences may contribute to international variations but are not likely to explain all variations in cancer differences encountered.

f. False. The three overlapping stages of carcinogenesis are initiation, promotion, and progression.

g. True.

h. True.

i. True.

j. False. Sunburn and increased duration of exposure to ultraviolet radiation from sunlight or artificial sources increase the risk for skin cancer.

k. False. Tobacco contains more than 60 known carcinogens present in both mainstream and secondhand smoke.

l. False. Red meat intake is associated with higher incidences of colon and prostate cancer but not breast cancer.

2. a. The process by which normal cells recognize the presence of other cells near them.

b. The cycle through which cells divide into daughter cells. Cell cycle consists of four phases: quiescence (GI), DNA synthesis (S), RNA and protein synthesis and mitotic spindle (G2), and mitosis (M).

c. The rapid proliferation of cells into those that resemble their forebears with fully mature, specialized function and morphology.

d. An alteration in adult cells characterized by changes in size, shape, and organization.

e. Abnormal cellular division not necessary for normal cell growth and development.

f. Cells that show normal cell growth patterns, even though the new tissue growth is not necessary.

g. Cells that serve no useful function, do not exhibit contact inhibition, and spread to and grow in other body locations.

3. a. B, b. M, c. M, d. B, e. M, f. B, g. B, h. M, i. B, j. M, k. M

4. a. Biopsy
b. Cytology, Papanicolaou smear
c. Endoscopy
d. Tumor imaging (computed tomography scans, radiographs)

5. Biotherapy is a new form of cancer therapy and is still considered experimental. Although giving the patient hope is important, informing the patient of potential side effects is equally necessary. The ethical dilemma is striving for balance between informed choices and maintaining a sense of hope. Ethically,

the question becomes, "If biotherapy may have only a moderate effect on the tumor, and side effects are often debilitating, should patients be encouraged to undergo biotherapy?"

6. a. A group of glycoproteins produced by T lymphocytes in response to viral infections or other stimuli. Function: cause changes in viral RNA and protein synthesis, inhibit function of several oncogenes, and activate natural killer cells.

b. Group of biologic factors. Function: stimulate and increase a number of other immune cells and other cytokines.

c. Group of glycoproteins. Function: stimulate the development of hematopoietic cell lines.

d. Synthetic (manmade) antibodies. Function: serologic detection of tumor cells and cytotoxic destruction of tumor cells.

7. a. May halt abnormal cell growth at the molecular level.

b. Demonstrated anti-cancer effect on advanced non–small-cell cancer, head and neck cancer, colorectal cancer, and other solid tumors.

c. Replaces diseased bone marrow with healthy bone marrow, rescues healthy bone marrow, protects bone marrow from effects of intensive solid tumor therapy, and replaces diseased stem cells with healthy stem cells.

8. Screening programs, assessing and determining risk potential, identifying individuals and families at risk (case finding), teaching regarding warning signs and prevention, community role modeling, improving public attitudes regarding early detection and prevention, allaying misconceptions, and conducting research on risk behaviors and attitudes.

9. a. The client's risk for skin cancer is higher than most because of her light complexion, risk for occupational exposure to radiation, and tendency to sunbathe. She should wear protective sunscreens and protective clothing at work, routinely check her skin for lesions or moles, and be alert to changes in their appearance.

b. He should institute ways to minimize exposure to possible carcinogens (e.g., chemical fertilizers) by wearing protective clothing, using a mask, or avoiding chemicals altogether). Given his family history, he is at risk for colon cancer, and the family should take steps to decrease their fat and red meat intake.

c. The triad of diabetes, hypertension, and obesity places this client at risk for endometrial cancer. Being childless and beginning menopause late in life also increase her risk. Because these risk factors cannot be altered, she should have yearly pelvic examinations and Pap screens.

10. a. False. The most radiosensitive tissue in the body is the bone marrow. Cells in the mitosis phase of the cell cycle are the most sensitive to radiation. The bone marrow has a high proliferative cell turnover rate.
   b. True. As a side note, radiotherapy is typically delivered in multiple small doses (fractionation) over a period of weeks to reduce normal cell injury or death.
   c. True.
   d. False. An individual who stands 2 m away from the source of radiation receives one fourth as much exposure as when standing only 1 m away. Standing 3 m away means the person receives one ninth as much exposure as when standing only 1 m away. This is the law of inverse-square.
   e. False. Hair loss is only temporary and occurs in the treatment area approximately 3 weeks after the initiation of radiotherapy.
   f. False. Skin should be kept dry, especially in folds where moisture collects. Because the skin is extremely vulnerable to the effects of radiation, the skin should be kept clean, dry, and protected from irritants, including lotions and ointments.

11. Preoperative radiation is often used to decrease the tumor bulk of a large mass, thus improving the potential for removal of the entire tumor during surgery. In contrast, smaller tumors are approached first with surgery and then postoperative radiation to eradicate any residual tumor.

12. Paclitaxel (Taxol)
   Benefits: death of rapidly dividing malignant cells.
   Risks: concurrent administration with other drugs may increase incidence of side effects. Thrombocytopenia is a major concern in this case.

   Dexamethasone
   Benefits: reduces inflammation, stimulates appetite.
   Risks: may mask signs of infection; side effects of special interest include nausea, petechiae, muscle wasting, and increased susceptibility to infection.

   Filgrastim (Neupogen, G-CSF)
   Benefits: stimulates proliferation of granulocytes, improves immune function, reduces incidence of infection.
   Risks: No real problems with other drugs on the profile.

   MS Contin
   Benefits: morphine preparation effective in reducing chronic pain.
   Risks: respiratory depression, sedation, constipation.

   Ondansetron
   Benefits: prevention and treatment of nausea and vomiting.
   Risks: can increase fatigue and cause constipation, dry mouth, and elevated liver enzymes.

Ginseng
   Benefits: improves physical stamina, appetite, sleep pattern.
   Risks: increases risk of bleeding. Has estrogenlike effects; thus this medication may be contraindicated for patients with breast cancer.

13. a. Teach the patient to report signs and symptoms of infection (i.e., elevated temperature, redness, swelling, drainage, soreness), and to avoid crowds and people with colds. Teach the importance of good hand washing and use of techniques for dressing changes. Discuss the importance of a diet high in vitamins and protein to help the healing process.
   b. The most obvious advantage of a central line is the elimination of painful needle punctures for chemotherapy and blood samples, which are required in order to monitor the CBC during therapy. The primary disadvantage is the threat of infection in an immunosuppressed patient.

14. a. Nursing diagnosis: Ineffective protection related to bleeding potential secondary to thrombocytopenia. Activities: bleeding precautions, which include avoiding razors, aspirin products, and invasive procedures; using a soft-bristled toothbrush; and wearing shoes.
   b. Nursing diagnosis: Risk for infection related to neutropenia secondary to chemotherapy.
   c. Activities: infection precautions, which include avoiding crowds, fresh fruits, vegetables, or flowers; meticulous hand washing; measures to keep the skin intact; and monitoring temperature.

15. Patients who seek unconventional therapies are often dissatisfied with the present therapy and/or are faced with intolerable side effects or poor prognosis. The best approach is to remain supportive and advocate for the patient. Nurses can encourage patients to discuss their frustrations. Avoid conveying personal attitudes about a patient's decision, and let patients know that they will be supported by the health care team if they need future care. Furthermore, nurses have a responsibility to discuss both the potential advantages and disadvantages of such methods and may refer patients to the American Cancer Society for literature.

16. First and foremost, the patient should be involved in the planning stages of pain management. The patient must determine what is an acceptable outcome. For example, the patient in this case may want to be as alert as possible and thus may find a pain level of 3 (on a scale of 1 to 10) acceptable. This information would be helpful in planning analgesic therapy and other noninvasive interventions.

406

CHAPTER 24

Assessment of the Respiratory System

1. Similarities: All terms refer to breathing. Differences: Ventilation involves the movement of air from the atmosphere through the upper and lower airways and into the alveoli. Ventilation is correlated with inspiration. Respiration involves both oxygen uptake and elimination of carbon dioxide, a process that occurs at the alveolar-capillary membrane. The term respiration is commonly used to describe the number of inspiratory/expiratory cycles per minute. However, true respiration occurs at the cellular and alveolar level, where oxygen moves into the pulmonary vasculature and carbon dioxide moves out of the body by expiration. Breathing consists of both ventilation and respiration.

2. Possible analogy: Compliance is like a rubber band. Compliance refers to the ability of the lungs to expand, or stretch, when intraalveolar pressure increases, and then return, or recoil, to their previous position. Similar to a rubber band, when pressure is applied (someone pulls on it), a rubber band has the ability to stretch. When the pressure is released, the rubber band recoils to its former shape (elasticity).

3. Movement of gases is a function of pressure gradients. Possible analogy: Three children are playing a game of push and shove. When Tommy and Johnny overpower Barbara with their greater strength, Barbara is forced over the game line. Similarly, when the partial pressure of oxygen is greater in the alveoli than in the pulmonary circulation, oxygen moves to the other side. When the partial pressure of carbon dioxide is greater in the pulmonary circulation, carbon dioxide moves where the pressure of carbon dioxide is lower (alveoli). This process effectively allows the uptake of oxygen by the body and elimination of carbon dioxide.

4. The mechanism that drives normal breathing in the patient with chronic obstructive pulmonary disease (COPD) is the level of carbon dioxide (CO_2) in the bloodstream. Increases in CO_2 will lead to increased respiration to "blow off" the excess CO_2. This occurs because chemoreceptors in the medulla are sensitive to changes in blood pH and CO_2 levels. Conversely, decreases in CO_2 will lead to decreased respiration to retain CO_2 in the bloodstream. The patient with COPD chronically retains carbon dioxide. The brain's receptors no longer respond to elevations in CO_2. Rather, the patient's peripheral chemoreceptors respond to low oxygen levels to maintain respiration. Therefore, if oxygen levels are increased (without concurrent decreases in CO_2), apnea may result.

5. Possible age-related changes: skeletal changes (e.g., kyphosis) may result in an increase in the anteroposterior diameter of the thorax. Pulmonary function studies may show decreased compliance related to decreased lung elasticity. Diminished lung sounds may be present because of thickening of the alveoli, and dyspnea may occur from exertion related to decreased diffusion of oxygen.

6. Initially, distinguishing between the two types of chest pain may be difficult. Pain assessment alone may not definitively distinguish between the two because chest pain in either case may be similar. For example, an individual with a dull, constant ache in the chest could have a lung tumor or a myocardial infarction. A detailed history and investigation of the patient's symptoms is necessary to differentiate between a cardiovascular cause and a pulmonary cause of chest pain.

7. Bronchoscopy: maintain NPO status until gag reflex returns, place in semi-Fowler's position on either side to enhance postural drainage, monitor for signs of laryngeal edema or spasms, monitor sputum for signs of hemorrhage. Mediastinoscopy: Because this is a surgical procedure, postprocedural care is similar to any surgical procedure involving general anesthesia. Maintain NPO status until fully awake, monitor for signs of pneumothorax. Laryngoscopy: nursing care for laryngoscopy is similar to bronchoscopy; greater emphasis is placed, however, on monitoring for signs of laryngeal edema or spasm.

8. a. Palpation, b. inspection, c. auscultation, d. percussion, e. palpation, f. inspection, g. auscultation, h. palpation, i. percussion, j. auscultation

9. Additional data needed: (1) time of day dyspnea occurs. Is the dyspnea constant or episodic? Is the dyspnea associated with seasonal factors or weather changes? Is the dyspnea correlated with body position (e.g., recumbent)? (2) Any factors that help relieve the dyspnea. Is the patient taking any medication? Is anxiety a factor? Has the patient been exposed to any environmental irritants, including smoking? Is the dyspnea associated with activity, and to what degree? Has the patient's ability to perform activities of daily living been assessed? A detailed assessment is imperative to facilitate problem identification and appropriate treatment. For example, medication alone could be the cause of bronchoconstriction with resultant dyspnea. Moreover, the treatment of asthma is obviously quite different from the treatment of a disease such as lung cancer. All these questions and assessment parameters should be carefully analyzed to gain a clear, holistic picture of the patient and his condition.

10. a. No significance. Bronchovesicular breath sounds are normally heard over the sternum and between the scapulae.
    b. Whispered pectoriloquy and bronchophony.
    c. The loud, clear sound indicates consolidation (pneumonia) where lung tissue is more dense.

407

Vocal sounds are transmitted more effectively with increased lung tissue density. Increased fremitus results when sound passes through more dense lung tissue, as in the case of pneumonia. Percussion sound transmission is affected by lung density. As lung density increases, percussion sounds are flattened or dulled, as opposed to hyperresonant sounds, which occur with air trapped in the thoracic space.

d. Bronchial breath sounds are normal only when heard over the trachea. The high-pitched, loud nature of bronchial sounds heard over the left lower lobe indicate more lung density and probably correlate with this patient's pneumonia.

11. a. True.
    b. False. The oblique and lordotic views visualize specific parts of the chest, but pronated chest view does not exist.
    c. False. This definition refers to fluoroscopy. Computed tomography permits visualization of cross sections of the lung.
    d. True.
    e. False. Ventilation/perfusion lung scans provide a visual image of the distribution of ventilation and perfusion in the lungs. A pulmonary angiograph visualizes the pulmonary vascular system.
    f. True.
    g. True.
    h. False. Indirect laryngoscopy may be used to remove foreign objects, but direct laryngoscopy is used for taking a biopsy of tumors.
    i. True.

12. a. TV, b. IRV, c. ERV, d. RV

CHAPTER 25

Upper Airway Problems

1. Examples: How much drainage is present? How often is he changing the nasal pad? Is the red drainage bright red, pink, or brown? Is the patient taking aspirin? How active is he? Has he been doing any heavy lifting? Has he been blowing his nose or sneezing?

2. a. Excessive or repeated swallowing may indicate increased bleeding from the nose.
   b. Diminished visual acuity related to double vision may indicate damage to the optic nerve.
   c. Patients who have undergone sinus or nasal surgery have increased thirst because of mouth breathing.
   d. To prevent bleeding; increased pain may indicate infection of the involved sinus; tarry stools may be caused by swallowed blood. In addition, patients should be taught to report bright red blood.

3. Persons with a history of bacterial endocarditis are at increased risk of redeveloping infective endocarditis during the course of pharyngitis. Bacterial endocarditis

is primarily caused by streptococcal organisms. To prevent reinfection antibiotic therapy must therefore be completed.

4. Examples of necessary teaching: Patient may have anorexia related to inability to smell, nausea related to postnasal drainage and swallowing of old blood, and mouth dryness. Nutritional considerations include frequent oral care to improve taste; emphasis on food appearance and appeal to patient because smell may be diminished; and high-calorie, nutritious liquids.

5. Examples: Are bleeding or signs that indicate complications such as infection (e.g., swelling, redness over area, increased pain, warmth) present? If not, the nurse should reassure the patient that pain is a normal postoperative expectation and explain that a protective membrane has formed over the operative site where the tonsils once resided. Between the fourth and eighth postoperative day, the membrane breaks away and new tissue forms. The patient should also be advised to contact the nurse if the pain continues or increases in intensity.

6. Higher numbers in the TNM staging system indicate progressive degrees of tumor involvement. T refers to the size and extent of the tumor; in this case T3 indicates a larger tumor. N refers to nodal involvement, and the 0 indicates that regional lymph nodes are free of cancer cells. M refers to metastases; in this case no "known" distant spread is present.

7. Answers will vary. Examples may include maintaining eye contact when talking with me; explaining plans, equipment, and procedures in terms that I can understand; talking "to" me rather than "over" me; demonstrating patience when I am trying to communicate; using creativity to find ways to help me communicate my needs; attending to my nonverbal cues of pain and fear; anticipating my needs for reassurance and emotional support; and keeping my family informed of my progress.

8. Care of the tracheostomy alone involves precautions to avoid circulatory compromise to the skin flaps (tracheostomy ties tied at the side of the neck) and shoulder-strengthening exercises because the sternocleidomastoid muscle is dissected and the trapezius muscle atrophies. When radical neck dissection is also present, more complex wound care is required. Laryngectomy alone involves general incisional care, whereas radical neck dissection wound care requires careful assessment of the skin flaps because complications such as dehiscence, fistula formation between the pharynx and subcutaneous tissues, and carotid artery rupture can occur.

9. Answers will vary. Considerations may include (1) tracheal-esophageal prosthesis: less obvious to others, requires skilled care, risk of fistula stenosis,

more normal speech. (2) Esophageal speech: less-pleasing voice quality, degree of comfort with "burping" technique, more digestive difficulties during learning process, requires motivation and persistence, longer learning period. (3) External speech aids: more obvious to others, less-pleasing voice sound, no need to learn special speaking techniques.

10. Data suggest that the patient has a strong support system, which may enhance his coping ability. He adjusted to a prosthetic limb and has continued to enjoy social relationships. Because he has been successful in the past at adapting to adverse circumstances, he is likely to be successful in adapting to this situation. On the other hand, his apparent value of social relationships may make this adjustment more difficult given the nature of the surgery. The foot disfigurement is not readily apparent to others, but the facial and visual alterations will be outwardly visible. Interactions with the client should nonetheless focus on how he adjusted to former losses, noting his successes and strengths. Discussions may center on how he helped high school teenagers cope with the physical and emotional changes associated with growing up.

11. Several subtle behaviors indicate that the client may not be dealing with the vocal changes and alterations in his physical appearance. He has not yet set up an appointment with the speech therapist (avoidance behavior?). It may be too soon for him to face the reality of the vocal changes. He seems to have developed some sort of communication system with his family that is currently meeting his needs. Although the nurse notes that all seems well, the fact that his wife is apparently caring for the laryngeal stoma may indicate that he cannot or will not deal with the stoma himself. More information is needed before conclusions can be made about his psychological adjustment.

12. Some experts believe that inflation of the tracheostomy cuff during food intake prevents aspiration. Others believe that cuff inflation causes a bulge in the esophagus and makes swallowing difficult. Nursing assessment of the patient's ability to swallow will determine which method to use. Methylene blue dye can be swallowed initially. If the dye does not appear in tracheal secretions, proceeding with the meal is safe.

CHAPTER 26

Lower Airway Problems

1. a. R, b. O, c. R, d. R, e. P, f. O, g. R, h. P, i. O

2. a. False. Viral pathogens typically cause acute bronchitis. Bacterial pathogens can cause bronchitis as a primary or secondary infection.
   b. False. These drugs may minimize symptoms associated with influenza A virus infection.

c. True.
d. True.
e. True.
f. False. Only approximately 15% of the dose is delivered by these methods.
g. True.
h. False. Cyanosis occurs when 5 g or more of deoxygenated hemoglobin is present.
i. True.

3. Droplets of medication are contained in the spacer, which prevents them from being ineffectively dispersed in the mouth. Aerosol droplets are dispersed more fully and evenly into the airways. Patients receive a more correct dose of medication because traditional coordination of breathing with release of medication is not as imperative as with standard inhalers. The number and volume of puffs is often reduced, thereby reducing cost.

4. Possible factors: (1) general population and overcrowding, (2) increased number of immigrants to the United States, (3) increased number of homeless persons, and (4) increased incidence of HIV-positive individuals and persons with AIDS.

5. A positive reaction to a tuberculosis skin test does not necessarily mean that the individual has active tuberculosis. The patient could have been exposed to the disease but have no evidence of infection or could have the infection without active disease. Paradoxically, an individual with a negative tuberculosis skin test may have tuberculosis that is not clinically active. Consequently, sputum cultures and chest radiographs are most beneficial in confirming the actual status of patients.

6. Because all three drugs can potentially cause hepatitis and liver dysfunction, liver function studies are imperative. Baseline liver function studies should be conducted and repeated at regular intervals. The patient should be instructed on the importance of avoiding alcohol, which may increase the risk for liver side effects.

7. All are infections from fungus found in the soil, classified as deep mycoses because they involve deeper tissues and internal organs, and generally produce manifestations that are mild and self-limiting but can become disseminated. Disseminated infections are difficult to treat, although they may respond to antifungal medications such as ketoconazole. Collaborative management and nursing care are similar for all patients with fungal infections.

8. a. Milking or stripping chest tubing is unwise, especially in patients with fragile lung tissue (e.g., emphysema). The surgeon should be consulted regarding this procedure. Research indicates that stripping increases the negative pressure on

the pleural space and may cause persistent pneumothorax.

b. The nurse should check patency of the system and make sure the patient is not lying on the tubing. The patient should be encouraged to cough and change position to see if fluctuation is reestablished. If the tubing is not patent, the surgeon should be notified. Fluctuation ceases when lung reexpansion has occurred.

9. a. Time is required for adjustment to one lung. Otherwise, nursing care measures related to promotion of breathing, nutrition, and comfort do not vary between the two patients. No chest tubes are required after pneumonectomy because the lung is removed. However, a greater risk for mediastinal shift toward the "good" lung exists; monitor closely for tracheal deviation. A subcutaneous air leak in the patient with a thoracotomy could indicate inadequate chest tube function, whereas in the patient with pneumonectomy it could mean a serious leak in the bronchial stump. After lung removal the patient should be positioned supine or on the operative side to prevent drainage from the bronchial stump into the "good" lung. Activity may be restricted at first because vital capacity is lowered. The patient with a thoracotomy is probably most comfortable in the semi-Fowler's position, and although a chest tube is in place, activity is not generally restricted. Fluid overload is a greater concern with lung removal because the remaining lung takes 2 to 4 days to adjust to the increase in blood flow.

b. Pain medication needs to be administered. Pain may be interfering with the patient's ability to cough and breathe deeply. Fear of respiratory depression is generally unfounded in postoperative patients. If respiratory depression is suspected, the physician should be notified and reduced dosages of medications may be in order. Generally, undermedicating is counterproductive to postoperative recovery.

10. a. To interfere with the toxic mediators thought to trigger the cascade of events occurring with acute lung injury/acute respiratory distress syndrome.

b. Increasing the FiO_2 improves arterial oxygen saturation only when an intrapulmonary shunt is not responsible for oxygen desaturation.

c. Alveoli that would otherwise collapse on expiration are held open, thus increasing the opportunity for gas exchange across the alveolocapillary membrane.

d. Improves oxygenation by opening consolidated, dependent lung regions.

e. Improves oxygenation by reversing hypoxic pulmonary vasoconstriction in ventilated lung units.

f. Prevents movement of the endotracheal tube either in or out of the established position.

g. To determine if volume expanders or anti-hypotensive agents are needed.

11. a. Every milliliter of the intravenous fluid contains 40 U of heparin. To deliver 1000 U/hr, the intravenous infusion must run at 25 ml/hr.

b. Partial thromboplastin time (PTT) values for patients on anticoagulant therapy are generally maintained at two to three times the normal value. Normal PTT is 30 to 45 seconds. A PTT of 55 seconds is below the desired levels for anticoagulation. The physician should be notified and kept informed of daily PTT levels.

12. Because a tension pneumothorax is often the result of a closed pneumothorax, these two conditions share some of the same clinical manifestations. In contrast, an open pneumothorax is a sucking wound that causes a characteristic sucking sound at the wound site with each respiration. Tracheal deviation toward the unaffected side during inspiration is also characteristic of an open pneumothorax. A tension pneumothorax may also cause tracheal deviation as intrapleural pressure builds, causing mediastinal shift. Signs and symptoms of shock are indicative of a tension pneumothorax. The classic distinguishing manifestation of flail chest is paradoxic chest movement and movement of the mediastinum toward the unaffected side with inspiration and return to the midline on expiration.

13. a. This is an expected finding indicating that the desired level of suction is being attained.

b. Constant bubbling in the water seal bottle may indicate an air leak in the chest tube system. The nurse should begin at the insertion site and progressively move down the tubing to check for air leaks. If the bubbling continues, the physician should be notified.

CHAPTER 27

Chronic Respiratory Problems

1. Hypoxia, not elevated CO_2, is driving his respiratory effort. This is known as the hypoxic drive. Maintaining low-dose oxygen therapy is important to maintain his hypoxic respiratory drive. Continuous oxygen therapy is, however, essential for adequate relief of hypoxemia and pulmonary hypertension.

2. High-calorie, high-protein foods that are easily chewed are ideal. The meal plan should include frequent, small feedings that contain nutritious vegetable or cream soups, pureed meats, milk shakes or ice cream, puddings, crackers and cheese, and cream sauces or gravy over cooked vegetables. Adding mayonnaise, peanut butter, and other rich spreads to crackers or fruit will also enhance nutrition.

3. Status asthmaticus is an extension of an acute asthmatic attack. If measures that typically diminish signs and symptoms are ineffective, status asthmaticus is suspected. Patients with status asthmaticus are

often unable to talk. Wheezing and adventitious lung sounds typically present during asthmatic attacks are absent because of minimal air movement in and out of the lungs. The patient will appear cyanotic and may exhibit pulsus paradoxus and altered levels of consciousness.

4. a. The patient should be questioned briefly about the presence of wheezing. Absence of wheezing could signal status asthmaticus, which is a medical emergency.
   b. First, the patient should be instructed to take or repeat Proventil inhalant 4 to 6 puffs every 10 minutes for three doses. Ideally, the nurse should stay on the phone during this period. If no improvement occurs, the nurse should ask the patient how much prednisone she has taken. An additional 20 mg of prednisone may be taken if the patient's prescribed dose of 40 mg was taken earlier. The nurse should also determine if the patient is alone and inform her that the nurse will contact the physician. Have the patient stay near the phone and assure her that the nurse will call her back. Instruct her to seek emergency care immediately (call 911) if no significant improvement occurs after 20 to 30 minutes.
   c. 122 pounds equals 55.45 kg; 55.45 multiplied by 6 mg equals 332.7 mg
   d. 55.45 kg multiplied by 0.5 mg equals 27.7 mg/hr
   e. Each milliliter of fluid contains 2 ml of aminophylline. The patient is to receive 27.7 mg/hr. Thus 13.8 ml will deliver 27.7 mg of the drug. The infusion should be run at 14 ml/hr.
   f. Aminophylline has a short half-life that is even shorter in people who smoke. Therefore turning off the aminophylline for an extended period will dramatically reduce the therapeutic blood levels and could precipitate an asthmatic episode.

5. Health care reimbursement plans may impose restrictions on certain individuals with chronic diseases. These restrictions may create ethical dilemmas regarding access to health care. Some might argue that extending the life span of patients with cystic fibrosis (or any other chronic disease) places an economic strain on an already compromised health care system. In addition, individuals who are faced with a chronic illness such as cystic fibrosis may ultimately see life extension as prolonging anguish and suffering. Others may see it as their only hope for continued life.

6. Monitor for and report signs of rejection; plan activity schedule to enhance pulmonary function; teach patient regarding drug therapy.

7. a. To maintain positive end expiratory pressure and oxygenation, in-line closed suctioning is preferred. In-line suctioning also prevents contamination of the suction line.
   b. If ventilator alarms continue to sound despite no identified cause, the patient should be disconnected from the ventilator and manually ventilated. The nurse should elicit help from a co-worker who can consult a respiratory therapist for further evaluation of the machine.
   c. The nurse should assess for subcutaneous emphysema and evaluate symmetry of chest excursion. Blood gas analysis is advisable. A possible pneumothorax should be suspected and the physician should be notified of these changes.

8. A sounding pressure alarm means that the pressure required to deliver the set volume is exceeding the pressure limit. The patient could be coughing, resisting the machine, or experiencing an accumulation of secretions. The nurse should check for these three possibilities by assessing the patient for respiratory distress (inspection/auscultation), assessing the ventilator for function and settings, and inspecting the tubing for kinks.

9. Initiate prescribed sedation infusion such as morphine before the ventilator is disconnected, provide comfort measures to the patient, offer emotional support to the patient and family members, and encourage hospice involvement.

CHAPTER 28

Assessment of the Cardiovascular System

1. Example of analogy: The transportation system helps visualize the heart and major vessels. The heart can be compared to a major metropolitan area with major highways leading into the city, representing the vena cava and aorta. The city airport symbolizes the pulmonary system, and city suburbs represent the four heart chambers. Discussion of cardiac function with this analogy includes ideas such as the movement of traffic in and out of the city and visiting the airport (getting oxygen). Traffic may be described as greatest on the freeway leading away from the city (high-pressure side) versus less traffic at the airport (low-pressure system).

2. Many of the interview questions and assessment techniques will be the same for both individuals regardless of age. However, for the older adult the assessment will focus on response to exercise because age-related changes in the cardiovascular system are significantly more pronounced in response to activity. The older person will be asked about any incidents of mental confusion, lethargy, or weakness because these are early signs of cardiac disease in older adults. Caution will be exercised when palpating the carotid artery (older adults may have significant atherosclerosis and compromised circulation) and when checking for postural hypotension (a common finding in older adults).

411

3. Example: Preload is similar to a rubber band with stretching ability. The degree of stretch before letting go of the rubber band is called preload. In cardiac terms, preload is the degree of myocardial stretch before contraction. The degree of stretch is determined by the volume of blood stretching the ventricle during relaxation. When the normal rubber band is stretched, it is capable of a strong snap (contraction). If, however, the rubber band is overstretched, over time it will be less capable of a significant snap. Similarly, if the left ventricle is excessively stretched (as with ventricular hypertrophy caused by coronary artery disease), ventricular contraction will be less effective, leading to decreased cardiac output.

4. The 50-year-old's cough and dyspnea could be associated with cardiac disease, but further information is needed to rule out lung disorders. The 55-year-old patient has orthopnea, which is associated with advanced heart failure. The 58-year-old patient exhibits paroxysmal nocturnal dyspnea, which is related to the diseased heart's inability to compensate for an increase in blood volume when in a recumbent position.

5. Additional data include location, quality, and intensity of the pain. Did it radiate? Was it sharp, dull, or stabbing? Has he ever had this type of pain before? Did he have any other symptoms, such as shortness of breath or nausea? Did the pain stop when he began to rest?

6. h → f → c → i → a → g → d → j → b → e → k

7. a. 4, b. 1, c. 0, d. 2, e. 3, f. 0, g. 2, h. 3, i. 4, j. 2 and 3

8. a. 0, b. +, c. 0, d. +, e. 0, f. +, g. 0, h. 0, i. 0

9. a. Yes. Creatine phosphokinase MB is only found in myocardial tissue.
   b. No. Could reflect pulmonary problem(s).
   c. Yes. Related to decreased cardiac output.
   d. Yes. Suggests increased venous pressure related to congestive heart failure, volume overload, and tricuspid valve regurgitation.
   e. No. Pathologic in the elderly with congestive heart failure, but not necessarily in young adults.
   f. No. Could be caused by many other problems.
   g. Yes. S_4 often accompanies hypertensive cardiovascular disease, acute myocardial infarction, coronary artery disease, and angina.
   h. No. Characteristic of decreased circulation but not necessarily a diagnostic indicator of cardiac disease.
   i. Yes. Classic sign of congenital heart defects.
   j. No. May have many causes.
   k. Strongly suggestive, but may indicate chronic obstructive pulmonary disease, cardiac tamponade, or constrictive pericarditis.
   l. Yes. Indicates stenotic valve.
   m. Strongly suggestive, but not necessarily a definitive indicator of cardiac disease; may indicate primary renal disease but is likely associated with congestive heart failure and hypertension.
   n. Yes. Indicative of bundle branch block and mitral stenosis.
   o. Strongly suggestive but not definitive because this may be a normal finding in some individuals; abnormal if fixed on expiration and inspiration, indicating right bundle branch block, pulmonary hypertension.
   p. No. May be related to increased stroke volume associated with fever, exercise, anemia, and hyperthyroidism.

10. Although the central venous pressure is within normal range, it is showing a continuous increase (trending upward). Therefore the nurse in charge made the most appropriate decision by notifying the physician. An upward trend in a myocardial infarction patient could be very important, signaling increasing problems with left ventricular contractility.

11. a. Teaching needs to be directed at both the patient and his wife. An example is, "It is normal to feel apprehensive about the procedure and possible results. Let me tell you about the catheterization and what to expect. Please stop me at any time if you have questions. The physician and other experienced professionals will be with you in the room. There will be monitors and other equipment to help visualize your arteries, and there are many activities taking place. This is normal. The procedure is generally not painful, but you may feel some pressure in the groin area, a flushing sensation for about 30 seconds when the dye is injected, or some nausea. It is important that you report any sensations you are experiencing. The staff will keep your wife informed, and there is a waiting area close by."
    b. An assessment after cardiac catheterization must include evaluation of the femoral area, noting any bleeding from the insertion site. The site should be assessed for signs of inflammation or swelling. Pedal pulses must be assessed to determine patency of the artery and to detect any complications, such as thrombus formation.

12. The six cardinal clinical manifestations of altered cardiovascular status are dyspnea, chest pain, palpitations, edema, syncope, and excessive fatigue.

CHAPTER 29

Coronary Artery Disease and Dysrhythmias

1. a. False. Hypertension is a modifiable risk factor for CAD.
   b. False. Hormone replacement therapy is no longer recommended because research studies found an

increase in cardiovascular events in women taking hormone replacement therapy.
  c. True.
  d. False. Cigarette smokers have the highest incidence of CAD, followed by pipe and cigar smokers.
  e. True.
  f. True.
  g. False. Cholesterol accumulates within vessel walls and produces a fatty streak that protrudes into the lumen of the artery, impeding circulation.
  h. True.
  i. True.
  j. False. Patients having an acute myocardial infarction may describe their pain as mild indigestion, tightness, excruciating, or viselike. Aching and stabbing are not generally used as descriptors for acute myocardial infarction pain.
  k. True.

2. a. Creatine kinase
  b. Stress test
  c. Complete blood count
  d. 12-lead electrocardiogram
  e. Myoglobin
  f. Cardiac catheterization
  g. Serum troponin
  h. C-reactive protein

3. a. Antiplatelet agent. Blocks the formation of thromboxane A_2, inhibiting platelet aggregation.
  b. Antiplatelet agent. Prevents platelet aggregation by blocking adenosine diphosphate–induced platelet binding.
  c. Thrombolytic. Activates thrombolytic processes to lyse the clot that is occluding the lumen of the coronary artery.
  d. Glycoprotein IIb/IIIa receptor inhibitor. Blocks the binding of fibrinogen to the platelet, preventing platelet aggregation and clot formation.
  e. Anticoagulant. Binds to antithrombin III, inactivating coagulation factors Xa, IXa, and thrombin, thereby blocking the conversion of fibrinogen to fibrin.
  f. Nitrate. Causes vasodilation of the coronary arteries, reducing the amount of blood returning to the heart from the venous system, decreasing preload. Nitrates also decrease the workload of the heart and demand of the myocardium for oxygen and increase collateral blood flow to ischemic parts of the myocardium.
  g. Block $beta_1$ receptors, causing a decrease in force of contraction, slowing of heart rate, and slowing of impulse conduction.
  h. Calcium channel blocker. Inhibits the influx of calcium through the slow calcium channels to slow heart rate, decrease myocardial oxygen demand, and decrease the force of contraction.
  i. Angiotensin-converting enzyme inhibitors. Decrease preload and afterload and the overall workload of the heart.

  j. Opioid analgesic. Blunts the sensation of pain, promotes vasodilation, and decreases preload.
  k. Cholesterol-lowering agent. Increases receptor activity that removes low-density lipoprotein from the blood and blocks its production.

4. a. C, b. B, c. F, d. A, e. D, f. E

5. a. Delivers greater concentration of oxygen to the heart and decreases myocardial demand.
  b. Thrombolytic agents open the blocked coronary artery and must be given within 4 to 6 hours for maximal benefit. Some benefit may be possible up to 12 hours.
  c. Anxiety is common in patients with acute coronary syndromes. Anxiety increases the patient's myocardial oxygen demand at a time of decreased oxygen supply.
  d. The partner may have fears about the effects of sexual activity on the patient's heart.
  e. Thrombolytics increase the risk for bleeding because these agents break up clots.

6. An abnormally wide QRS complex indicates that the impulse is traveling abnormally through the ventricular portion of the conduction system. A major implication is bundle branch block, in which the contraction of one ventricle stimulates the contraction of the other ventricle.

7. Both are benign dysrhythmias that originate in the sinoatrial node and have a gradual onset. Both are associated with ischemia and may increase the risk for development of congestive heart failure. Sinus bradycardia, however, may be beneficial after myocardial infarction because the slower rate reduces myocardial oxygen demand. The primary difference in these two dysrhythmias is their etiology. Sinus tachycardia is caused by increased automaticity and sympathetic tone (as with alcohol, caffeine, tobacco, fever, pain), whereas sinus bradycardia is caused by increased vagal tone (as in athletes, secondary to vomiting or carotid stimulation). Either can result in decreased cardiac output with similar clinical manifestations (chest pain, weakness, dizziness, shortness of breath). Pharmacologic management is often necessary for both, and drug selection differs for each dysrhythmia.

8. The nurse can differentiate by assessing for various manifestations of sick sinus syndrome and other causes of confusion. The patient has a history of sick sinus syndrome; therefore his apical heart rate should be assessed for evidence of a tachycardia-bradycardia–type rhythm, which is characteristic of the disorder. Other potential causes of confusion in this situation may include alterations in the patient's blood sugar or hypoxia related to the pneumonia. All these parameters need to be assessed.

413

9. Premature ventricular beats (PVBs) are more significant in the man who recently had a myocardial infarction. Although the PVBs are occurring only occasionally, they reflect ventricular irritability from the myocardial injury and may progress to more dangerous PVBs, such as multifocal or bigeminal beats. In the absence of heart disease, occasional PVBs are relatively insignificant and may be a function of age in the other patient.

10. (1) Decreased cardiac output. (2) Ineffective tissue perfusion (cardiovascular) related to decreased cardiac output. (3) Anxiety (moderate to severe) related to antidysrhythmic medications, perceived threat to well-being.

11. The three-letter code VDD means the pacemaker is (1) capable of pacing the ventricle (V); (2) can sense the electrical activity in both the right atria and right ventricle (D); and (3) can either be inhibited from pacing or triggered to pace, depending on the patient's intrinsic rate (D).

12. Loss of sensing means that the pacemaker does not sense the patient's heartbeat and thus begins pacing. This would be evident on the electrocardiographic tracing with the appearance of pacing beats in addition to the patient's own rhythm. The danger in this situation is that the pacemaker may pace during the vulnerable period, causing a dangerous dysrhythmia such as ventricular tachycardia. To correct this problem the pacer's sensitivity to the patient's intrinsic heart rhythm needs to be increased.

13. a. I, H; b. L, A; c. A, C, F, E, G; d. B, K, E, F, G; e. D, J, K, F; f. K, H

14. Sinus tachycardia. Both atrial and ventricular rates are 10 beats/min and regular. PR interval, 0.20 seconds; QRS, 0.04 seconds. Unique characteristics: rate more than 100 beats/min. Cause: compensatory mechanism in response to hypoxic conditions. In this patient factors include anemia and increased metabolism associated with hyperthyroidism. Treatment: treat underlying cause. In this case treatment may include blood transfusion and antithyroid medication.

15. Sinus bradycardia. Both atrial and ventricular rates are 40 beats/min, regular. PR interval, 0.20 seconds; QRS, 0.04 seconds. Unique characteristics: rate less than 60 beats/min, syncope with very slow rates. Cause: increased parasympathetic stimulation. In this case the patient was possibly straining to have a bowel movement, causing vagal stimulation; digoxin would also slow the rate. Treatment: atropine.

16. Atrial fibrillation. Atrial rate cannot be counted because of its fibrillation (no P wave); irregularly irregular; ventricular rate, 110 beats/min; PR interval, not measurable; QRS, 0.04 seconds. Unique charac-

teristics: pulse deficit, loss of synchronous atrial kick with greater signs of decreased cardiac output. Cause: rapidly firing ectopic foci in the atria often secondary to CAD, pericarditis, and thyrotoxicosis. In this patient likely idiopathic with no underlying cardiac disease. Excessive alcohol consumption may be a contributing factor. Treatment: drugs to control fast ventricular rate, including digoxin and diltiazem; cardioversion may be attempted by using antidysrhythmics such as procainamide and amiodarone; electrical cardioversion may be necessary.

17. Bigeminy (premature ventricular beat). Atrial rate, 40 beats/min, regular; ventricular rate, 70 beats/min, irregular. PR interval, 0.20 seconds; QRS, 0.04 seconds. Unique characteristics: wide, bizarre QRS complexes. Cause: irritable ventricular focus associated often with congestive heart failure, digoxin toxicity, electrolyte imbalance, hypoxia, and stimulants. In this patient, possible factors include congestive heart failure and hypokalemia, which could result from diuretic therapy.

18. Ventricular fibrillation. Neither atrial nor ventricular rates measurable. No P waves, variable QRS complexes. Unique characteristic: chaotic rhythm, no vital signs. Primary cause in this situation is severe CAD. Treatment: CPR, immediate defibrillation; epinephrine may enhance effectiveness of defibrillation.

19. Mobitz II, 3:1 heart block. Atrial rate, 60 beats/min, regular; ventricular rate, 40 beats/min, regular. PR interval, variable; QRS, 0.08 seconds. Unique characteristics: progressive lengthening of the PR interval before a QRS complex is dropped. Cause: atrioventricular block of impulses often associated with CAD, acute coronary syndrome, cardiomyopathy. Treatment: atropine may increase the atrial rate but not necessarily the ventricular rate; may require permanent pacing.

20. a. 4, b. 2, c. 2, d. 1, e. 2, f. 2, g. 1, h. 4, i. 2, j. 2, k. 4, l. 1

CHAPTER 30

Heart Failure, Valvular Problems, and Inflammatory Problems of the Heart

1. a. A, b. C, c. A, d. B, e. C, f. B, g. B, h. A, i. B, j. A, k. B

2. a. Mitral valve prolapse, b. tricuspid stenosis, c. aortic regurgitation, d. mitral stenosis, e. aortic stenosis, f. mitral regurgitation

3. Acute pericarditis: Pathophysiology: inflammatory process of the visceral or parietal pericardium. Clinical manifestations: Pericardial friction rub; severe precordial chest pain; pain intensified by coughing, swallowing, or breathing deeply; fever; leukocytosis;

414

bradycardia. Collaborative management: treat symptomatically for fever, malaise, and pain; salicylates; nonsteroidal antiinflammatory drugs; treat underlying problem.

Chronic pericarditis: Pathophysiology: fibrosing of the pericardial sac from trauma or neoplastic disease; pericardium tightens around heart and decreases its ability to pump. Clinical manifestations: dyspnea, fatigue, congestive heart failure. Collaborative management: pericardiectomy, digitalis, diuretics, low-sodium diet.

Myocarditis: Pathophysiology: inflammatory disease producing myocardial cell injury from drug hypersensitivity, toxicity, or infection. Clinical manifestations: fever, lymphadenopathy, pharyngitis, myalgias, pericardial pain, elevated erythrocyte sedimentation rate and cardiac enzymes, mild to moderate leukocytosis, electrocardiographic changes, congestive heart failure. Collaborative management: bed rest, digitalis, immunosuppression, treatment of cause if known.

4. a. Metabolic needs of the body are not being met even though cardiac output remains normal or above normal.
   b. Cardiac output falls below normal, compromising the metabolic needs of the body.
   c. Failure of the left ventricle followed by pulmonary congestion and edema.
   d. Right ventricular failure, which frequently follows left ventricular failure and results in systemic venous congestion and peripheral edema.
   e. Damming of blood in vessels proximal to the heart.
   f. Inability of the heart to maintain cardiac output.

5. a. Immediately place the patient in high Fowler's position, then notify the physician.
   b. He is developing pulmonary edema.
   c. Relief of anxiety, relief of hypoxia, decrease of venous return, and improvement in cardiovascular function.

6. a. Examples: furosemide, hydrochlorothiazide, spironolactone. Advantages: decreases volume overload and preload, increases urine output.
   b. Examples: nitroglycerin, nitroprusside. Advantage: decreases cardiac workload, improves cardiac output.
   c. Examples: enalapril, captopril. Advantage: blocks aldosterone, prevents vasoconstriction.
   d. Examples: digitalis, dobutamine. Advantage: increases force of cardiac contraction, increases cardiac output.
   e. Examples: propranolol, atenolol. Advantage: decreases heart rate, allowing more complete emptying of heart; decreases myocardial oxygen demand.
   f. Examples: verapamil, nifedipine. Advantage: decreases systemic vascular resistance, reduces left ventricular hypertrophy.

7. a. Administer oxygen, position for maximum ventilation, teach relaxation techniques.
   b. Assess for edema, teach regarding fluid and sodium restrictions, monitor effectiveness of diuretics.
   c. Organize activities, teach to balance rest with activity, use interventions to promote sleep, gradually progress activities.
   d. Provide a calm, quiet environment; position in semi-Fowler's position or position of comfort; monitor for changes in cardiac status.
   e. Teach regarding signs of fluid overload, fluid or sodium restrictions, and prescribed medications.

8. a. Factors that may be contributing to the elevated digitalis level: hypothyroid condition, diuretic therapy, hypokalemia and hypomagnesemia, possible renal insufficiency.
   b. Insufficient cardiac output decreases renal perfusion, which activates the renin-angiotensin system to correct perceived hypovolemia, leading to sodium and water retention. The increase in fluid volume helps increase renal perfusion but increases the workload of the heart. Failure of the heart to adequately pump the increased fluid leads to further renal compromise; therefore a direct relation between heart failure and renal compromise exists.
   c. Administer oxygen for dyspnea, place in position for maximal ventilation, balance rest with activity, assess for complications and effectiveness of treatments; teach regarding sodium and fluid restrictions.

9. Pulmonary edema should be suspected in any patient with heart failure who develops profound dyspnea, pallor, audible wheezing, cyanosis, restlessness, anxiety, tachycardia, or decreased oxygen saturation levels.

10. a. Mitral stenosis, mitral regurgitation (insufficiency), aortic stenosis, aortic regurgitation (insufficiency), or tricuspid stenosis
    b. Mitral stenosis, aortic stenosis, or aortic regurgitation (insufficiency)
    c. Aortic regurgitation (insufficiency)
    d. Mitral valve prolapse and aortic regurgitation (insufficiency)
    e. Aortic regurgitation (insufficiency)
    f. Mitral stenosis
    g. Mitral regurgitation (insufficiency)
    h. Aortic regurgitation (insufficiency)

11. Teaching includes information about the procedure itself; where the family may wait during surgery so that the surgeon may find them when the surgery is completed; about the ICU/CCU; and what to expect postoperatively: intubation and ventilation, suctioning techniques, closed chest drainage, pacer wires, intravenous access, elastic stocking, incision, indwelling urinary catheter, coughing and deep

415

breathing after extubation, and visitor regulations. All questions should be answered.

12. a. False. The surgeon will be concerned because alcohol intake and use of tobacco may affect both the safety and the outcome of the surgery.
   b. True.
   c. True.
   d. False. Both the electrocardiogram and cardiac enzymes are important. Surgery will not be performed until the cardiac status is stable.
   e. False. The patient's perception is not less important than other considerations. The patient's perception may dictate how well the patient adjusts to, or denies, the illness as well as affect response to the surgery.

13. First, the idea that she is having open heart surgery should be corrected because an incision into the heart is not necessary. New vessels will be attached to the outside of the heart where her present heart vessels are. The machine is a bypass pump that supplies oxygen and maintains circulation to the body while the heart is being operated on. The pump allows for the administration of medications that may be needed during surgery and assists with cooling of the body, which decreases the amount of energy needed by her body during the surgical procedure. To prevent anxiety over the cooling procedure, the patient should be reassured that she will be warmed to normal temperature after the surgery.

14. a. Perform hourly circulation checks of all pulses in both extremities until the balloon is removed; do not allow the patient to flex his hip on the affected side; use a well-padded leg restraint if the patient is unable to cooperate.
   b. To prevent migration of the balloon, do not elevate the head more than 30 degrees.
   c. Keep the dressing over the balloon insertion site clean and dry and change the dressing every 24 to 72 hours with aseptic technique.

15. a. Electrolyte imbalance, especially potassium; hypotension; hypovolemia; P_{O_2} values for possible hypoxia.
   b. Indicators of shock, such as hemorrhage.
   c. Hypothermia. Shivering increases metabolism and therefore oxygen demand.
   d. Possible clotting of tube. Inability to drain fluid can result in cardiac tamponade.
   e. Hypoxia or brain embolization.
   f. Shock or hypovolemia, which may result in acute renal failure.

16. a. The left ventricle is fibrotic and thickened as a result of infiltrates. The ventricle loses its ability to stretch, thereby decreasing compliance. Cardiac output is decreased by the heart's inability to fill,

and heart failure ensues. As myopathy increases, so does heart failure.
   b. Management will focus on decreasing the workload of the heart, improving contractile efficiency, and managing symptoms and complications until a donor heart is available or the patient's condition deteriorates and heart transplantation is no longer a consideration.

CHAPTER 31

Vascular Problems

1. All these conditions involve circulation, are progressive, and begin with atherosclerosis (plaque development), which narrows arteries and leads to increased peripheral vascular resistance and subsequent secondary hypertension. Both atherosclerosis and hypertension contribute to the development of heart disease (coronary artery disease, myocardial infarction, and congestive heart failure). Arterial occlusion or narrowing can contribute to cerebral vessel occlusion or narrowing, causing a cerebrovascular accident, or stroke. These conditions are closely interwoven, each augmenting the other's development. Diabetes inhibits macrocirculation caused by altered glucose and fat metabolism and results in subsequent development of atheromatous plaque.

2. a. S, b. P, c. P, d. S, e. S, f. P, g. P, h. S, i. S, j. P

3. a. Beta-blockers are contraindicated in patients with chronic obstructive pulmonary disease because they can cause bronchoconstriction.
   b. Furosemide decreases sodium and water reabsorption, thus decreasing blood volume and blood pressure. Nifedipine is a calcium channel blocker that relaxes arteries, reduces arterial spasms, and enhances vasodilation.
   c. Monitoring for hypokalemia and postural hypotension with furosemide. Monitoring for hypotension, fatigue, edema, and headache with nifedipine. Both drugs can cause nausea. Blood pressure is monitored closely because both drugs can cause hypotension.
   d. Captopril acts by inhibiting the conversion of angiotensin (a potent vasoconstrictor) to angiotensin II, thus blocking release of aldosterone and decreasing sodium and water retention. The result is the same as for furosemide, but the actions are different.
   e. Hypotension, dizziness, and fatigue. The combination of furosemide, nifedipine, and captopril can lead to hypotension. Captopril can also cause increased potassium levels, although this is unlikely because the patient is also receiving furosemide.
   f. Teaching should include the need to monitor for drug side effects, rise slowly from a lying position, avoid foods high in potassium, minimize salt

416

and alcohol intake, and maintain regular follow-up and compliance with prescribed medication regimens.

4. Increasing pain, diminished or absent pulses, change in skin color, temperature, drainage, paresthesia, decreased limb movement. Edema is not usually present.

5. Allowing a moderately wet dressing to dry before removal causes debridement of necrotic tissue. This may be sufficient to promote healing and may avert surgical debridement.

6. The stump is supported with a pillow during the immediate postoperative period. Support along the outer aspect of the limb prevents outward rotation. Both abduction and adduction are avoided to prevent abnormal hip rotation and misalignment. Elevating the leg is avoided to prevent flexion contracture. The prone position is encouraged to stretch the hip flexor muscles.

7. Thromboangiitis obliterans, or Buerger's disease, involves both small and medium arteries and veins. It is an inflammatory process involving the hands and feet and is similar to arterial occlusive disease in that intermittent claudication occurs. Unlike the other two arterial diseases, Raynaud's disease occurs primarily in the hands and has been linked to cold weather and emotional stress. Raynaud's disease is caused by arterial spasm. Throbbing pain, tingling, and tricolor changes occur (pallor to cyanosis to redness).

8. a. Heart disease and obesity contribute to both arterial and venous insufficiency as a result of increased workload on the heart muscle and ultimate effects on blood flow.
   b. Many factors can contribute to endothelial damage and hypercoagulability that increases the potential for thrombus formation in veins. Venous blood flow involves capillaries and veins that are considerably smaller than arterial vessels; thus hypercoagulation disorders interfere more readily with venous blood flow. However, arteries are not exempt from thrombus formation in association with atherosclerosis. Acute arterial occlusion can occur as a result of a dislodged thrombus (embolism), which is often caused by deep vein thrombosis.

9. Both arterial and venous insufficiency are frequently a consequence of underlying cardiac disease. Decreased arterial blood flow commonly results from atheromatous plaque development and increased blood pressure, which places an increased workload on the heart. Venous insufficiency can be caused by cardiac disease, which involves clot formation caused by venous pooling that may result from dysrhythmias or decreased venous return, as in congestive heart failure.

10. a. False. Heparin prolongs the clotting time to prevent clot extension and new clot formation. It does not dissolve existing clots.
    b. False. Streptokinase is a synthetic protein that acts as a thrombolytic. It is useful in dissolving existing clots in emergency situations.
    c. False. The partial thromboplastin time is used to monitor the anticoagulant effects of heparin therapy, and the prothrombin time is used to monitor Coumadin therapy.
    d. False. Patients on Coumadin therapy should consume only moderate amounts of vitamin K because vitamin K promotes clotting and can counteract the effects of Coumadin.

11. a. Patient A is exhibiting signs and symptoms of deep vein thrombosis. Characteristic symptoms include sharp pain at rest, during activity, or both; warmth of the extremity; and obvious edema. Collateral vessels are often engorged. Patient B has arterial occlusion, as evidenced by the aching, cramping sensation exaggerated by activity and relieved by lowering the extremity. Other characteristic symptoms include coolness, dryness, shiny appearance, and diminished hair growth. Peripheral pulses are diminished.
    b. Symptoms of limb-threatening ischemia include severe pain at rest with sudden onset, numbness, tingling, decreased capillary refill, absent or diminished peripheral pulses, marked pallor or mottling, and coolness. Neither patient exhibits limb-threatening ischemia at this point.
    c. Homans' sign is helpful in confirming a diagnosis of venous thrombosis, although it may be absent in a significant number of people. Dorsiflexion of the foot causes increased resistance or pain.
    d. (1) Ineffective tissue perfusion (lower extremity); (2) Risk for impaired skin integrity; (3) Activity intolerance; (4) Impaired mobility; (5) Deficient knowledge; (6) Pain.
    e. Similarities: both need to be taught to avoid constrictive clothing, crossing legs at ankles or knees, astringents such as alcohol, and pressure or massage; both patients require close monitoring of circulation parameters. They need to understand the importance of skin care. Differences: patient A is encouraged to (1) engage in aerobic exercise and Buerger-Allen exercises, (2) avoid direct heat application, (3) keep the environment warm to avoid chilling and vasoconstriction, and (4) place leg in a slight dependent position to increase arterial blood flow. Patient B will be treated with bed rest for approximately 5 to 7 days with his leg elevated to enhance venous return. Care includes antiembolism stockings and moist heat to decrease inflammation. Calf circumference should be monitored.

417

f. Stasis ulcers are generally found on the medial aspect of the ankle and cause moderate pain, edema, and pigment changes, leading to a brawny appearance. Stasis ulcers (commonly occurring on the heel, lateral malleolus, and toes) are more common than ischemic ulcers (which are more painful and have a pale, gray base). Less edema is present than with venous ulcers, and pulses may be diminished or absent.

12. a. The patient probably has an acute arterial occlusion created by a thrombus originating in the left side of the heart as a result of myocardial infarction. The sudden onset of pain, absence of pulses, poikilothermia, and numbness of the leg all suggest acute arterial occlusion.
    b. Much of the nursing care is similar, with the exception of care associated with anticoagulant therapy.
    c. The patient's value is high normal, indicating that clotting time is not within therapeutic range for anticoagulant therapy. The goal of heparin therapy is an increase in the partial thromboplastin time to one and one-half to two times the normal value. The heparin drip rate will likely be increased.

13. Acute coronary syndrome: Monitor vital signs and hemodynamic parameters such as pulmonary artery pressure and pulmonary capillary wedge pressure to assess ventricular contractility. Closely monitor for cardiac dysrhythmias. Assess cardiac rate and rhythm, lung sounds, and pain. Renal failure: Monitor urine output and input and output ratio, blood urea nitrogen, and creatinine. Assess for signs of fluid volume deficit, including mucous membranes, vital signs, hemoglobin and hematocrit, and level of consciousness. Stroke: Conduct neurologic checks focusing on mentation, speech, movement of extremities, and muscle strength.

CHAPTER 32

Assessment of the Hematologic System

1. Because the patient has no kidney function, he is unable to secrete erythropoietin in response to blood loss. Erythropoietin stimulates the production of erythrocytes. He will have greater difficulty compensating for his blood loss than people with kidney function and will require a greater degree of intervention.

2. Elevated neutrophil and monocyte counts are associated with bacterial infections. An infection could alter the outcome of the patient's surgery. The surgeon needs to be notified immediately because the patient's surgery will be canceled if infection is present.

3. This is very significant information. Aspirin prevents aggregation of platelets and may increase the risk for bleeding. The surgeon needs to be notified so that the patient's clotting time can be obtained and monitored more closely for potential bleeding.

4. Their blood counts may be fairly similar. The younger patient may demonstrate a higher leukocyte count in response to the infection. The older patient may have a lower hemoglobin level because of her age. Both women will have similar platelet counts.

5. a. To detect anemia, to monitor response to treatment for anemia, to detect blood loss.
   b. To differentiate between anemias.
   c. To obtain information regarding the cause of anemia.

6. a. False. Both fever and night sweats are common in hematologic diseases.
   b. False. Iron-deficiency anemia is associated with dry skin, dry hair, and brittle nails.
   c. False. Enlarged lymph nodes may reflect a disease process; therefore any enlarged lymph node requires further evaluation.
   d. True.
   e. False. An abdominal assessment is important because enlargement of both the liver and spleen may occur in hematologic diseases.

7. a. C and G, b. A, c. B, d. E, e. B, f. F, g. D, h. A, i. D

8. a. Identification and evaluation of congenital and acquired deficiencies in the coagulation system, monitoring the effectiveness of heparin therapy.
   b. Monitoring effectiveness of warfarin therapy and screening for vitamin K deficiency and disseminated intravascular coagulation.
   c. Evaluation of rejection of transplanted organs.
   d. Identification of specific coagulation deficiencies.
   e. Diagnosis of sickle cell disease and thalassemia.
   f. Evaluation of microcytic anemia.
   g. Visualization of the lymphatic system to detect disease.

9. Explain that the site where the needle is inserted will be anesthetized before the procedure. The patient will have a brief, sharp pain as the marrow is removed. Assure the patient that a nurse will remain with her during the entire procedure to offer support and comfort.

CHAPTER 33

Hematologic Problems

1. a. Examples of similarities: same type of red blood cell deficiency, exertional dyspnea, fatigue. Examples of differences: etiology, medical treatment, and prognosis.
   b. Assessment parameters are similar, and patient problems are similar: activity intolerance, potential for infection, potential for bleeding, and knowl-

edge deficit regarding treatment and follow-up care. Teaching will vary because each type of anemia has a different cause.

   c. Most patients have similar clinical manifestations and consequently require similar nursing care; teaching varies depending on cause and treatment and the knowledge base of the patient and caregiver.

2. a. Aplastic
   b. Chronic blood loss
   c. Megaloblastic
   d. Thalassemia
   e. Iron-deficiency
   f. Aplastic
   g. Acquired hemolytic
   h. Hereditary spherocytosis
   i. Chronic blood loss

3. a. True.
   b. False. Transfusion therapy is the treatment of choice for thalassemia. Drug cessation applies to hemolytic anemia.
   c. True.
   d. True.
   e. False. It is an autosomal dominant trait, which leads to swelling of red blood cells.
   f. False. Persons with G6PD deficiencies have anemia only when exposed to oxidant drugs, during infections, or during the newborn period. Response to therapy is generally good.
   g. False. Hemoglobin S sickles when the oxygen tension is decreased.
   h. True.

4. Examples: explanation of the condition; events that may trigger episodes, such as dehydration, infection, overexertion, cold weather changes, intake of alcohol, or smoking; how to recognize the onset of crises; whom to contact for assistance and when.

5. (1) Thrombotic: most common; sickled cells occlude blood vessels, producing pain. (2) Aplastic: temporary decrease in erythropoiesis generally caused by continual red blood cell stimulation, usually caused by infection, results in rapid worsening of anemia because of the short life of red blood cells. (3) Splenic sequestration: shock condition related to pooling of blood with sudden increase in the size of the spleen.

6. Other patient needs: the patient's anxiety, activity intolerance needs, assessing the patient's and family's degree of coping and assisting as needed, assessing for possible sexual dysfunction, including family and significant other in teaching.

7. a. Nail condition: assess for brittleness and concavity. Tongue: assess for atrophy, shininess, redness, and smoothness of surface. Mouth: assess for cracks at corners that may be painful.

   b. Advise patient to take iron with meals to help prevent gastrointestinal irritation, warn the patient that iron may turn her stools black; report symptoms of diarrhea or nausea to the physician.

8. Neurologic abnormalities such as peripheral neuropathy, disorders of balance, and neurologic degeneration.

9. They measure different clotting pathways. Prothrombin time measures the adequacy of the extrinsic coagulation pathway, and partial thromboplastin time measures the intrinsic coagulation pathway.

10. The procedure itself for administering these products does not vary. Both are administered by basic intravenous administration procedures. However, the monitoring and storage differ. A platelet count is obtained 1 hour before and 1 hour after administration of platelets to assess effectiveness. Platelets cannot be stored as long as whole blood. Both infusions require careful handling to prevent cell damage.

11. No, further data are needed. For example, the presence or absence of blood in stool and the presence of excessive menstrual bleeding in female patients also help detect bleeding.

12. a. Neutropenia
   b. Vitamin K deficiency, hemophilia, thrombocytosis, or disseminated intravascular coagulation
   c. Hemophilia
   d. disseminated intravascular coagulation
   e. Vitamin K deficiency
   f. Neutropenia
   g. Hemophilia

13. a. Causes activation of intrinsic clotting system by release of factor XII after vessel damage and platelet aggregation
   b. Causes factor VII activation
   c. Similar to sepsis with activation of intrinsic clotting system
   d. Proteolytic enzymes in snake venom activate factors II and X

14. As the depletion of clotting factors II, V, VIII, platelets, and fibrinogen occur, fibrin degradation products are formed by fibrinolysis. Fibrin degradation products are similar to anticoagulants in that they increase the potential for hemorrhage. Consequently, bleeding follows clotting in disseminated intravascular coagulation.

15. The patient has been adequately taught; however, the nurse should ascertain his level of understanding, answer any questions that he may have, repeat any teaching that is needed, and include the family and significant others in teaching.

16. a. The patient should be reassured that DDAVP, the drug being used to treat his condition, does not carry the risk of transmitting HIV/AIDS.
   b. The response would be different. He would need to be reassured about the very remote possibility of contracting HIV by antihemophilic factor. Donors are thoroughly screened and factor VIII concentrates are heat-treated to kill the HIV virus.

17. a. Examples: acute forms of leukemia primarily affect younger persons, whereas chronic forms of leukemia are more common in middle-aged to older persons.
   b. Examples: fever, infection, and bleeding are common to acute leukemia; anemia is common to acute lymphoblastic leukemia, acute myeloblastic leukemia, and chronic lymphocytic leukemia; weakness and fatigue are more common in the chronic conditions.
   c. Examples: increased in chronic states, variable in acute states.

18. Examples: chemotherapy is used for all forms of leukemia. Bone marrow transplant is more useful than chemotherapy for acute myeloblastic leukemia and chronic myelogenous leukemia. Chemotherapy is not as effective for chronic conditions. Chemotherapy is highly beneficial for children with acute lymphoblastic leukemia. Chemotherapy only minimally affects survival with chronic myelogenous leukemia.

19. Examples: prevention of complications such as hemorrhage or infection; provision of supportive therapy, such as comfort, hydration, and hygiene; monitoring of effectiveness of therapy; teaching regarding the disease process, the effect of the drug(s), potential side effects of the drug, and possible drug outcomes; and teaching regarding follow-up care and home care.

20. Information regarding the availability of community resources within her geographic location need to be included.

21. Differences: the person with Hodgkin's disease is probably much younger than the patient with non-Hodgkin's disease because the former most often affects young adults; therefore their care will vary depending on their developmental needs. The patient with Hodgkin's disease may voice greater concern over treatment-induced sterility. The patient with non-Hodgkin's disease may be more concerned over treatment schedules that could interfere with life routines. Similarities: both may undergo radiation and/or chemotherapy; consequently monitoring for and dealing with the side effects of therapy will be similar for both. Teaching will be similar for both regarding medications, monitoring of blood counts, symptoms that require immediate reporting, the need for follow-up care, and community resources

available. Care for both will depend on the stage of their disease and the type of treatment plan followed.

22. The nurse should assure the patient that stage II does not imply terminal disease. Staging allows the comparison of persons with Hodgkin's disease and their response to treatments so that the most appropriate treatment course can be prescribed for persons with similar disease. The patient can be appropriately reassured that treatment cure rates have been as high as 80% for persons with stage II disease and that no reason exists to believe that he will not be among that 80%.

23. Infectious mononucleosis is a self-limiting disease in which recovery generally occurs spontaneously. With rest, full recovery is most likely even though she may be fatigued for several weeks.

CHAPTER 34

Assessment of the Renal System

1. a. F, b. B, c. E, d. G, e. D, f. A, g. C

2. a. False. The distal and collecting tubules are responsible for electrolyte balance.
   b. True.
   c. False. The cortical hormone is aldosterone, not angiotensinogen.
   d. False. Glucose is 100% reabsorbed. Only 96% of calcium is reabsorbed.
   e. True.
   f. False. The kidneys actively secrete H^+ ions in the distal tubule but passively secrete them in the proximal tubule.

3. The kidneys maintain homeostasis by regulating acid-base balance; retaining or eliminating fluids or electrolytes; and excreting metabolic waste products, drugs, and toxins.

4. a. The kidneys perform several functions to increased blood pressure. They sense low blood pressure and release renin, which sets the angiotensin-aldosterone system into motion. Sodium and water are reabsorbed, resulting in increased blood pressure. Prostaglandins are released in an attempt to increase blood pressure.
   b. Secretion of potassium by the distal tubule is increased and reabsorption by the proximal tubule is decreased to bring the potassium level back to normal.
   c. Erythropoietin, which is produced by the kidneys, stimulates the production of red blood cells to correct anemia.

5. a. Examples: "Do you leak urine continually or only with stress, such as coughing, laughing, or lifting?" "Is your urine leakage preceded by a feeling of bladder fullness?" "Do you have any chronic

health conditions?" "What concerns you most about this problem?"

 b. Examples: "Do you urinate in small or large amounts?" "Is urination associated with pain?"

 c. Examples: "How often do you urinate at night?" "How much fluid do you drink at night?" "In a 24-hour period?" "Does your urinating at night represent a change from your normal urination patterns?"

 d. Examples: "Do you have to strain to start your urinary stream?"

6. Patient A's renal status will be normal if he has had no renal trauma or disease. Because of his age, patient B may have decreased glomerular functioning, decreased reabsorption, and decreased ability to concentrate urine. As a result, patient B's blood urea nitrogen, serum creatinine, and blood glucose levels may vary from normal.

7. Instruct the patient to use a sterile container (provided by the facility) and to touch only the outside of the container to maintain sterility. For women: keep labia separated throughout collection and clean meatus from front to back. For men: retract foreskin if uncircumcised and cleanse glands. Both men and women need to collect the specimen after the urinary stream has started.

8. A creatinine clearance test involves collecting urine for a 24-hour period and measuring both the total volume and total amount of creatinine excreted. It provides a rough estimate of glomerular filtration rate. Serum creatinine is a blood test that provides information about the kidneys' ability to excrete creatinine. Both are tests for renal function.

9. The serum creatinine level is normal; therefore renal function is likely normal. The blood urea nitrogen level is elevated. Because nutritional status affects blood urea nitrogen, the patient's malabsorption is likely the cause of the elevation.

10. a. This is a painless and noninvasive procedure used to identify abnormal structures, masses, or fluid accumulation. You may be asked to drink a lot of water before the test because a full urinary bladder assists with outlining other structures.

 b. This is a painless and noninvasive x-ray procedure. The test is helpful in determining the size and location of your kidneys. A laxative or enema may be given before the examination to provide better visualization.

11. Because the patient only needs to lie flat for 4 hours if no evidence of bleeding is present, the nurse should assess the puncture site. If no bleeding is apparent, the patient may be allowed to move about in bed but should remain on bed rest until 9:00 AM the next morning.

12. Tests A and B require the use of an intravenous dye, whereas test D can be performed with or without dye. Test C is different because it requires injection of a radioactive isotope rather than a dye. Tests B and D provide data regarding renal circulation, whereas test C provides data about renal blood flow. Test A provides no data about either circulation or blood flow. Tests A, B, and C require prior preparation. Test D may or may not require prior preparation depending on whether dye is used.

CHAPTER 35

Kidney and Urinary Tract Problems

1. The commonality is their increased risk for urinary tract infection. The nurse is overdistending her bladder by ignoring her need to void. The 78-year-old woman has a portal of entry for pathogens by her indwelling catheter, and the 67-year-old man has a partial obstruction, with urinary retention and stasis, from prostate enlargement.

2. The nurse has covered the majority of necessary teaching but omitted informing the patient about the need for increasing her fluid intake to 3 to 4 liters of fluid per day, avoiding the use of contraceptive jellies at this time, and urinating after sexual intercourse.

3. a. Assessment of vital signs for fever, tachycardia, tachypnea, and hypertension; assessment of abdomen for tenderness over the bladder; assessment for flank pain; amount of urine voided; and further information regarding her normal urinary patterns.

 b. While demonstrating empathy, the nurse should explain that kidney function is temporarily altered by pyelonephritis but generally returns to normal after treatment. Any misconceptions need to be corrected and the importance of follow-up care stressed.

4. The patient's peak levels need to be monitored because gentamycin is toxic to the kidneys. His urine needs to be assessed for presence of proteinuria and hematuria because gentamycin can affect glomerular permeability. Eosinophils in the urine may need to be monitored if allergic interstitial nephritis is suspected because gentamycin can cause this condition as well.

5. a. False. Acute glomerulonephritis can follow acute poststreptococcal pharyngitis, but it is an immune-complex disease, not an infection of the kidney.

 b. True.

 c. True.

 d. False. Urine specific gravity is increased, not decreased. Increased serum creatinine and decreased urine output are associated with acute glomerulonephritis.

6. Antibiotics such as penicillin are given to eliminate residual streptococcal bacteria and prevent new streptococcal infections, subsequently reducing the antibody-antigen reaction that is injuring kidney tissues. Antibiotics are of no value in the treatment of the antigen-antibody reaction itself.

7. a. Restrict sodium intake, restrict fluid intake, monitor for edema, and administer diuretics as prescribed.
   b. Monitor blood pressure, administer antihypertensives as prescribed, and restrict fluid intake.
   c. Teach regarding medications, prognosis, diet, and follow-up care.

8. The nurse can best address the patient's concerns by explaining that chronic glomerulonephritis is a slowly progressive disease; therefore symptoms are not always readily noticeable. Persons with no prior disease or predisposing infection can be unaware that their kidney function is deteriorating.

9. Renal insult (acute glomerulonephritis, allergic reaction, etc.) → increased glomerular permeability → proteinuria and decreased serum protein levels → decreased serum osmotic pressure → generalized edema.

10. a. Similarities: protein is lost in urine. Serum protein is decreased. Edema may be present. Patients may have fatigue or lethargy, nausea and vomiting, and electrolyte imbalance. Sodium restriction may be required. Serum potassium level may be elevated. Diuretics may be necessary. No specific treatment is recommended. Differences: nephrotic syndrome is generally accompanied by increases in lipids, cholesterol, and phospholipids. Chronic renal failure from nephrotic syndrome is a greater risk than acute glomerulonephritis. Antibiotics may be helpful in reducing the streptococcal bacterial count, thus the resultant antigen-antibody response that occurs with acute glomerulonephritis.
    b. Excess fluid volume, risk for infection, and deficient knowledge.

11. a. Malignant nephrosclerosis
    b. Diabetic neuropathy
    c. Renal artery stenosis
    d. Benign nephrosclerosis

12. Assessing for bladder distention at least every 8 hours and monitoring for signs of systemic fluid overload, urinary retention, oliguria or anuria, anorexia, vomiting, or lethargy.

13. a. He has urinary retention with overflow.
    b. The nurse should first use noninvasive measures to help the patient void, such as running water or helping him stand to void. If these measures fail, catheterization may be necessary on this one occasion to relieve his urinary retention and prevent bladder spasms or other complications.
    c. Renal damage can occur from back pressure of urine up the ureters and into the kidneys.

14. a. Coudé
    b. Either a Malecot or Pezzer
    c. Robinson
    d. Whistle-tip

15. Reposition the patient or assist him to a standing position, run water in a nearby sink, pour warm water over his perineum, or place his hand in warm water to stimulate urination.

16. Maintain adequate hydration consisting of at least 2500 ml of fluid per day; remain active to prevent urinary stasis; eat a low-purine diet to maintain an alkaline-ash urinary pH to prevent stone formation; see his physician regarding use of bicarbonate, citrate, or allopurinol as preventive measures.

17. Percutaneous lithotripsy is a surgical procedure in which the calculi are retrieved by an endoscope passed through a small incisional tract. Extra corporeal shock wave lithotripsy involves use of external sound waves to fragment calculi so that they can be excreted in the urine. Laser therapy involves use of a urethroscope to break up calculi with a laser beam.

18. Their care will essentially be the same: interventions addressing risk for general postoperative complications, risk for renal complications such as hemorrhage, postoperative pain, indwelling catheter care and monitoring (if present), and urinary retention or burning on removal of the catheter.

19. The patient should be advised to report to her health care practitioner right away regarding her hematuria for further evaluation. Painless intermittent hematuria is the most common symptom associated with renal cell carcinoma and early treatment is essential.

20. Presence of bleeding or pain. His present data (vital signs, etc.) need to be compared with his baseline data to determine if the patient is bleeding or developing signs of shock or if he is in pain.

21. Explaining the expected changes in anatomy and appearance of the stoma, reassure the patient that normal activities of daily living need not change, focusing on recovery and adaptation, encouraging the patient to express fears and concerns, and correcting misconceptions.

22. a. Ileal conduit or ileal loop
    b. Continent urostomy

23. Assess the pouch to determine if it fits properly. Reassure the patient that changing her pouch earlier is okay if necessary. If it leaks by the fifth day, she should change the pouch on the third or fourth day.

24. a. Stress incontinence
    b. Overflow incontinence
    c. Urge incontinence

25. Perineal (Kegel) exercises strengthen pelvic muscles. They will help prevent the woman from developing stress incontinence from pelvic muscle relaxation, which can occur with the aging process and as a result of childbirth.

26. The woman's concerns are justified. Polycystic kidney disease is a bilateral disorder in which cysts are diffusely scattered throughout the renal parenchyma, producing ischemia. Polycystic kidney disease undergoes relentless progression to end-stage renal failure in a high percentage of cases.

CHAPTER 36

Kidney Failure

1. Similarities: in both cases, the kidneys lose their ability to maintain the internal environment of the body. Differences: the time period for development of each condition. Chronic renal failure develops over months to years. Acute renal failure can occur within hours to days. Acute renal failure generally has a better prognosis than chronic renal failure when treatment is initiated early. Chronic renal failure is nonreversible.

2. Risk factors include potential renal toxicity from chemicals used in his job. His sore throat 3 weeks ago may have been caused by streptococcus, predisposing him to glomerulonephritis, which can cause permanent kidney damage. His positive family history for diabetes mellitus and hypertension are risk factors for chronic kidney failure.

3. a. Prerenal acute renal failure, because it is related to decreased renal perfusion secondary to hemorrhagic hypovolemia.
   b. Serum potassium of 5.6 mEq/L.
   c. Hyperkalemia and subsequent cardiac dysrhythmias or arrest.
   d. Pulmonary compromise (crackles), hypertension, peripheral edema, fluid and electrolyte imbalance.

4. a. Cool extremities and normal blood pressure suggest decreased tissue perfusion, most likely related to recent coronary insult. Her elevated serum creatinine and blood urea nitrogen levels are suggestive of acute renal failure, which can occur after cardiac compromise and decreased renal perfusion.

   b. Urine output; vital signs, especially blood pressure; changes in urinalysis findings, including urine sodium and specific gravity; changes in serum creatinine, blood urea nitrogen, and serum potassium; lung sounds; peripheral fluid status; cardiac status.
   c. Nausea, vomiting, cardiac dysrhythmias, Kussmaul's breathing, drowsiness, confusion, edema, congestive heart failure, pulmonary edema, and sustained hypertension.
   d. It is a slow ultrafiltration process; therefore it will not place unnecessary stress on her already compromised heart, especially because she does not have significant electrolyte abnormalities or azotemia.
   e. Energy will be provided by fats and carbohydrates, thus sparing body protein. This diet decreases nitrogenous waste production, which can further injure the kidneys. Moderate fat is preferred in this case because of her cardiac disease.
   f. Signs and symptoms of returning renal failure, such as fluid retention or decreased urine output; any dietary restrictions; activity limitations.
   g. Her hypertension needs to be controlled to prevent renal hypoxia from decreased blood flow to her kidneys.

5. a. True.
   b. True.
   c. False. Na$^+$ reabsorption from the proximal tubule is decreased.
   d. True.
   e. False. Lethargy and confusion are caused by electrolyte imbalance and the inability to excrete metabolic wastes.

6. a. B, b. C, c. D, d. A, e. B, f. C, g. D, h. B, i. C, j. C, k. A, l. B, m. A

7. a. Systemic lupus erythematosus, which places her at increased risk for renal disease secondary to immune complex glomerulonephritis.
   b. She most likely has renal insufficiency.
   c. The kidneys are unable to concentrate urine; therefore patients urinate larger volumes of urine than normal, necessitating getting up at night to urinate.
   d. It will be 40% to 50% of normal, or 62 to 75 ml/min.
   e. Serum creatinine will be at least 1.2; blood urea nitrogen will be approximately 25 (values will vary for individual patients).

8. a. Primarily blood pressure, lung sounds, edema, and weight. Dyspnea, heart rate, and respirations secondarily.
   b. Serum creatinine, blood urea nitrogen, glomerular filtration rate, and serum electrolytes.
   c. Hemodialysis by a temporary access site to reestablish fluid and electrolyte balance and acid-

423

base balance and to prevent complications such as pulmonary edema or hyperkalemia.

d. He most likely has symptoms related to the rapid removal of intravascular fluid volume. The rate of fluid removal and ultrafiltration pressure should be reduced to prevent symptoms associated with hypovolemia.

e. How to palpate for a thrill or bruit to determine patency of his site; dietary restrictions if necessary; the schedule, expected actions, and side effects of prescribed medications; dialysis schedule; and information regarding follow-up care.

9. a. Ultrafiltration, b. osmosis, c. diffusion

10. a. B, b. B, c. A and C, d. B, e. B, f. B

11. a. 1. Cause: rapid water removal. Action: intravenous administration of 0.9% NaCl.
2. Cause: shift in fluid and acid-base balance. Action: administer prescribed intravenous antiemetic.
3. Cause: change in acid-base and fluid balances. Action: rest, sleep, administer prescribed mild analgesic.
4. Cause: use of heparin. Action: apply pressure to venipuncture site.

b. 1. Cause: contamination of peritoneal equipment. Action: administer prescribed antibiotics, stop use of dialysate, obtain sterilized equipment.
2. Cause: absorption of dialysate fluid in abdomen. Action: monitor, administer prescribed insulin if necessary.
3. Cause: large fluid volume in abdomen. Action: reposition for comfort, use diversional activities, administer mild analgesic.

12. Demonstrate respect for the woman's decision to discontinue treatment. Provide opportunities for her and her family to share their feelings and concerns, provide emotional support to both her and her family, and ensure her physical comfort and safety as death approaches.

13. a. Chronic, b. hyperacute

14. Potential complications: electrolyte imbalance, infection, rejection, hypertension. Clinical manifestations of rejection: oliguria, anuria, increased serum creatinine and blood urea nitrogen levels, hypertension, hypervolemia.

15. Monitor for and report signs of rejection, teach about collecting urine specimen, preserve dialysis access site.

16. Organs and tissues are in very short supply and the demand is great. The demand far outweighs the supply.

17. A non–heart beating donor is a person who has been declared dead by traditional cardiopulmonary criteria rather than brain death criteria. A deceased donor is a person who has been declared brain dead.

18. Ideally, the drug could be administered both orally and intravenously, would increase neutrophil counts, would selectively suppress T lymphocytes, could be developed from embryonic tissue rather than foreign protein, would inhibit the action of T lymphocytes as immune cells. Other ideal qualities are possible.

19. a. True.
b. True.
c. False. The postoperative care of a live donor is similar to that provided after a nephrectomy procedure.
d. False. Dehydration is avoided; however, it is to prevent renal hypoperfusion, not hyperperfusion.
e. True.
f. False. The first priority is medication teaching. Patients and their families must be able to explain the action, dosage, and potential effects of all medications before discharge.

CHAPTER 37

Assessment of the Endocrine System

1. A furnace thermostat is an example of an analogy. Low calcium level in the blood (low room temperature) stimulates the parathyroid gland (furnace turns on). Parathyroid hormone is released (warm air is released from the furnace), which causes calcium absorption to increase (room temperature increases). As calcium level in blood rises (thermostat registers increased room temperature), the parathyroid is inhibited or "turned off" (furnace is shut off).

2. Both hormones are controlled by a feedback loop; however, regulation of thyroid hormone is much more complex, involving interactions among the hypothalamus, anterior pituitary, and thyroid gland. For example, to maintain normal levels of thyroid hormone, the feedback loop sends a message to the hypothalamus and anterior pituitary, inhibiting release of thyroid-releasing hormone and thyroid-stimulating hormone, respectively. The control of antidiuretic hormone is similar but does not involve the use of hormones that stimulate or inhibit its release. Instead, when serum osmolality is increased, the posterior pituitary is stimulated to release antidiuretic hormone, which acts on the kidney to promote reabsorption of water. This response "turns off" the system because osmolality has returned to normal.

3. The concept of intrinsic rhythmicity means that the hormone (for example, acetylcholine) is regulated by daily sleep-wake patterns that cause the hormone to rise and fall.

4. Factors such as stress or infection can cancel out the effect of the negative feedback mechanism, causing an increase of acetylcholine.

5. a. Hyponatremia, possible syndrome of inappropriate secretion of antidiuretic hormone
   b. Decreased stress response
   c. Decreased response to sodium restriction
   d. Impaired glucose metabolism
   e. Increased incidence of hypothyroidism
   f. Loss of calcium from bone, osteoporosis

6. All patients with a suspected endocrine disorder should undergo a thorough head-to-toe examination. However, general areas significant to endocrine assessment regardless of the specific hormonal imbalance include (1) history of nutritional/fluid intake and output, (2) assessment of appearance and body features, (3) ability to perform activities of daily living and energy level, (4) sexual and reproductive history, and (5) tolerance to stressors.

7. All these findings are significant; however, they carry even greater meaning under some of the following circumstances.
   a. Weight loss is significant if the loss is unexplained or accompanied by other signs and symptoms, such as fatigue and nervousness.
   b. A family history of diabetes mellitus is relevant because the disorder has a genetic predisposition. In addition, older adults with a family history of diabetes may be at even greater risk because reduced insulin sensitivity occurs in older adults.
   c. Postural hypotension may signal fluid and electrolyte alterations (resulting from hormonal dysfunction). It warrants further investigation.
   d. Decreased libido may be associated with depression or stress. However, further data are necessary to rule out a hormonal imbalance as the cause.
   e. Because hormonal imbalances can affect metabolism and the central nervous system, nervousness and irritability are significant findings, especially when accompanied by other physical signs and symptoms.

8. A person with diabetes insipidus responds to water deprivation by exhibiting no increase in urine osmolality because antidiuretic hormone is not being produced. In contrast, the same patient given exogenous antidiuretic hormone (vasopressin) shows an increase in urine osmolality, demonstrating that the source of the problem is the abnormally low secretion of antidiuretic hormone from the pituitary and that renal impairment is not the cause.

9. Exocrine function of the pancreas is related to the external secretion of pancreatic juices by the pancreatic duct into the duodenum, where they play a major role in digestion. Endocrine function of the pancreas relates to the internal secretion of insulin and glucagon, which play a primary role in carbohydrate metabolism.

10. a. False. Estrogen in men and testosterone in women are not under feedback control.
    b. True.
    c. True.
    d. False. Iodine is necessary to the production of thyroid hormone.
    e. False. The adrenal medulla produces epinephrine and norepinephrine.
    f. False. An elevation of serum calcium causes an increase in the release of calcitonin by the thyroid, with a subsequent decrease in parathyroid hormone.

11. a. S, b. S, c. I, d. S, e. I, f. S

12. a. E, b. E, c. U, d. E, e. U, f. U, g. E, h. E

13. Fatigue, mental sluggishness, forgetfulness, and constipation may all be signs of hypothyroidism; however, these symptoms are not uncommon findings in the aging process. Patient A's symptoms may be caused by her age or lifestyle changes. On the other hand, she may have an underlying endocrine disturbance. Unfortunately, endocrine disorders in older adults with symptoms such as these are sometimes misdiagnosed or overlooked. In contrast, age would generally not be viewed as an etiologic factor for patient B, who is experiencing extreme fatigue, lethargy, weight gain, and constipation. She will likely receive further assessment more quickly than will patient A.

14. Endocrine abnormalities can begin with subtle changes in appearance or bodily function. The patient's symptoms should warrant further investigation because they may be associated with a hormonal imbalance.

CHAPTER 38

Pituitary, Thyroid, Parathyroid, and Adrenal Gland Problems

1. Women: prolactin causes irregular menses, oligomenorrhea/amenorrhea, infertility, galactorrhea, dyspareunia, and decreased libido. Men: prolactin decreases libido, causes impotence, decreases sperm count, and causes gynecomastia.

2. After complete removal of the anterior pituitary gland (hypophysectomy), patients require lifelong cortisol replacement therapy as well as thyroid hormone, gonadal steroids, and possibly antidiuretic hormone. After adenectomy, patients do not necessarily have a disruption in glucocorticoid secretion but will be monitored for signs and symptoms of deficiency. Teaching plans are similar for these patients except regarding drug therapy.

425

3. SIADH → increased antidiuretic hormone = increased total body water = hypoosmolar state → water intoxication → decreased urine output and increased specific gravity → dilutional hyponatremia. On the other hand, diabetes insipidus → decreased antidiuretic hormone = decreased water reabsorption = hyperosmolar state → cellular dehydration → increased urine output and decreased specific gravity → hypernatremia.

4. SIADH: Hypertonic saline is used to replace sodium loss. It is administered along with a loop diuretic to increase serum sodium levels. It is administered cautiously to prevent overly rapid shift of fluids from intracellular space to extracellular space. Diabetes insipidus: With normal blood pressure and loss of pure water, free water is given orally or as D5W. If the patient is hypotensive and hyponatremic, 0.9% saline solution is given to restore vascular volume. Careful replacement occurs over a 48-hour period to prevent a hypoosmolar state, causing water to shift from extracellular space to intracellular space.

5. Thiazide diuretics (plus a low-sodium diet) produce a state of mild hypovolemia. In turn, sodium chloride and water are reabsorbed in the proximal kidney tubule, resulting in less water going to the collecting ducts where antidiuretic hormone should normally be (but is not). Consequently, less water is excreted.

6. a. During transsphenoidal pituitary surgery normal antidiuretic hormone secretion may be disrupted as a result of surgical trauma. This places the patient at risk for developing diabetes insipidus, which can lead to fluid volume depletion.
   b. Diabetes insipidus should be suspected because the patient's urine output is excessive and his urine specific gravity is low, even though his vital signs are essentially normal. His weight and serum sodium level would be useful information to help support the presence of diabetes insipidus.
   c. The nurse should be concerned about possible cerebrospinal fluid leakage. Nursing actions, in order of priority, are (1) assess drainage for appearance of a halo ring. If halo ring is present, send specimen to laboratory for glucose analysis. (2) Elevate the head of the bed. (3) Instruct the patient to remain on bed rest. (4) Assess the patient every 4 hours (at least) for nuchal rigidity or headache and vital signs, especially temperature.
   d. These manifestations may indicate secondary hypothyroidism subsequent to tumor removal and trauma to the pituitary gland. Reduction in secretion from the anterior pituitary leads to decreased thyroid hormone. Although signs and symptoms do not necessarily reflect adrenal hyposecretion, it is a possibility and warrants further investigation because reduction in acetylcholine can follow pituitary tumor removal.

7. a. Given the patient's signs and symptoms, and knowing that oat cell carcinomas can be associated with SIADH, the nurse would be correct to expect a low Na^+ level and an increase in total body water. The patient's weight gain, malaise, and lack of edema indicate water intoxication. General malaise without other more serious signs of central nervous system disruption indicate mild hyponatremia (120 to 125 mEq/L).
   b. The patient will likely show increased central nervous system symptoms related to water intoxication and swelling of brain cells. Clinical manifestations may include lethargy, headache, and decreased level of consciousness.
   c. SIADH involves an increase in the release or effect of antidiuretic hormone, causing water retention. This event results in increased glomerular filtration and lack of sodium reabsorption by the renal tubules; hence sodium is lost in the urine. The change in serum osmolarity (hypoosmolar state) causes cellular water intoxication. Interstitial edema is not present because hyponatremia and natriuresis are present.
   d. The 3% NaCl saline solution is used to replace sodium. As a hypertonic solution, it also draws fluid into the vascular space from the intracellular fluid compartment. Furosemide is a high loop diuretic used to remove excess water. Because sodium is also lost, dietary sodium should be increased.

8. a. Family history of endocrine disorders, evidence of goiter, reports of visual disturbance, history of intolerance to heat, and result of any recent thyroid studies.
   b. No. Ophthalmopathy may occur before, at the same time, or after the onset of hyperthyroidism in Graves disease.
   c. It seems paradoxic that thyroid-stimulating hormone is low in hyperthyroidism, in which thyroid hormone is above normal levels. The negative feedback mechanism that regulates thyroid hormone levels explains this apparent contradiction. In the case of Graves disease, certain immunoglobulins are thought to stimulate the thyroid gland, causing excess synthesis and release of thyroid hormone. When thyroid hormone levels become elevated, the negative feedback system operates to turn off the release of thyroid-stimulating hormone at the pituitary level.
   d. Dexamethasone inhibits the release of thyroid hormone and also the conversion of T4 to T3 in the periphery.
   e. A cooling blanket and tepid baths are valid choices for lowering body temperature. Of course, the physician should be consulted regarding use of the cooling blanket because rapid lowering of the temperature produces chilling and increases metabolic rate, which may be detrimental to the

426

patient. Use of aspirin is not a wise choice, however, because salicylates ultimately increase free thyroid hormone levels. Consequently the practitioner is unlikely to prescribe aspirin. Acetaminophen is the drug of choice.

9. a. B, b. B, c. B and C, d. B, e. B, f. B and C, g. A

10. Statements a, d, and e are correct.

11. a. Thyroid storm etiology: Thyroid storm can be precipitated by stress (infection, trauma, surgery). Clinical manifestations: hyperthermia, hypertension, tachycardia, delirium, tremors, or restlessness. Nursing care priorities: lower metabolic rate, maintain cardiac output, maintain normal body temperature, decrease any external stressors.
    b. Myxedema coma etiology: Associated with hypothyroidism and can be precipitated by sedatives, narcotics, exposure to cold, and external stressors such as surgery or infections. Clinical manifestations: classic symptoms of hypothyroidism plus coma, severe hypothermia. Nursing care priorities: provide respiratory and cardiac support, maintain normal body temperature, monitor fluid status.

12. Primary hypothyroidism occurs with thyroid dysfunction and reduction of thyroid hormone. Decreased thyroid hormone levels "turn off" the negative feedback mechanism, allowing increases in thyroid-stimulating hormone, which stimulates the thyroid to produce more thyroid hormone. As a result, thyroid enlargement (goiter) occurs. In contrast, hypothyroidism is caused by dysfunction of the pituitary, which results from a lack of thyroid-stimulating hormone. Thus the thyroid is not stimulated, and goiter formation does not occur.

13. Decreased weight, increased appetite, reduction of facial puffiness, and reduction in fatigue are primary signs that treatment is effective.

14. Much of the teaching will be the same as for younger patients. Teaching will include the fact that initial doses of thyroid hormone replacement may precipitate cardiovascular problems such as angina or congestive heart failure, especially in older adults who may have compromised circulatory function. The increase in metabolic rate and myocardial oxygen consumption can trigger chest pain and congestive heart failure. The nurse will instruct the patient to report chest pain, edema, or shortness of breath.

15. Injury to parathyroid glands during surgery can lead to reduction in parathyroid hormone and resultant reduction in serum calcium levels. Calcium deficiency can cause tetany, respiratory obstruction, and death.

16. Respiratory distress can be caused by several factors, including recurrent damage to the laryngeal nerve, tracheal compression related to hemorrhage, tissue swelling, and tetany. The nurse should assess for hoarseness, check the dressing for bleeding or tightness, assess the patient's ability to swallow, note any tingling or numbness around the mouth or of toes or fingers, or the presence of Chvostek's and Trousseau's signs. Nursing actions include loosening the dressing, elevating the head of the bed, locating a tracheostomy set and intravenous calcium gluconate, and immediately informing the physician of findings.

17. Hypersecretion: Low self-esteem (disturbed body image), imbalanced nutrition, activity intolerance, sexual dysfunction, ineffective coping, anxiety, decreased cardiac output, risk for injury. Hyposecretion: activity intolerance, low self-esteem (disturbed body image), ineffective individual coping, sexual dysfunction, imbalanced nutrition, anxiety, risk for injury, impaired elimination (bowels). Other nursing diagnoses may also be appropriate.

18. Hypersecretion: Caloric adjustments are advised for patients with hyperthyroidism (increased calories) and adrenal hypersecretion (decreased calories). Sodium restriction is recommended for individuals with hyperpituitarism and adrenal hypersecretion, and perhaps hyperthyroidism related to congestive heart failure and edema. Glucose and sugar adjustments may be required in persons with hyperpituitarism and adrenal hypersecretion because of associated effects on carbohydrate metabolism. Hyposecretion: Caloric adjustments are recommended for individuals with hypothyroidism (decreased calories) and adrenal hyposecretion (increased calories). Persons with hypopituitarism and hypothyroidism may need fluid and sodium restrictions. Individuals with hypoparathyroidism will require increased calcium intake and associated reduction in phosphates.

19. Both hypersecretion and hyposecretion of the pituitary can interfere with thyroid and adrenal function. In other words, the higher the disorder in the hypothalamic-pituitary-thyroid-adrenal chain, the greater the endocrine dysfunction.

20. Examples of desired outcomes: Patient describes anxiety level as decreased or tolerable and identifies one or more anxiety-reducing strategies; discusses nature of the disorder, related signs and symptoms, and how the disease will affect activities of daily living; verbalizes positive aspects of self and describes body characteristics and functions that are reversible; describes strategies to cope with body characteristics and functions that are not reversible.

21. Anxiety often causes hyperventilation, which can exaggerate hypocalcemia because respiratory

alkalosis may occur ("blowing off" carbon dioxide). The patient should be assured that the situation is reversible, and the nurse should stay with the patient until her anxiety level is reduced and hyperventilation has ceased.

22. Nursing diagnoses: (1) Excess fluid volume. Nursing actions: restrict fluids as ordered, monitor intake and output, provide low-sodium diet, provide potassium replacements, monitor daily weight. (2) Risk for infection. Nursing actions: monitor temperature every 4 hours, assess for signs of infection, institute preventive sterile technique for intravenous procedures. Other nursing diagnoses are also appropriate.

23. Iatrogenic refers to treatment induced. Cushing's syndrome occurs when a patient takes large doses of exogenous glucocorticoids for their therapeutic antiinflammatory effects. Side effects are produced that mimic Cushing's syndrome. The greater the dose, the greater the possibility of side effects.

24. Tachycardia, palpitations, throbbing headaches, elevated blood glucose level, nausea, vomiting, tremors, hypertension (especially paroxysmal hypertension), nervousness, anxiety.

CHAPTER 39

Diabetes Mellitus and Hypoglycemia

1. Both patients are at increased risk for developing type 2 diabetes mellitus. Patient B has more control over her risk factors than patient A because she can change her sedentary lifestyle and lose weight if she chooses. If patient A's autoimmune disease is well controlled, it may delay the onset of diabetes.

2. a. F, b. C, c. A and C, d. F, e. D, f. E, g. B, h. F

3. Relative insulin deficiency means that the insulin being produced is either ineffective or inadequate to meet the individual's needs. Absolute insulin deficiency means the person is not producing an adequate amount of insulin to control blood glucose levels. Both conditions result in abnormal glucose metabolism and subsequent diabetes mellitus.

4. a. Examples: hyperglycemia, elevated serum triglycerides, increased ketone production
   b. Examples: failure of glucose uptake, failure of amino acid uptake, weakness
   c. Examples: elevated free fatty acids, weight loss

5. a. She may be in the early stages of diabetic ketoacidosis.
   b. An elevated blood glucose level coupled with headache, nausea, polydipsia, polyuria, tachycardia, hypotension, and fatigue.
   c. Positive serum acetone, serum osmolarity between 300 and 350 mOsm/L, serum bicarbonate less than 15 mEq/L, decreased arterial pH, and change in serum electrolytes with an increased anion gap.
   d. Careful monitoring, reporting of abnormal data, preventing complications, and providing emotional support for both the patient and family.
   e. HHNC is a continuation of insulin deficiency but more severe because of the oliguria and failure to eliminate glucose. The serum glucose level becomes extremely high, resulting in hyperosmolality. As a result, intracellular and extracellular dehydration occur, leading to central nervous system dysfunction, shock, and hypoxia. HHNC is not associated with ketosis or acidosis, as is diabetic ketoacidosis.
   f. The patient with HHNC is lethargic to comatose and displays signs of severe fluid deficit, including polyuria followed by oliguria. Serum glucose levels are greater than 600 mg/dl, serum osmolarity is greater than 350 mOsm/L, serum acetone is undetectable, serum bicarbonate is normal, arterial pH is greater than 7.3, and anion gap is normal.
   g. Frequent monitoring of blood glucose, intake and output, vital signs, mental status, serum potassium, arterial blood gases, serum electrolytes, and serum ketones as the patient's condition warrants, as well as preventing complications and offering emotional support.

6. The patient is most likely hypoglycemic. The assessment findings, coupled with headache, fatigue, and blurred vision, indicate too much insulin and/or a low blood glucose level. The patient should be given 10 to 15 g of a quickly absorbed carbohydrate such as fruit juice and monitored until his blood glucose stabilizes.

7. a. Diabetes mellitus alters blood vessels and nerves. Smoking further decreases circulation to the lower extremities. Persons with diabetes who smoke place themselves at increased risk for loss of sensitivity to pain or pressure in the lower extremities. Injury or infection could ultimately lead to the need for foot or limb amputation.
   b. The patient has diabetic retinopathy, which can be progressive and lead to blindness from microaneurysm in the retinal vessels, retinal hemorrhage, or proliferative retinopathy.
   c. The presence of hypertension is the factor that most often accelerates diabetic nephropathy, proteinuria, and renal disease.
   d. Extensive nerve damage (peripheral polyneuropathy) has already occurred once the diabetic patient has an abnormal monofilament examination. The patient is at increased risk for paresthesias, numbness, and pain.

8. Sensory impairment leads to painless trauma and the potential for foot ulceration. Motor impairment contributes to muscle wasting, resulting in foot

deformity. These conditions can lead to fractures or amputation from infection and sepsis.

9. Patient A needs more insulin because her regular insulin will only be effective for 6 to 8 hours. Patient B may not require insulin at 1730 because Lente is an intermediate-acting insulin with effects lasting up to 16 hours.

10. An insulin pump may be helpful because the patient has a variable eating schedule. It requires time and interest, but this patient is an ideal candidate if she is committed to assisting with her own care.

11. The nurse should determine if the patient has discussed her problem with her health care provider. If not, the patient needs to be encouraged to do so because she may be developing resistance to her prescribed insulin.

12. Example: hemoglobin A1c is a marker for blood glucose control and reflects the average blood glucose level over a period of time. Once glucose is attached to hemoglobin it remains throughout the life span of the red blood cell (erythrocyte) and is not affected by age, sex, duration of diabetes, or very recent blood glucose levels. It reflects overall blood glucose control for the past 3 months and is used in conjunction with home blood glucose monitoring to assess adequacy of blood glucose control.

13. Intensive insulin therapies better mimic the physiology of the pancreas, decrease nocturnal hypoglycemia, and provide better glycemic control, which ultimately decreases the incidence of micro-vascular complications.

14. a. A, b. B, c. D, d. A, e. D, f. C, g. B

15. Many plans are possible; however, the plan should contain five bread, four meat, two vegetable, three fruit, two skim milk, and two fat exchanges.

16. Daily living patterns and family patterns that may influence the patient's adjustment to the disease still need to be assessed.

17. a. False. The glycosylated level will be twice that of normal.
    b. True.
    c. True.
    d. False. Urine ketone testing is recommended for blood glucose levels of 240 mg/dl or higher.
    e. False. Not all goals are met by selecting correct foods. Other goals, such as including specific food preferences, making adjustments to dietary patterns, planning menus for weight loss, and independent management of the diet are not demonstrated by correctly selecting menu items.

f. False. Knowing exactly what to teach and how much to teach the patient with diabetes is a problem confronting nurses because no two patients have exactly the same knowledge level or teaching requirements.
    g. False. Regular or short-acting insulin should always be drawn up first so that it will work rapidly when needed.
    h. True.

18. Insulin should not be administered if the patient is unable to take in food or fluids because it places her at risk for hypoglycemia from insulin excess. However, her health care provider should be notified immediately. If the provider is not available, the local emergency department or urgent care facility must be contacted for further advice.

19. Yes, the nurse should intervene because the patient may not understand why rotating sites is necessary. Insulin injection sites need to be rotated to prevent poor absorption of the medication and tissue injury.

20. Atrophy or scarring can occur at injection sites. This can cause erratic or inadequate insulin absorption from the loss of healthy subcutaneous tissue.

21. a. Because of the presence of risk factors, screen for diabetes, hypertension, atherosclerotic heart disease, and peripheral vascular disease. Secondary prevention.
    b. Counsel the patient and her husband about monitoring their child for diabetes so that the condition, if it develops, can be detected early. Tertiary prevention.
    c. Encourage the man to begin a hobby that requires physical activity such as walking or golfing. Primary prevention.
    d. Suggest or provide access to dietary support and nursing or medical care by home health or volunteer assistance. Secondary prevention.

22. The patient needs to be monitored for both hyperglycemia and hypoglycemia because of her NPO status before, during, and immediately after surgery and for her hormonal response to surgery. Her usual diet needs to be initiated as soon as possible. Her blood glucose and urine acetone levels need to be monitored, and the possible need for additional insulin must be considered.

23 a. The nurse should suspect reactive hypoglycemia related to ingestion of her lunch.
    b. The nurse should check the patient's blood glucose level and vital signs, give her something to eat to increase her blood glucose if low, and report the incident to the physician.

24. Answers will vary depending on the students' fears, knowledge, and so forth.

429

CHAPTER 40

Assessment of the Gastrointestinal, Biliary, and Exocrine Pancreatic Systems

1. Similarities: Both have anatomic sphincters that prevent reflux and are affected by vagal stimulation and mechanical distention. Peristaltic contractions occur in both the esophagus and stomach to move food. Differences: Enzymes are secreted in the stomach but not in the esophagus. The esophagus does not have a secretory function. Mechanical digestion takes place in the esophagus, whereas chemical digestion occurs in the stomach.

2. Differences exist primarily in the digestive enzymes required to facilitate breakdown of these nutrients. The breakdown of carbohydrates begins in the mouth through the action of salivary amylase. The breakdown of protein begins in the stomach through the action of gastric pepsin. Further breakdown of both protein and carbohydrates occurs in the small intestine. Different pancreatic and intestinal enzymes work on protein and carbohydrates to break them down for absorption.

3. Knowing that the patient had an upper gastrointestinal series first, the nurse needs to determine if the patient has excreted all the barium from the barium enema. Enemas or laxatives may be required to clear the colon before the barium enema can take place. Generally, if both an upper gastrointestinal series and barium enema are ordered, the barium enema is scheduled first so that barium is not in the colon when the barium enema needs to be performed.

4. Carcinoembryonic antigen is a protein commonly present in patients with colorectal tumors. Its use as a diagnostic tool is limited because other factors can cause an elevation. However, it is used to determine if the patient is responding to therapy or if the tumor is growing. In this case, the elevation after chemotherapy suggests that the tumor is increasing in size or has returned.

5. a. The finding is below normal (3.2 to 4.5 g/dl). This may mean that the person is malnourished or has a condition in which protein is being wasted or poorly absorbed.
   b. This finding is below normal (9.0 to 11.5 mg/dl). Low calcium levels may occur in persons with severe pancreatitis or steatorrhea.
   c. Normally, bilirubin should not be found in the urine. Biliary stricture, inflammation, or stones may cause bilirubin to be excreted in the urine.
   d. Elevated serum lipase, an enzyme secreted primarily by the pancreas, is a specific indicator of pancreatic disease.
   e. Alkaline phosphatase is elevated, suggesting a biliary problem. However, bone and liver also secrete this enzyme in response to inflammation or disease. Therefore it is not considered a specific test for pancreatic or biliary disease.

6. The tests are similar because they both involve passage of an endoscope down the esophagus. The primary difference is that the endoscopic retrograde cholangiopancreatography views the pancreatic and biliary ducts, whereas the esophagogastroduodenoscopy is only capable of visualizing the duodenum and structures above. Preprocedural and postprocedural care is essentially the same.

7. a. False. As persons age, saliva decreases, making susceptibility to infection greater.
   b. True.
   c. False. Chronic gastritis is common in older adults but is generally related to *Helicobacter pylori*.
   d. False. Chronic constipation is a common complaint of older adults, but contractions of the large intestine have been found to be unchanged as long as the person remains physically active.
   e. True.

8. Additional data are needed and include the following.
   a. Nutritional status: use of alcohol; usual eating habits; food preferences and allergies; 24-hour dietary recall; financial resources; and other gastrointestinal symptoms such as flatulence, pain, and weight loss.
   b. Abdominal pain: duration and location of pain, presence of fullness or distention.
   c. Energy level: is energy the same as it was before the onset of anorexia?
   d. Elimination pattern: use of laxatives, suppositories, usual stool patterns.

9. Data that need to be reported: abdomen firm with tenderness noted over the left lower quadrant; bowel sounds hyperactive throughout; reddened, visible hemorrhoids; and small white plaque on the lower gum line that cannot be removed by a tongue blade. Significance of findings: nonremovable white plaque found on mucous membranes may indicate cancer (leukoplakia). Distention may indicate gas or fluid accumulation. Tenderness may indicate infection or obstruction. Hyperactive bowel sounds may signal infection or obstruction. Hemorrhoids may bleed and cause slow blood loss and discomfort.

CHAPTER 41

Mouth and Esophagus Problems

1. a. Gingivitis: encourage frequent brushing and flossing; teach the need for regular dental checkups.
   b. Candidiasis: encourage frequent oral hygiene; encourage the intake of buttermilk or yogurt to maintain normal oral flora.
   c. Parotitis: teach oral hygiene techniques; encourage adequate fluid intake.

d. Herpes simplex: teach patient to avoid ultraviolet light; assist patient with identifying methods to reduce stress.

2. Clinical manifestations: Although the pathophysiology of the two conditions is quite different, the symptoms produced are very similar. Both conditions cause pain from gastric reflux, which results from increased intraabdominal pressure. Other findings common to both are heartburn, regurgitation, frequent use of antacids, weight loss, changes in meal patterns, presence of odynophagia, and reflux aspiration. Nursing care: Nursing diagnoses and corresponding interventions are primarily related to pain, knowledge deficit, and risk for ineffective airway clearance. Treatment: These conditions share similar secondary prevention strategies, such as weight management, diet, and lifestyle modifications to reduce gastric reflux. Treatment is similar and includes antacids, histamine receptor antagonists, and other antireflux agents. Patients with gastroesophageal reflux have more dietary restrictions than patients with hiatal hernia. Activities that increase intraabdominal pressure are restricted for both patients.

3. a. Risk = 2. Gastroesophageal reflux disease does not place the patient at high risk, although repeated episodes of inflammation change epithelial tissue and are associated with an increased risk for adenocarcinoma of the esophagus.
   b. Risk = 2. Chewing tobacco correlates with premalignant oral lesions. However, research is inconsistent in demonstrating a causative link to oral cancer. No correlation to ethnicity or race has been identified.
   c. Risk = 2. Asians have a high incidence of esophageal cancer. Chronic malnutrition may be a factor.
   d. Risk = 3. Combination of long-term smoking and heavy alcohol use places this person at high risk for esophageal and oral cancer. Incidence of esophageal cancer is higher in men and African-Americans.
   e. Risk = 3. Statistics suggest a high incidence of esophageal cancer in the Chinese. A higher incidence is also found in men and individuals with a deficient diet.
   f. Risk = 2. A clear link has been identified between long-term tobacco and alcohol use and both oral and esophageal cancer. Risk will increase if lifestyle remains the same.
   g. Risk = 1. High-risk factors are absent.
   h. Risk = 3. Symptoms suggest an esophageal condition. Long-term smoking and alcohol history are both risk factors.

4. The nurse should ask questions that evaluate the patient's lifestyle habits such as: "Have you made any changes in your diet since your initial diagnosis (e.g., reduction in fatty foods, caffeine, chocolate)?" "Do you use nicotine? If so, have you made any headway in eliminating or reducing smoking?" "What other medications do you take, either prescribed or over the counter (e.g., calcium channel blockers, theophylline, nonsteroidal antiinflammatory drugs, all of which may lower the pressure of the lower esophageal sphincter, which promotes reflux)?" "Are you taking measures to reduce your reflux (e.g., eating small meals, avoiding food 2 to 3 hours before bed, elevating the head of the bed)?" and "Have you tried any other over-the-counter medications with noted improvement?"

5. a. Additional data: Is the patient experiencing pain? If so, what is the quality, duration, and relation to eating? Does the patient have more difficulty with solids or liquids? Is the gag reflex present? Has dysphagia been progressive? Does she tolerate some foods more than others? Have any strategies been successful in managing difficulty swallowing?
   b. The patient's history of multiple sclerosis, a neuromuscular disorder that affects esophageal motility. The chief complaint is consistent with achalasia.
   c. Encourage the patient to experiment with different food consistencies. Suggest small, semisoft meals. Avoid extremes of temperature in food preparation. Experiment with different positions during mealtime. Try using the Valsalva maneuver while swallowing.

6. Diagnoses 1: Insufficient data are presented to validate this diagnosis. A more appropriate diagnosis is Anticipatory grieving related to decreased life expectancy, poor prognosis. The student should focus on cues for depression and encourage the patient to verbalize his feelings. Diagnosis 2: At this point the patient's nutritional status can only be assessed rather than promoted because the patient is NPO for 4 to 5 days. The effects of NPO status, such as *Altered oral mucous membranes* or *Potential complication: fluid and electrolyte imbalance,* would be better nursing diagnoses. Nasogastric tube care does not include irrigating, to avoid disrupting sutures at the anastomotic site(s). Tube feedings are not initiated unless the patient is unable to resume oral fluid and foods, which are introduced in small amounts, because the patient's stomach size has been reduced. Diagnoses 3 and 4: Although the nursing diagnoses are accurate, respiratory care is of highest priority at this time. Leakage of the anastomosis is a high risk 5 to 9 days after surgery. Leakage at the suture line will be evidenced as bloody drainage in the nasogastric tube, not the chest tube. The student should assess for signs and symptoms of shock, fever, and inflammation.

CHAPTER 42

Stomach and Duodenum Problems

1. a. C; b. A; c. C and D; d. A and E; e. A, C, and D;
   f. B, C, and D; g. A; h. A; i. B; j. C; k. E

2. Both types of ulcers have a genetic predisposition, similar clinical manifestations, and comfort measures. Consequently, clearly differentiating them on the basis of history and physical examination is quite difficult. An endoscopic procedure is required to make a differentiating diagnosis.

3. a. Advantages: good buffering effect, no constipation, and low Na^+ content, which may be important in patients with hypertension. Disadvantages: does not decrease pepsin activity or influence prostaglandin synthesis, as do aluminum hydroxide preparations. Liquid preparations have a shorter duration of effect. The frequency of administration is problematic for some patients.
   b. Advantages: inhibits hydrochloride secretion by binding to H_2 receptors and blocking the release of histamine, least expensive of the H_2 receptor antagonists, effective, few side effects, excellent record of safety. Disadvantages: risk for misuse or overuse because nonprescription strength is available over the counter.
   c. Advantages: excellent healing effects.
   d. Disadvantages: causes constipation (may add to constipating effects in patients also taking Maalox) and should not be combined with acid-suppressing agents.

4. a. Incorrect. Research has not conclusively correlated small, frequent feedings with improved ulcer management. Snacks at bedtime are discouraged because food can increase nighttime acid secretion. Overeating should be avoided.
   b. Incorrect. Ibuprofen, aspirin, and other nonsteroidal antiinflammatory drugs are quite irritating to the gastric mucosa. Patients who need to continue daily nonsteroidal antiinflammatory drug use need to explore other options with their physicians.
   c. Correct action and rationale.
   d. Correct action and rationale.
   e. Correct action and rationale.

5. The best explanation is B.

6. a. First action: elevate the head of the patient's bed and turn his head to the side to prevent aspiration.
   b. Other actions: monitor vital signs at least every 15 minutes, establish at least one large-bore intravenous access site for fluid replacement therapy, prepare for insertion of a nasogastric tube and tap water lavage, place suction equipment at bedside, remain with the patient and provide comfort measures such as adequate warmth.

c. Iced solutions decrease body temperature but are ineffective at inducing vasospasm and resultant decreased bleeding. Iced saline may cause cardiac dysrhythmias.
   d. Thermal coagulation: Heater probes are inexpensive, portable, and provide consistent results, whereas a laser is expensive and rarely portable, although it provides excellent results. Injection therapy: Sclerosing agents are easier to administer and the least expensive approach. Surgery: invasive with a higher mortality rate than other methods of treatment.

7. a. Active bleeding or occult blood (causes gastric drainage to appear reddish or have a coffee ground appearance) and the presence of melena or signs of fluid volume depletion (dry oral mucous membranes, decreasing blood pressure, tachycardia).
   b. She has endured considerable stress as a result of her own injuries and the knowledge that her family members were seriously injured, both of which contribute to stress ulcer development.

8. Avoid eating highly processed or cured foods, eat plenty of fruits and vegetables that contain vitamin C, have regular checkups, and report any persistent symptoms such as weight loss or abdominal discomfort to her health care provider.

9. Stage II means that the tumor has invaded part, but not all, of the stomach lining. The tumor has not spread to the lymph nodes or other organs of her body.

10. The nurse was correct to advise the patient to stop eating at that time. Small, frequent meals are encouraged after gastric surgery to prevent gastric distention. However, the head of the patient's bed should not have been lowered. Lying flat can result in the reflux of gastric acid and food into the esophagus and exacerbate nausea and vomiting.

11. Encourage the patient to eat a diet high in protein, moderate in fat, and low in carbohydrates while totally avoiding refined sugars. Discourage the patient from taking fluids with meals because fluids increase the total volume ingested. Instruct the patient to lie on his or her left side for 20 to 30 minutes after eating to delay gastric emptying.

12. Cyclizine is the drug of choice because it is effective in relieving postoperative nausea and vomiting. Metoclopramide is an effective drug; however, it is most effective when used before chemotherapy. The consequence of using metoclopramide would be that the patient might not receive the most effective relief from her nausea, which is caused by the surgery.

13. Malabsorption: Signs and symptoms result from failure to assimilate one or more essential ingested nutrients (fats, protein, and carbohydrates) from primary (e.g., lactase deficiency) or secondary (e.g., pancreatic disease) causes. Classic sign is steatorrhea, excess loss of fat in the stool, and concurrent fat-soluble vitamin deficiency. Avoidance of source of problem (e.g., wheat) or addition of essential enzymes is the treatment.

Protein-calorie malnutrition: Inadequate intake of fats, carbohydrates, and protein related to serious illness, aging, or inability to access food, causing negative nitrogen balance and impairment of cellular function of all body organs and tissues. Treatment includes identifying persons at risk, monitoring for deficiency, and replacement of losses.

14. a. False. High-density formulas are quite hypertonic, contributing to diarrhea.
    b. True.
    c. True.
    d. False. Peripheral glucose solutions are generally 10% solutions or less.
    e. False. Blood glucose levels may be checked as frequently as every 4 hours when total parenteral nutrition is initiated and until endogenous insulin production adjusts to the increased glucose load.
    f. True.

CHAPTER 43

Intestinal Problems

1. a. Encourage increases in dietary fiber intake, fluid intake, and activity. Teach patient to maintain a daily schedule for defecation; encourage avoidance of laxatives.
   b. Monitor severity of diarrhea, estimate fluid loss, teach that over-the-counter kaolin and pectate products may be useful, encourage avoidance of very hot or very cold foods, encourage use of sitz baths and protective ointments, report continued diarrhea to physician.

2. Encourage a diet with increased fiber; encourage the intake of at least 2500 ml of fluid per day; after optimal time for defecation has been established, use a glycerin suppository to stimulate defecation; offer psychological support and encouragement.

3. The nurse should explain that heat does decrease pain; however, heat also increases circulation to the abdomen. If his appendix is inflamed the increased circulation could cause it to rupture. The nurse should ask his permission to remove the heating pad and offer an alternative but appropriate method of pain control.

4. Statement c indicates the need for further teaching. No evidence supports the need to eliminate these foods from her diet.

5. Example: outpouchings formed in weakened areas of the bowel wall producing diverticula. The diverticular sac became inflamed and swollen. The pressure caused the sac to rupture, leaking feces into the abdominal cavity, which is normally a sterile environment. The leakage resulted in an infectious process within the abdominal cavity known as peritonitis. The infection is treated with intravenous antibiotics and a nasogastric tube to relieve abdominal pressure. Her nutrition is being managed with intravenous solutions.

6. a. Similarities: both conditions are inflammatory bowel diseases with no known prevention or cure. They have a familial link; neither has a psychogenic origin. Diagnostic methods are similar. Both result in diarrhea and may lead to anorexia, weight loss, weakness, fever, increased white blood cell count, and iron-deficiency anemia. They are treated with similar medications. Differences: the location and extent of bowel lesions, the appearance of the bowel mucosa, the complications associated with each, the number and type of stools produced per day, the intensity and location of pain produced, the area of bowel removed for surgical intervention.
   b. Nursing care for these patients is similar, including assessment, nursing diagnoses, and specific nursing actions to detect complications, promote comfort, promote rest and nutrition, and teach the patient how to live with his condition.

7. a. Examples: assist with repositioning, encourage use of relaxation techniques, offer medications to decrease bowel motility as prescribed.
   b. Serve fluids chilled; offer a variety of fluids; encourage a high-protein, high-carbohydrate diet; encourage avoidance of raw fruits and vegetables; teach avoidance of alcohol, caffeine, and high-fat foods.
   c. Assure patient that this is not an emotional illness, encourage participation in all decisions related to management of the disease, encourage verbalization of fears and concerns, focus on positive aspects of progress.

8. Continue to monitor the patient. Paralytic ileus is a common complication of bowel surgery. However, if peristalsis does not return after the patient begins to ambulate, findings need to be reported because they may indicate abscess formation or obstruction.

9. a. Advantages: the anal sphincter is left intact, allowing some bowel control and a normal method of defecation; results improve for up to 12 months after surgery, reducing bowel movements to between three and eight daily; psychologically superior to other types of ileostomies. Disadvantages: two-stage procedure requires more than one surgery, fecal incontinence may be

433

persistent, complications such as pouch inflammation do exist.

   b. Persons older than 55 years may have age-related anal sphincter deterioration, which increases the risk for greater fecal incontinence.

10. a. The integrity of the stoma is the most significant factor influencing the patient's ability to manage his colostomy.

   b. The nurse should reassure the patient that the stoma looks as expected after surgery. The serosanguineous drainage is expected, and the site is generally swollen because of surgical manipulation. The redness of the stoma is a sign of adequate circulation, which is desirable.

   c. The nurse should thoroughly cleanse the skin with soap and water and then apply nystatin powder to the irritated skin, allowing time for the skin to dry before further treatment and pouch application. A skin sealant should be used to protect the skin from the pouch adhesive. A pouch with a skin barrier (wafer) attached can then be applied. These interventions will promote healing.

   d. The nurse should acknowledge the patient's fears and explain that people who have ostomies commonly have fears related to sexual activity. The nurse should suggest community support groups and offer pamphlets that address this issue.

11. Because of the smaller diameter of the bowel lumen, small bowel obstructions tend to develop more rapidly than large bowel obstructions. The pain from a small bowel obstruction is higher in the abdomen, and vomiting is usually present early in the course of the obstruction. Both small and large bowel obstructions tend to manifest with high-pitched bowel sounds, but large bowel obstructions tend to produce borborygmus sounds, which this patient did not exhibit. Given that the patient's signs and symptoms began suddenly, a small bowel obstruction should be suspected. Hyponatremia and hypokalemia can develop rapidly with small bowel obstructions because of fluid shifts.

12. a. The presence of a sliding abdominal hernia places the patient at constant risk for strangulation and bowel obstruction. Symptoms such as nausea, vomiting, and abdominal distention cause concern because they indicate intestinal obstruction.

   b. Bowel obstruction is a concern for this patient because lesions of the distal colon generally grow circumferentially, thus narrowing the intestinal lumen. His symptoms indicate at least partial obstruction based on his change in bowel habits (pencil-shaped stools), abdominal discomfort, and the presence of occult blood in his stool.

13. Examples: monitor vital signs and urine output for early signs of shock; carefully monitor abdominal girth and bowel sounds every 2 to 4 hours; use nonpharmacologic measures for controlling pain,

such as positioning or relaxation; monitor closely for electrolyte imbalances; institute oral and nasal care every 2 to 4 hours.

14. a. True.

   b. False. Bowel preparation does cleanse the colon and suppresses bacterial growth, which helps prevent but does not totally eliminate the possibility of postoperative bacterial infections.

   c. False. Incisional pain can interfere with lung expansion and predispose the patient to atelectasis or pneumonia.

   d. True.

   e. False. Sexual dysfunction is a common complication of pelvic lymph node dissection.

   f. False. Chronic renal disease is not associated with hemorrhoid development.

   g. False. Blood loss from hemorrhoids is generally small; however, blood loss over a long period of time, even though small, may produce loss of iron stores.

   h. False. Anal abscesses (not fissures) most often occur from the obstruction of gland ducts in the anorectal region by feces.

CHAPTER 44

Gallbladder and Exocrine Pancreatic Problems

1. Differences: Cholecystitis refers to acute or chronic inflammation of the gallbladder. Cholelithiasis refers to stones within the gallbladder. Choledocholithiasis refers to the formation of stones in the common bile duct. Relations: These disorders have similar risk factors, affect the gallbladder, and can occur in succession. Cholecystitis generally precedes cholelithiasis; cholelithiasis generally precedes choledocholithiasis.

2. Example: when bile salts, lecithin, and cholesterol are out of balance, cholesterol precipitates out of solution. Mucin glycoprotein traps cholesterol particles and supersaturates the bile, which decreases bile motility and contributes to stasis, allowing the formation of gallstones.

3. a. Cholecystogastrostomy
   b. Choledochotomy
   c. Cholecystectomy
   d. Choledochoduodenostomy
   e. Cholecystostomy
   f. Choledochojejunostomy
   g. Choledocholithotomy

4. a. Biliary colic can occur in the mid-epigastrium or right upper quadrant or radiate to the back or right shoulder. Such pain is called "referred" pain.
   b. Fever, chills, and biliary colic. These signs indicate that a stone may be lodged in the duct system.
   c. It does not differ.

434

d. An abdominal incision may be necessary if empyema is present, requiring external biliary drainage; if chronic decompression of the biliary tract is needed; or if the common bile duct requires exploration.

5. a. Both patients will require pain medication, but patient A may have less pain for a shorter period of time than patient B.
   b. Both may have nausea or vomiting during the immediate postoperative period. Foods and fluids are not allowed until they can be tolerated. A well-balanced diet is encouraged for both patients during their recovery period or a reduced-calorie diet if weight is a issue.
   c. Both patients will need essentially the same teaching, although patient B will need to know how to care for his abdominal incision. Both require teaching regarding any dietary restrictions, prescribed medications, and follow-up care.
   d. Patient A may have fewer restrictions. He will be able to return to work and full activities in as little as 7 days. Patient B's activities and return to work may be restricted for 6 weeks after surgery because of his abdominal incision.

6. Primary sclerosing cholangitis should be suspected on the basis of the patient's history, clinical manifestations, and diagnostic laboratory studies. Liver transplant is the only curative treatment for this disorder, although ursodeoxycholic acid has been shown to improve the biochemical abnormalities of primary sclerosing cholangitis. Teaching: the disease process and its possible outcomes, including eventual liver transplantation; methods to reduce itching; the need for maintaining a low-fat diet to decrease diarrhea or steatorrhea; and the need for taking fat-soluble vitamin supplements.

7. The patient's history of intermittent abdominal pain, which is quite different from that of cholecystitis.

8. The person with hemorrhagic pancreatitis has an acutely inflamed pancreas with hemorrhage and marked tissue necrosis as well as extensive fat necrosis throughout the abdominal and thoracic cavities. He is likely to develop abscesses and infection and complications such as fat emboli, hypotension, and shock. Organ failure occurs in 50% of patients. The patient with interstitial pancreatitis has a better prognosis because the gland retains its normal anatomic features even though it is diffusely swollen and inflamed. Neither hemorrhage nor necrosis occurs, and healing does eventually occur.

9. a. Pain status, breath sounds, general appearance, level of consciousness, appearance of stools, presence of nausea or vomiting.
   b. 1. Elevated, between 300 to 800 U; 2. elevated; 3. elevated; 4. elevated.

c. Her pancreatitis is most likely caused by gallstones because her alkaline phosphatase level is elevated and she has no history of alcohol abuse.
d. Example: ultrasonography is a diagnostic procedure used to determine if the pancreas is enlarged from fluid collection or has fluid-filled sacs called pseudocysts.

10. a. G, b. C, c. A, d. H, e. E, f. B, g. D, h. F, i. A, j. D, k. G, l. C, m. F, n. B

11. a. To reduce pain, rest the pancreas, and relieve ileus.
    b. To treat hyperglycemia if present from disease process or total parenteral nutrition.
    c. To maintain nutritional status while the patient is NPO and to promote healing.
    d. To ensure adequate fluid volume, monitor renal function, and calculate the need for intravenous fluids.

12. a. Encourage side-lying, knee-chest position; avoid use of opiates for pain control (they may cause sphincter of Oddi spasms); maintain nasogastric suction.
    b. Monitor electrolytes daily, weight daily, fluid output, and vital signs.
    c. Monitor lung sounds, bowel sounds, and for hypocalcemia.
    d. Maintain total parenteral nutrition, weigh daily, and monitor skin and mucous membranes.
    e. Provide simple explanations, answer questions, and explain diagnostic tests.

13. Manifestations of these conditions are similar, with abdominal pain being a major symptom. Both can cause nausea, vomiting, and anorexia. Patients with chronic pancreatitis are more prone to weight loss and malnutrition from the prolonged course of the illness. Patients with chronic pancreatitis also develop ascites and diabetes mellitus and may have normal serum amylase and lipase levels.

14. Examples: *Chronic pain, Imbalanced nutrition: less than body requirements,* and *Health-seeking behaviors.* Other diagnoses are also appropriate.

15. a. True.
    b. False. The pain is steady in character, not intermittent.
    c. False. Pancreatic duct obstruction, not bile duct obstruction, causes diarrhea and steatorrhea.
    d. True.
    e. False. Most tumors are inoperable at the time of diagnosis, and few patients are eligible for surgical management of their pancreatic cancer.
    f. True.
    g. True.

CHAPTER 45

Assessment of Hepatic System

1. (1) Total bilirubin: Total bilirubin measures both conjugated and unconjugated bilirubin. Unconjugated bilirubin is a byproduct of red blood cell hemolysis and is not water soluble. Thus if unconjugated bilirubin is increased, hepatocellular disease or increased breakdown of red blood cells is suspected, as in cases of anemia. The liver is responsible for conjugating bilirubin into a water-soluble form. Thus if conjugated or direct bilirubin is elevated, hepatocellular or obstructive disease of the biliary tract is suspected. (2) Urinary bilirubin is also diagnostically helpful. Because unconjugated bilirubin is not soluble in water, even excess amounts will not be excreted in the urine. Thus jaundice created by excessive red blood cell breakdown will not be accompanied by bilirubin in the urine. Jaundice associated with obstructive or hepatocellular disease will result in excretion of excess conjugated bilirubin.

2. Liver dysfunction impairs carbohydrate, protein, and fat metabolism. It may affect maintenance of normal blood glucose levels; production of albumin and breakdown of proteins for energy; breakdown of fatty acids and formation of triglycerides; and production of bile salts for absorption of fats, cholesterol, and fat-soluble vitamins. Consequently, liver dysfunction has major nutritional implications. Patients with liver disorders require increased amounts of carbohydrates and protein (unless increased ammonia levels are present). Fat intake is often restricted because of decreased production of bile salts and impaired fat metabolism.

3. Examples: "Have you traveled out of the country recently?" "Are you sexually active?" "Do you use any prescription, over-the-counter, or street drugs?" "Have you received a blood transfusion in the recent past?" "Do you use alcohol?" "Has your pattern of bowel elimination changed?" "What do you do for a living and where do you work?" "Have you had any body part pierced or a tattoo recently?"

4. Because patients undergoing a liver biopsy may have problems with clotting, hemorrhage is a possible complication. Nursing measures include close monitoring of the prothrombin time and the puncture site and identifying signs of hypovolemia and shock (changes in vital sign pattern, concentrated and/or decreased urine output). The patient is instructed to lie on the right side (liver side) to diminish the possibility of bleeding. Peritonitis can also occur as a result of accidental puncture of a biliary canniculi; therefore the patient is monitored for fever and other signs of infection.

5. Both liver biopsy and paracentesis can be complicated by hemorrhage, hypovolemia, and shock. Nursing assessment for paracentesis includes all the parameters outlined for post–liver biopsy care. In addition, paracentesis can lead to protein loss, which may further compound hypovolemia. Potassium may be lost if large amounts of fluid are aspirated. Therefore nursing care includes monitoring serum potassium levels and observing for signs and symptoms of hypokalemia.

6. (1) Risk for injury related to changes in level of consciousness and cognition. (2) Ineffective protection related to impaired clotting. (3) Excess fluid volume related to decreased colloidal osmotic pressure. (4) Risk for impaired skin integrity related to fluid volume excess. (5) Activity intolerance related to weakness and fatigue. (6) Imbalanced nutrition: less than body requirements related to impaired metabolism of nutrients, anorexia.

7. a. C, b. B, c. D, d. A

8. a. Examples: "Do particular foods or fluids tend to aggravate or increase your abdominal pain?" "What did you eat yesterday? Is this your typical eating pattern?" "For you, what is a normal amount of alcohol consumption?" "What medications do you take?" "What factors either increase or decrease the itching?" "Have you been having any elimination problems, such as diarrhea or constipation?" "What is the color of your stools?" "Have you been dizzy; weak or fatigued; or had swelling of the hands, feet, legs, or abdomen?" "Have you had any changes in coordination or memory?"

   b. The liver plays a primary role in the detoxification of many medications, such as barbiturates, analgesics, and sedatives. In addition, a number of drugs can be hepatotoxic and may be the causative factor in liver dysfunction. Because the patient has a history of depression and leukemia, he may be on drug therapy.

   c The patient may be losing weight, given his anorexia and nausea. Weight gain therefore suggests he may be retaining fluid, possibly in the form of ascites.

   d. All the patient's laboratory values, with the exception of NH3, are abnormal and indicate altered liver function. The elevated PT indicates inability of the liver to produce clotting factors (vitamin K). The slightly elevated total bilirubin level validates the presence of jaundice. The elevated ALT is specific for liver dysfunction because high concentrations of this enzyme occur in the liver and only small concentrations occur in skeletal and heart muscle. The AST and LDH are less effective than other tests in supporting the presence of liver dysfunction because they can be elevated in acute coronary syndrome, anemia, and neoplasm/leukemia. Alkaline phosphatase can also be elevated with metastatic bone disease and leukemia. Care must be taken when interpreting the liver enzymes because of the patient's medical history.

CHAPTER 46

Hepatic Problems

1. a. B, b. H, c. K, d. E, e. C, f. L, g. I, h. M, i. J, j. A, k. G, l. D, m. F

2. Answers will vary, but should include information such as that alcohol liver damage is related to amount versus type of alcohol consumption (e.g., beer can be as harmful as hard liquor); signs and symptoms of liver disease develop late because the liver has the ability to carry out its functions until a large portion of the liver is damaged; damage can be reversed and the liver can regenerate if alcohol consumption is stopped early in the disease process.

3. The nurse needs to explain that malnutrition, especially low-protein intake, contributes to the shift of fluid into the abdomen. However, high-protein intake is contraindicated in persons with Laënnec's cirrhosis because they cannot adequately metabolize protein. This occurs from structural damage and the routing of blood around the liver. Consequently, the liver cannot metabolize ammonia produced from the breakdown of protein. Therefore protein intake is restricted to avoid a toxic buildup of ammonia.

4. The nurse should suspect prodromal portosystemic encephalopathy. The irritability and pain are also of concern because many sedatives and analgesics are metabolized by the liver. The nurse needs to communicate these findings to the physician, anticipating that a serum ammonia level will need to be obtained and the patient will be treated with low-dose analgesia.

5. a. Rationale: May assist with respiratory exchange and help relieve the patient's breathing difficulty.
   b. Rationale: Bed rest is usually required for patients with dyspnea and fatigue. If the patient also has peripheral edema, alternating pressure mattresses or flotation pads may help prevent skin breakdown.
   c. Rationale: Potassium replacement is given for hypokalemia. If hepatorenal syndrome develops, decreased renal function occurs, impairing the excretion of potassium and placing the patient at risk for hyperkalemia.
   d. Rationale: The patient is at greatly increased risk for bleeding because of poor vitamin K absorption, impaired production of clotting factors, and thrombocytopenia. Esophageal varices and hemorrhoids can easily rupture, causing excessive bleeding.

e. Rationale: Patients with cirrhosis have increased caloric needs but poor appetites; therefore measures need to be taken to increase calories without increasing volume, such as providing butter, ice cream, gravies, and so forth.

6. Direct toxins such as poisonous mushrooms cause structural damage to the liver by directly affecting hepatic cells (necrosis). Altered metabolic liver function follows. In contrast, indirect toxins such as methotrexate may disrupt metabolic liver function, which is then followed by structural liver alterations.

7. a. False. It is a chronic necroinflammatory (not infectious) liver disorder.
   b. True.
   c. False. Viral hepatitis as a whole, not specifically hepatitis B, is the most frequently reported infectious disease in the country.
   d. True.
   e. False. Jaundice is associated with a disturbance in bilirubin metabolism, not bile metabolism.
   f. False. Persons with serum bilirubin concentrations greater than 10 mg/dl or liver failure require hospitalization.
   g. False. Hepatitis B and A are vaccine-preventable diseases. Prophylaxis for hepatitis C is not as effective as that for hepatitis B or A.
   h. False. Patients need 3000 ml/day.
   i. True.
   j. True.

8. Focal hepatocellular disorders involve localized alterations. Examples are abscesses and tumors. Diffuse liver disorders involve major portions of the liver. Examples of diffuse disorders are hepatitis and cirrhosis.

9. 1: d. Acute pain (basic need on Maslow's hierarchy of needs)
   2: c. Deficient fluid volume (potentially life threatening)
   3: a. Alteration in nutrition (potentially life threatening)
   4: b. Impaired oral mucous membranes (important, but not life threatening)

10. The patient has most likely sustained blunt trauma to the liver (no penetrating wound). His assessment findings also suggest the possibility of shock, renal trauma, fractured ribs, or pneumothorax. Blunt trauma to the liver carries a high mortality rate, especially if other organs have sustained injury. The patient's prognosis is guarded.

11. The incidence of chronic liver disease such as hepatitis and nutritional cirrhosis are more common in countries other than the United States because of crowded living conditions, poor sanitation, and nutritional deficiencies. The chronic nature of such

liver disorders is a predisposing factor to primary liver cancer.

12. a. Patients undergoing liver surgery are at increased risk for hemorrhage because of the vascularity of the organ.
    b. If insufficient drainage of the surgical defect is present, subphrenic abscess may occur. Infection is more common in patients with cirrhosis and carries a high mortality rate.
    c. Portal hypertension occurs from surgical alteration in venous blood flow in the remaining liver. It is generally transitory because over time, the remaining liver has the potential to compensate for the increased blood flow.

13. Monitor for and report signs of infection, rejection, and occlusion of vessels. Monitor hemodynamic status and liver function tests (to detect improving or deteriorating liver function). Maintain immunosuppressive therapy and antibiotic/antifungal therapy as prescribed.

CHAPTER 47

Assessment of the Nervous System

1. a. The <u>neuron</u> is the basic structural and functional unit of the nervous system.
   b. The <u>axon</u> is specialized for the transmission of information away from the cell body to adjacent neurons.
   c. In the resting state all neurons possess a potential for action and are said to be <u>polarized</u>.
   d. When a neuron is stimulated, membrane permeability to sodium significantly <u>increases</u>.
   e. A strong stimulus <u>does not</u> give rise to a larger action potential.
   f. The presence of myelin causes nerve fibers to be called <u>large</u> fibers.
   g. Large fibers have a <u>greater</u> conduction velocity than small fibers.
   h. Transmission across a synapse is essentially a <u>chemical</u> process.
   i. Chemicals allowing <u>excitatory</u> transmission are acetylcholine, norepinephrine, dopamine, and serotonin.
   j. Nerve endings <u>can</u> regenerate.
   k. Passage of substances into the brain is <u>slower</u> compared with other body organs.
   l. The blood-brain barrier <u>inhibits</u> entry of plasma protein.

2. a. O, b. F, c. T, d. P

3. a. C, b. A, c. D, d. E, e. B

4. a. C, b. G, c. D, d. H, e. F, f. A, g. E, h. B

5. a. aphasia, b. dysarthria, c. ataxia, d. apraxia, e. stereognosis, f. anosmia, g. homonymous hemianopia

6. a. B, b. F, c. C, d. D, e. G, f. A, g. E

7. a. I, b. VIII, c. III, d. V, e. XII, f. II, g. VI, h. V, i. IX and X, j. II, k. VII, l. IX, m. XI, n. III, o. IV and VI

8. Patient A is exhibiting expressive aphasia, which results in the inability to control verbal, expressive speech. She understands verbal language but cannot respond verbally herself (Broca's aphasia). Patient B cannot clearly receive and interpret words, although she can clearly verbalize her own thoughts. This is known as receptive aphasia (Wernicke's aphasia).

9. In the presence of increased blood pressure, the cardiovascular system generally compensates by vasodilation of blood vessels. In contrast, cerebral vessels constrict in response to increased blood pressure, so that blood flow decreases in an attempt to avoid tissue damage. Conversely, when blood pressure is decreased, the cardiovascular system compensates through vasoconstriction of blood vessels to increase blood pressure. Cerebral vessels dilate to increase blood flow, ensuring adequate oxygenation of the brain.

10. Example: The two examinations are quite similar. Both use dye to help visualize cerebral arteries. Images are taken throughout the examinations. Digital subtraction angiography uses a computer to store the images taken before and after the dye. The computer removes images found both before and after the dye, leaving a clearer image of blood vessels and possible abnormalities.

11. The patient's sluggish pupillary reaction may suggest increasing intracranial pressure or irritation to cranial nerve III. Other data suggestive of cranial nerve irritation include her visual field defects (difficulty moving eyes in the lateral fields), slight ptosis, and diminished facial sensation. These data suggest irritation to cranial nerves II, IV, and VI. Motor function is intact, but sensation is augmented (hyperalgesia). Slight disorientation is noted with regard to time. Difficulty following commands and interpreting a proverb may also suggest increasing intracranial pressure. The pain on neck flexion and leg extension (nuchal rigidity and positive Kerning's sign) may be indicative of some form of meningitis. Relevant diagnostic tests that may help confirm her diagnosis include complete blood count and cerebrospinal fluid analysis.

12. Water-based dyes are absorbed into the bloodstream and require less rigid procedures after myelography. Oil-based dyes are removed after the test to prevent the dye from flowing above the level of the spine, which could cause meningeal irritation and severe headaches. Therefore the patient must lie supine for several hours if an oil-based dye is used. Otherwise, patients who had a water-based dye can resume an

upright position. Both approaches generally require that the patient take nothing by mouth for 4 to 8 hours before the procedure, and informed consent is necessary. Any reports of neck stiffness and pain on flexion of the neck should be immediately reported. Fluids are encouraged and the site is closely monitored for bleeding.

CHAPTER 48

Traumatic and Neoplastic Problems of the Brain

1. a. E, b. B, c. E, d. A, e. C, f. D

2. a. D, b. I, c. H

3. a. CP, b. T, c. M, d. S, e. A

4. Nurse A uses the term "obtunded," which could be misinterpreted. Without additional data to describe the patient's level of awareness, this patient could be anywhere from semiconscious to comatose. Nurse B has inappropriately used the term stupor. The remainder of the documentation does not coincide with the usual definition of the term. Therefore whether the patient is in a conscious but confused state or a semiconscious state is unclear. Both nurses should avoid using such terms as obtunded and stuporous. These terms are often defined differently by different people. To communicate clearly about the patient's level of awareness, documentation should focus on the patient's behavior by using descriptive terms and quotations.

5. Eye response = 3, verbal response = 3, motor response = 4

6. Patients may be at risk for injury if restraints are not applied when they are confused. However, restraints can further agitate the patient, causing increases in intracranial pressure and other injuries.

7. The documentation does not contain information regarding the presence or absence of initial body movements, head deviation, chewing, salivation, or pupillary or eye changes that may have preceded or occurred concurrently with tonic activity. The nurse failed to note the patient's color and presence or absence of incontinence. No mention was made of the duration of each phase of seizure activity or length of unconsciousness. No follow-up assessment of orientation level and general behavior was documented.

8. The physician or emergency department should be contacted immediately if the child develops forceful vomiting; diplopia or nystagmus; nasal bleeding or discharge; increased intensity of headache, especially when active; seizure activity; unusual behavior or change in speech; excessive sleepiness; and dizziness or disequilibrium.

9. Other needed information: any prescribed or over-the-counter medications (e.g., antidepressants, sedatives), use of alcohol, onset of confusion. A more complete neurologic assessment is needed, including vital signs, pupillary and sensorimotor signs, and reflexes. Additional laboratory data such as blood urea nitrogen, creatinine, calcium, phosphorus, and liver function studies would be helpful in ruling out possible systemic causes such as hypocalcemia (which often accompanies malnutrition and low albumin levels) and hypoxic encephalopathy (often associated with congestive heart failure and severe anemia).

10. Many nursing diagnoses are appropriate. Examples include ineffective breathing pattern related to increased intracranial pressure; ineffective cerebral tissue perfusion related to decreased arterial blood flow caused by increased intracranial pressure; disturbed thought processes related to hypoxia, increased intracranial pressure; risk for imbalanced nutrition, less than body requirements, related to chewing and swallowing difficulties caused by increasing intracranial pressure; risk for injury related to sensory and motor deficits; risk for disuse syndrome related to immobility and weakness; risk for impaired skin integrity related to immobility; ineffective thermoregulation (hyperthermia) related to increased intracranial pressure.

11. Analyzing a 3-day record of activities may not provide enough information to determine which factors are contributing to the patient's headache. However, some of the likely key factors in this case are the patient's stress level and eating habits. Alcohol may be a contributing factor, but the character of the headache indicates a migraine rather than cluster headache. Intake of peanuts and chocolate as well as work stress are important factors to consider if the patient has migraine headaches.

12. The patient is exhibiting signs and symptoms of diabetes insipidus, a complication of cranial surgery. An appropriate nursing diagnosis is fluid volume deficit related to impaired antidiuretic hormone secretion. Collaborative interventions that should be anticipated include fluid replacement and administration of synthetic antidiuretic hormone (aqueous vasopressin). Urine specific gravity and accurate intake and output need to continue to be monitored.

CHAPTER 49

Vascular and Degenerative Problems of the Brain

1. a. False. A stroke is a syndrome that is the result of many pathologic processes, not one particular disease. The syndrome does result in interrupted cerebral blood flow and sudden focal neurologic deficits.

b. False. Diabetes mellitus and hypertension are modifiable risk factors.

c. True.

d. False. Cerebral edema may peak by 72 hours and remain up to 2 weeks.

e. True.

f. False. Visual defects are common after stroke because visual pathways pass through most of the cerebral hemispheres.

g. True.

2. a. Cerebral infarction caused by emboli
   b. Reversible ischemic neurologic deficit
   c. Completed stroke
   d. Hemorrhagic stroke
   e. Transient ischemic stroke
   f. Stroke in evolution

3. Comprehension or receptive aphasia means the individual has difficulty interpreting words. Nursing interventions may include minimizing distractions, speaking simply and slowly, rewording messages, and using gestures to illustrate words. Expressive aphasia means the person understands but has difficulty verbalizing. Nursing approaches include using gestures, pictures, and writing utensils; praising and patience on the part of the nurse; and scheduling short periods of verbal exercises.

4. The right cerebral hemisphere plays a significant role in perception. The nurse systematically assesses visual fields to detect deficits such as hemianopsia; superficial sensations such as touch, temperature, heat, and cold; the patient's ability to recognize familiar objects by sight, smell, and touch; the ability to use objects correctly and discriminate right from left; and the patient's awareness of the left side of the body.

5. The brain must receive adequate blood flow to obtain nutrients such as glucose and oxygen. During ischemic events such as stroke and increased intracranial pressure, the brain must receive adequate perfusion to ischemic areas. Any attempt to decrease systemic blood pressure would reduce blood flow to the brain tissue and is therefore contraindicated. Maintaining blood pressure and increasing fluid volume with isotonic fluids are early treatment interventions to increase brain perfusion.

6. Specific nursing interventions universal to patients who have either a vascular (stroke) or degenerative (e.g., multiple sclerosis) disorder include: (1) Aspiration precautions, which include assessing the gag reflex; positioning the patient upright, with head and neck slightly forward and chin tucked; avoiding thin fluids and experimenting with thickeners and different types of foods; and checking mouth for pocketing of food. (2) Swallowing therapy, which includes teaching the patient to take small bites and chew food thoroughly; providing adequate time in an unhurried atmosphere; and monitoring tongue movements while eating. (3) Nutrition management, including a well-balanced, natural fiber, high-calorie diet, and monitoring weight.

7. Major strokes, regardless of type, are associated with a fairly typical onset and course of symptoms; thus the plan of care will be similar for all and will include (1) monitoring for cerebral perfusion, (2) preventing complications of immobility, (3) promoting independence, swallowing, continence, and (4) dealing with sensory-perceptual deficits. The primary difference involves medical management, which may vary depending on the underlying cause of the stroke. Nursing care responsibilities related to pharmacology vary according to the underlying etiology. For example, embolic stroke patients may be receiving anticoagulation therapy, whereas anticoagulants are contraindicated for patients with hemorrhagic strokes.

8. a. A cerebral aneurysm is a thin-walled <u>outpouching</u> or <u>dilation</u> of an <u>artery</u> in the brain.
   b. Between <u>20%</u> and <u>40%</u> of persons having <u>rupture</u> of a cerebral aneurysm die at the time of <u>rupture</u>.
   c. When a cerebral aneurysm ruptures, blood at <u>high</u> pressure is forced out into the <u>tissue</u>, usually into the <u>subarachnoid</u> space.
   d. The classic symptom of <u>hemorrhage</u> from either an aneurysm or arteriovenous malformation is the <u>sudden</u> <u>onset</u> of a violent <u>headache</u>.
   e. The focus of nursing care for patients with aneurysm or arteriovenous malformation is careful patient <u>monitoring</u> and implementation of aneurysm <u>bleeding</u> precautions.

9. a. False. Multiple sclerosis is a chronic, degenerative disorder. It is an autoimmune disorder but it is characterized by inflammation (not infection), demyelination, and scarring of the myelin sheath.
   b. True.
   c. True.
   d. False. A viral infection, not a latent bacterial infection, is theorized to initiate the autoimmune response occurring in multiple sclerosis.
   e. False. The inflammation decreases the thickness of the myelin sheath.
   f. True.
   g. True.
   h. False. Urinary tract infection is a common cause of morbidity (not mortality).

10. Examples: keep hallways and walking paths clear of objects; avoid uneven surfaces when walking; remove throw rugs; remind the individual to stand erect; during ambulation, stop periodically to slow gait; encourage the patient to maintain a wide-based gait, wear closed-heeled, supportive shoes when walking; and avoid pivoting, making turns in a wide arc.

440

11. The data suggest the patient is having a cholinergic crisis. The onset of increased weakness began 2 hours after the administration of Mestinon (during the drug's peak effect). No data are given to suggest an acute exacerbation of the disease (myasthenia crisis) from stress or infection.

12. A myasthenic crisis occurs in response to an acute stressor that exacerbates the disease. A cholinergic crisis occurs as a toxic response to the cholinesterase drug therapy and is exhibited by increased muscle weakness. Acetylcholine is allowed to build up, eventually exhausting muscular activity. If no improvement is seen with the administration of Tensilon, a cholinergic crisis can be assumed because blockage of cholinesterase does not necessarily improve the action of acetylcholine (because overstimulation has exhausted the muscarinic effects). If improvement is seen, then a myasthenic crisis exists.

13. Examples: (1) Risk for impaired gas exchange related to paralysis of respiratory muscles. (2) Fear related to progressive nature of the disease. (3) Impaired swallowing related to muscle weakness. (4) Impaired verbal communication related to muscle weakness.

CHAPTER 50

Spinal Cord and Peripheral Nerve Problems

1. a. Rotational
   b. Vascular
   c. Compression
   d. Contusion
   e. Hyperextension
   f. Transection
   g. Hyperflexion
   h. Concussion
   i. Laceration
   j. Penetrating

2. Example: A highway system can be used as an analogy. A busy highway (upper motor neuron) receives traffic from three main streets (pyramidal tracts). At points along the highway, exit ramps (anterior horn cells) allow traffic to connect with side streets off the main highway (peripheral nerves). These streets allow traffic to connect (synapse) with other roads, leading to a final destination (muscle group or lower motor neuron). If a roadblock occurs along one of the main streets, traffic cannot gain access to the highway (spinal cord), paralyzing traffic movement along the entire thoroughfare (upper motor neuron). If a traffic accident (injury) blocks traffic at one of the exits, traffic cannot reach the desired destination. Cities cut off from the flow of traffic become paralyzed from lack of outside stimulation (lower motor neuron disease).

3. a. C3: No voluntary movement; may have varying degrees of head and neck movement.
   b. C6: Some shoulder strength, elbow flexion, and good control of head and neck; some ability to grasp objects.
   c. T10: Full control of upper extremities; some degree of control over abdominal and trunk muscles.
   d. L2: Full control of upper extremities, abdominal and trunk muscles; will likely have hip flexion, knee extension, and ankle dorsiflexion; ambulation with leg braces possible.

4. a. True.
   b. False. Secondary injury begins within minutes, not hours.
   c. False. Neurogenic shock occurs when the cervical or high thoracic spine is injured.
   d. False. This definition applies to neurogenic shock. However, neurogenic shock involves the sympathetic, not the parasympathetic nervous system.
   e. True.
   f. False. Central cord compression refers to damage to the central part of the spinal cord often due to hemorrhage or edema. The definition given refers to posterior (dorsal) cord syndrome.
   g. False. The syndrome is know as conas medullaris syndrome. Cauda equina syndrome refers to damage to the lumbar and/or sacral nerve roots that comprise the cauda equina.
   h. True.
   i. False. This statement applies to patients with injuries between the levels of C5 and T1, not C1 and C4.
   j. True.
   k. True.
   l. False. These interventions appear to be the most successful strategy for preventing deep vein thrombosis.
   m. True.
   n. False. Positioning and exercise are the two primary interventions for managing spasticity.
   o. True.
   p. True.

5. Spinal neurogenic shock: Flaccid paralysis, loss of all sensation below C6, hypothermia, absent bowel sounds, bowel and bladder incontinence. Each of these clinical manifestations reflects the loss of all reflex activity below the level of injury and are jointly referred to as spinal shock. Hypotension and bradycardia represent the loss of vasomotor tone and interruption of sympathetic pathways referred to as neurogenic shock. Hypovolemia: A relative hypovolemia occurs with spinal shock because of the enlarged vascular space occurring with loss of sympathetic tone and vasodilation. Fluid pools in the venous system, which decreases blood return to the heart with a subsequent decrease in cardiac output. Normally, patients who are hypovolemic will be hypotensive, tachycardic, and cool to touch because

441

of low circulating volume. However, in this case, because the sympathetic and parasympathetic nervous systems are not communicating, the hypotension does not stimulate normal cardiac acceleration. Therefore not all assessment findings will be consistent with typical hypovolemia. Other parameters that do indicate low circulating volume are the patient's low urine output and weak peripheral pulses.

6. a. E, F, G; b. C; c. A; d. E, F, G; e. B; f. C

7. The nurse should listen attentively to the patient's mother and then assure her that her son is experiencing normal grieving. The nurse should convey this information to health care team involved in the patient's care and rehabilitation so that approaches can be identified to help the patient work through the grieving process. Nursing measures should include conversations and activities that help him focus on current issues and plans for rehabilitation rather than directly confronting him about his apparent denial.

8. a. The data suggest that patient A has an upper motor neuron injury as manifested by spastic paralysis, hyperreflexia, and spastic bladder. The reflex arc is not disturbed; therefore reflex activity causes spasticity. Urination can be triggered by tapping over the bladder, stroking the thigh or pouring warm water over the perineum. Patient B's lumbosacral injury has impaired the sacral reflex, which accounts for flaccid paralysis, areflexia, muscle atrophy, and flaccid bladder.
   b. Both patients will require teaching about self-catheterization. Patient B (flaccid bladder) will likely require ongoing intermittent catheterization. Although patient A (spastic bladder) can stimulate his bladder to empty by using trigger points, initially he may need occasional catheterization because the bladder may not empty completely. Both patients should be encouraged to increase their intake of foods and fluids that increase urine acidity and drink ample amounts of fluid to help prevent stone formation. Both need to know how to prevent and recognize bladder infection.

9. Suspecting autonomic dysreflexia, in order of priority the nurse should:
   a. Immediately elevate the head of the bed and assess blood pressure because hypertension is the classic indicator and can be dangerously elevated. The nurse should also assess pulse because bradycardia is usually present because of vasodilation above the level of injury.
   b. Above the level of the injury (C6), assess for sweating. Ask about nasal congestion, headache, or blurred vision.
   c. Below the level of the injury, assess for cool, mottled skin and piloerection (goose bumps).
   d. Catheterize the bladder immediately even if the patient states he recently voided. If catheterization does not improve the patient's symptoms (decreased blood pressure), the nurse should check the patient's rectum for stool by using Nupercainal ointment. If stool is present, steps to lower the blood pressure are usually taken before removing the feces because this stimulus could worsen the dysreflexia.
   e. Notify the physician or use unit protocol to administer an antihypertensive drug and monitor vital signs.
   f. Other possible causes should be assessed if the above stimuli are not present (e.g., skin breakdown, urinary infection, tight-fitting shoes, ingrown toenail).

10. a. will, b. rib cage, c. C2-8, d. effective, e. bradycardia

11. Primary spinal cord tumors usually arise from the substance of the cord and meninges or from the surrounding bone or blood vessels. As such these tumors compress the cord. Thus care of the patient is most like the care of patients with compression cord injuries.

12. Trigeminal neuralgia should be suspected. Other triggering factors are chewing, smiling, touching the face, a draft of air, shaving, or washing the face. Pain relief takes 4 to 6 weeks, but it will occur without loss of function.

13. Disturbed body image related to facial paralysis; risk for aspiration related to difficulty swallowing secretions; deficient knowledge regarding disease and steroid therapy; risk for injury related to excessive dryness of the eye.

CHAPTER 51

Assessment of the Musculoskeletal System

1. Similarities: contain same structural elements; both are covered with periosteum; both have blood and nerve supplies. Differences: located in different areas of long, short, and irregular bones; have different organizational matrixes; cortical bone contains Haversian canals, whereas cancellous bone has trabecular bars; cortical bones are very dense and hard, whereas cancellous bones are strong but light in weight.

2. Support: muscle wasting disease such as muscular dystrophy. Protection: skull fracture. Movement: sprained ankle, ligament tear. Hematopoiesis: anemia, hemorrhage. Mineral homeostasis: osteoporosis. Other examples of each are possible.

3. The patient may have had bone loss at the time of his fracture, impairing his ability to heal properly.

Diabetes mellitus is an endocrine imbalance that can interfere with healing. Both factors placed the patient at risk for nonunited fracture (nonunion).

4. a. spasm, b. treppe, c. twitch, d. tonic, e. fibrillation, f. isometric, g. isotonic, h. tetanic

5. Cartilage is a strong, flexible, and avascular material composed of fibers embedded in a firm gel. Different types of cartilage serve to reduce joint friction, cushion bone during weight bearing, and compose the intervertebral disks. Ligaments connect the ends of two bones to provide stability or attach to soft tissue to suspend structures.

6. a. Further data needed: use of dietary supplements such as calcium, vitamins, or minerals; exercise patterns; psychological stressors; exposure to environmental irritants; pain status; reason for taking ibuprofen and effectiveness; family history; history of current problem, including the patient's perception of her problem and the amount of dysfunction it causes.
   b. 1. Response: implement and maintain joint rest; monitor and report. Reason: suspect joint inflammation.
   2. Response: monitor for and use strategies to prevent skin breakdown; report; monitor. Reason: possible impaired circulation to extremities.
   3. Response: report; monitor. Reason: may indicate connective tissue disease.
   4. Response: maintain joint rest; monitor; administer analgesics as prescribed. Reason: indicates the presence of inflammation or trauma.
   5. Response: apply cold to prevent further swelling. Reason: consider rheumatoid arthritis or other joint disorder.

7. The patient's fingers on both hands deviate at the metacarpophalangeal, or proximal, joints toward the outside, or ulnar, aspect of his hand. A convex thoracic spinal curvature is present, and the patient's legs have reduced muscle mass as a result of disease or lack of use.

8. a. Sluggish or diminished reflexes; may be related to neuropathy or lower motor neuron lesions
   b. Crepitus; significant indicator of pathology within the joint
   c. Refers to partial joint dislocation; usually indicates a chronic problem such as arthritis
   d. Lack of muscle tone; indicator of paralysis or muscle disease

9. a. Explain that the blood test is for protein substances normally found in the serum. Low levels often occur in active inflammatory conditions, such as the one the patient is suspected of having. The blood test will help her practitioner diagnose and treat her condition properly.

b. Offer emotional support to help reduce the patient's anxiety. Explain that the presence of antinuclear antibodies means that her immune system is producing antibodies to some of her own cellular components. This does not mean that she has cancer; rather, it supports the diagnosis of an autoimmune process.
   c. The patient cannot be assured that he will not develop a headache; however, he can be reassured that the possibility of headache has been reduced because newer dyes used for the procedure are water based and do not generally cause headaches. This information may reduce the patient's fears, which can contribute to his risk for postprocedural headache.
   d. The patient should be queried about allergies to iodine or seafood. Expectations of the procedure should be explained to reduce the patient's fears and anxiety. The patient should be reassured that the area will be anesthetized and any postprocedural pain controlled.
   e. The patient should be taught that magnetic resonance imaging uses magnetic forces rather than x-ray beams, as the computed tomography scan does. Consequently, the images obtained by magnetic resonance imaging are clearer than those obtained by a computed tomography scan, which allows for a more accurate diagnosis.
   f. The patient should be warned that needle electrodes placed in the muscle are stimulated and may produce mild to moderate discomfort. The patient should be reassured that any discomfort is brief and infrequent.

CHAPTER 52

Trauma to the Musculoskeletal System

1. a. Avulsion is a bone fragment attached to a ligament that breaks away from the main bone. A comminuted fracture has several bone fragments.
   b. A malunion is a fracture that has healed with an angulation or deformity. When a fracture is nonunited, excessive mobility at the fracture site occurs, creating a false joint known as a pseudoarthrosis.
   c. A stress fracture is a microfracture, whereas a bowing fracture is a bending of the bone rather than a break.
   d. A spiral fracture encircles the bone. An impacted fracture occurs when bone fragments are pushed into one another.

2. She needs to dry her skin beneath the cast with a warm hair dryer after showering to prevent skin breakdown. If she notes a foul odor coming from beneath the cast, she should contact her health care provider for instructions because it may indicate infection or skin breakdown. She should not use sharp objects to scratch beneath the cast because they can tear skin, leading to breakdown and infection.

3. Risk for impaired skin integrity beneath the splint, sling, and so forth or at the pin sites; impaired mobility with ensuing potential complications of immobility; decreased independence; potential for discomfort related to positioning, muscle spasms, or fatigue, boredom, discomfort, or constipation.

4. a. True.
   b. False. Allografts are taken from cadaver bone; autografts are taken from the patient's iliac crest.
   c. False. Neurocirculatory checks must be made hourly for the first 24 to 48 hours after internal fixation of a fracture.
   d. False. Other assessments need to be made, including the presence of deformity and/or immobilization device, ecchymosis over or surrounding the injury, and indications of fear or anxiety.
   e. False. Any surgical wound places the patient at risk for infection. The appearance of the surgical site is a better indicator of infection than a dry, intact dressing.

5. a. Teach when patients show interest in learning; avoid teaching while patients are in pain; repeat teaching on several occasions; include family or significant others in all teaching; answer questions in terms patients can understand.
   b. Monitor the surgical site (if present) for signs of infection; maintain a high-protein diet to promote healing; monitor for signs of systemic infection.
   c. Allow patients to participate in self-care at their own pace; praise accomplishments; place toileting items within patient's reach; assess the immediate environment for obstacles to self-care and remove.
   d. Encourage ambulation as early as possible; encourage performance of any ordered exercises; perform passive range-of-motion exercises when necessary.
   e. Use distractions such as music to alter pain perception; assess pain status and medicate before pain becomes severe; allow patients to manage their own pain control, if feasible; reduce external stimuli and allow for adequate rest periods.

6. The nurse needs to assess for neurocirculatory compromise first. If no abnormalities are noted, the patient should be repositioned and the positioning of the cast reassessed. If the cast is chafing or rubbing his leg, the cast needs to be padded. If none of these measures is effective, the practitioner needs to be notified. An alternate pain medication may be needed or the patient may need more extensive assessment for complications.

7. Concepts learned about patients with fractures can be generalized to surgical patients; patients who are immobilized, such as the patient with a cerebrovascular accident or chronic illness; patients experiencing pain or discomfort; patients undergoing joint replacements.

8. Encourage activity, attend to hygienic needs, provide adequate pain control measures; be aware of the potential for complications and monitor for same; detect complications in a timely manner so that corrective treatment can be initiated early; attend to both the psychosocial and physical needs of the patient.

9. a. The patient may be developing compartment syndrome. The nurse needs to assess for a palpable pulse, edema, sensation and paresthesia, hand and finger movement, and capillary refill. The practitioner must be notified immediately if alterations exist.
   b. Potentially irreversible neurologic or circulatory damage.
   c. Goals: increased tissue pressure, restoration of blood flow, and preservation of limb function. These goals can be achieved by removing external compression from casts or dressings or by performing a decompressive fasciotomy or epimysiotomy.
   d. To detect urinary discoloration, which indicates the presence of myoglobin. Myoglobinuria is associated with acute renal failure as a result of muscle cell death.

10. a. The nurse should suspect fat embolism syndrome.
    b. Fat embolization syndrome is a medical emergency. The practitioner must be notified immediately. The patient will be transferred to a critical care area for fluid resuscitation, mechanical ventilation, and possible glucocorticoid therapy.
    c. The surgical reaming of the intramedullary canal for seating of the knee prosthesis placed the patient at increased risk for fat embolization because it may allow fat cells to enter the circulation.

11. a. Increased age has been correlated with less-successful rates of full recovery from hip fractures. The patient demonstrates no cognitive impairment or chronic or debilitating conditions, which are positive factors influencing his recovery. If he has no surgical complications, he has a greater likelihood of returning to a near-normal lifestyle. Conversely, if he has complications, his prognosis may be negatively altered.
    b. An intracapsular fracture occurs within the hip joint and capsule and often disrupts the blood supply to the femur. If this happens, necrosis of the femoral head occurs. An extracapsular fracture occurs outside the joint and capsule, below the lesser trochanter.
    c. Hip flexion is limited to 60 degrees for 10 days and 90 degrees for 10 days to 2 months. Adduction of the left leg beyond the midline is avoided for 2 months. He will be limited to partial weight bearing for at least 2 months.

444

d. Laboratory data within normal limits; pain controlled by oral analgesia; stable vital signs; ability to ambulate bearing partial weight with an assistive device; tolerating a regular diet; eager to return home with a positive outlook.

e. The patient may not be able to provide for all his needs. He may need assistance from relatives, friends, home health care providers, home health nurses, or meal services.

12. Home assessments: Whether she uses area rugs, which may be a safety hazard; if she needs assistance caring for her pet and if the pet poses a fall hazard; if she can reach all her cabinets, food, stove, and so forth; if she has a good relationship with any neighbors; if she has any perceived needs or limitations.

13. a. Prevention of surgical complications; management of pain related to fracture and surgical procedure; prevention of potential alterations in skin integrity related to altered mobility; prevention of neurocirculatory problems and infection; stabilization of fracture fixation.

b. Use of the logrolling technique to avoid twisting the spine, use of a special bed, the need for a postoperative corset or brace, no limitations of extremity movement.

14. a. Anterior cruciate ligament injury
b. Rotator cuff tear or strain
c. Anterior cruciate ligament injury
d. Meniscal or lateral tear or extension/flexion injury to knee
e. Anterior cruciate ligament injury
f. Torn rotator cuff
g. Meniscal tear
h. Torn rotator cuff
i. Anterior cruciate ligament injury

CHAPTER 53

Degenerative Disorders

1. The 24-hour urine sample is indicated to determine uric acid levels. If they are elevated, the diagnosis of gout is supported. Accurate diagnosis ensures accuracy of treatment. Allopurinol decreases the formation of uric acid, thereby reducing synovial tissue deposits and relieving pain and swelling.

2. Few similarities exist between these two disorders, although both are associated with joint pain and swelling. Gout is inflammatory and bacterial arthritis is infective. Gout is primarily treated by diet and medication, whereas bacterial arthritis is treated with antibiotics, rest, and surgical drainage if antibiotics are ineffective. Nursing care is, however, similar for both and involves promoting comfort and educating the patient.

3. a. Is the tick attached? How long has it been attached if known?
b. The tick can be pulled directly out with a pair of tweezers. Twisting should be avoided because it will detach the head from the body, leaving the head embedded in the tissues.
c. The patient is at risk for Lyme disease if the tick has been attached for more than 72 hours. If the patient thinks the tick has been attached for more than 72 hours, further medical evaluation and possible treatment with antibiotics are needed.

4. a. The patient should be assured that systemic lupus can exacerbate for a variety of reasons and may return in spite of all her efforts to control her disease. Emphasize that the exacerbation is not her fault.
b. The patient's concern about arthritis needs to be recognized. But she can also be reassured that the arthritic inflammation occurring with systemic lupus is nonerosive and not generally associated with deformity. The patient should be encouraged to use heat or cold to decrease discomfort. Analgesics should be offered as well.
c. The laboratory findings should be reported to the practitioner because proteinuria may indicate early renal involvement (acute glomerulonephritis).
d. The nurse should institute seizure precautions (central nervous system involvement may precipitate seizure activity) and closely monitor the patient's blood pressure. The effectiveness of the antihypertensive medications needs to be evaluated.

5. a. True.
b. False. The disease affects the proximal muscles first.
c. False. Both disorders can produce dysphagia, cardiomyopathy, and Raynaud's phenomenon.
d. True.
e. True.

6. a. Recurring infections are common. Antibiotics do not penetrate bone well. Access for antibiotic irrigation is difficult. Dead space must be eliminated to prevent recurrence.
b. Teaching will differ. The patient needs to be taught how to detect recurrent infection and how to self-administer antibiotic therapy, which may last as long as 6 months.

7. Use a back support when lifting; perform back-strengthening exercises on a regular basis; lift with his legs rather than with his back; maintain erect posture and good body alignment; discontinue smoking.

8. Degenerative disk disease is primarily a disease of persons older than 50 years and involves fibrous replacement of nucleus pulposus. The disk space is

445

narrowed and less flexible, producing chronic low back pain. A herniated intervertebral disk is the protrusion of the nucleus pulposus through a rupture in the annulus. If the disk places pressure on a nerve root or the spinal cord, pain, sensory or motor impairment, and decreased reflexes may be produced.

9. Neurologic function; monitoring for changes in motor and sensory function is vital to establish a baseline and detect the development of complications.

10. Teaching regarding the type of procedure to be performed and how instrumentation will function, if used; how surgery is staged; preoperative and postoperative expectations; assurance that pain control measures will be used; explanation of postoperative devices. The patient should also be asked about fears or concerns.

11. Actively performing finger extension exercises while soaking his hands in warm water and avoiding continual grasping activities (raking, hammering, etc.).

12. Answers will vary; students must think about their own feelings.

13. Disfigurement; loss of independence because of disability, immobility, or need for assistive device; loss of self-esteem; loss of income or inability to maintain standard of living; change in family or social roles.

14. By making the patient and significant other aware of community resources; offering less-expensive ways to modify their living spaces; enhancing the patient's understanding of medications that will control pain and thereby reduce disability.

CHAPTER 54

Osteoarthritis and Rheumatoid Arthritis

1. a. False. By age 50 years, more than 80% of the population have radiographic evidence of osteoarthritis.
   b. True.
   c. False. Regular moderate exercise does not appear to cause or increase existing degenerative joint disease in normal joints.
   d. True.
   e. False. Osteoarthritis is not an inflammatory disease. Elevated leukocyte counts indicate an inflammatory condition such as rheumatoid arthritis or gout.
   f. False. Just the opposite. Nonsteroidal anti-inflammatory drugs are superior to acetaminophen for pain associated with osteoarthritis.
   g. True.
   h. True.
   i. True.

2. Nursing interventions include managing pain; preventing infection; preventing complications associated with immobility (constipation, urinary retention, respiratory complications, altered skin integrity, venous stasis); monitoring for bleeding and hemoglobin and hematocrit counts in patients receiving anticoagulants; and teaching regarding activities, diet, medications, rehabilitation, and follow-up care.

3. a. Surgical management of the patient with osteoarthritis is indicated to relieve pain, improve function, or correct deformity.
   b. Surgical procedures for osteoarthritis include those that preserve or restore articular cartilage and those that realign, fuse, or replace joints.
   c. Procedures to restore or preserve cartilage include joint debridement, abrasion chondroplasty, and replacement of articular cartilage with grafts.
   d. Materials for prosthetic implants include metal, high-density polyethylene, ceramic, and other synthetics.
   e. A particular risk associated with total joint arthroplasty is infection, which usually necessitates removal of the prosthesis.
   f. Persons having knee or hip joint replacement are at risk for development of deep vein thrombosis and pulmonary or fat embolism.
   g. Without prophylactic coagulation, the frequency of deep vein thrombosis in persons undergoing hip replacement may be as high as 60%.
   h. Erythropoietin-alpha administered before joint replacement surgery is effective in stimulating erythropoiesis and reducing the need for allogenic transfusions by 50%.
   i. The venous foot pump is an alternative method of decreasing venous stasis and reducing the risk for deep vein thrombosis after joint surgery.
   j. Pain management is an important aspect of nursing care for patients after joint replacement.

4. a. False. Rheumatoid arthritis is thought to be an autoimmune process. However, it is thought that immunoglobulin G, not A, interacts with rheumatoid factor.
   b. True.
   c. True.
   d. True.
   e. True.
   f. False. Complications of rheumatoid arthritis are usually the result of systemic manifestations of the disease.
   g. False. The erythrocyte sedimentation rate is generally elevated in approximately 60% of patients with rheumatoid arthritis.
   h. False. The goals of pharmacologic therapy are pain relief and control of inflammation, but bone erosion cannot be reversed.
   i. True.
   j. True.

k. False. High cost and toxic effects are disadvantages of disease-modifying antirheumatic drugs. However, long onset of action is the other disadvantage.

l. True.

5 a. synovectomy, b. tendon transplant, c. arthrotomy, d. interposition, e. arthrodesis, f. arthroplasty, g. osteotomy, h. replacement

6. a. Similarities: clinical manifestations (joint discomfort, morning stiffness, joint swelling and enlargement); treatment modalities (salicylates, nonsteroidal antiinflammatory drugs, intraarticular steroid injections, adjunct analgesics), assessments, precautions, the need for a well-balanced diet and weight control, nursing diagnoses and interventions.

   b. Differences: diagnostic test results (osteoarthritis) produces few laboratory changes. Laboratory findings for the woman with rheumatoid arthritis will demonstrate active inflammatory response and positive rheumatoid factor. Patients with rheumatoid arthritis are encouraged to exercise their affected joints to reduce pain and prevent deformity, but patients with osteoarthritis must rest their joints to relieve pain. Patients with osteoarthritis may require surgical intervention (joint replacement, realignment, etc.) to relieve pain or correct deformity; however, surgical intervention will not benefit the patient with rheumatoid arthritis.

7. a. Promotes comfort; prevents fatigue
   b. Promotes comfort
   c. Promotes positive feelings of self; decreases fears and anxiety
   d. Prevents injury

8. a. Mobility in patients with rheumatoid arthritis ranges from mild joint dysfunction to severe disability. Nursing care is directed at maintaining function and preventing further disability.

   b. Pain is a hallmark of rheumatoid arthritis. Exercise and movement are difficult when a patient is in pain; weight bearing increases stress on inflamed joints and may cause more pain.

   c. Many patients with rheumatoid arthritis have an overwhelming feeling of exhaustion and an inability to complete their usual activities. Fatigue may also affect appetite and result in nutritional deficits.

   d. Rheumatoid arthritis produces disability and is also disfiguring. Loss of function results in loss of independence, which in turn leads to lifestyle changes that may result in low self-esteem.

CHAPTER 55

Assessment of the Reproductive System

1. Parallels in function: both function as endocrine glands, producing hormones important for reproduction. Testosterone, produced by the testes, is responsible for development of male genitalia and secondary sex characteristics. Similarly, estrogen, produced by the ovaries, is responsible for development of female genitalia and secondary sex characteristics, such as breast enlargement. Testosterone and estrogen depend on pituitary gland function and are essential for establishing and maintaining a reproductive state. The ovaries are responsible for producing mature ova, and the testes produce sperm.

2. Women who are postmenopausal and exhibit signs or symptoms of ovarian enlargement need immediate further assessment to rule out a cancerous process. Because the ovaries atrophy during menopause, any kind of mass, regardless of size, is abnormal and needs to be evaluated.

3. Prostatic specific antigen is secreted by the prostate in all healthy men. Because it can be elevated in both benign and cancerous prostate conditions, an elevated level does not always indicate cancer. It is helpful when monitoring treatment for prostate cancer and follow-up for recurrence.

4. Each step of the procedure should be explained so that the patient will know what to expect. The patient should be encouraged to ask questions and seek clarification if needed. The nurse should attend to the patient's verbal and nonverbal cues during the examination. Care should be taken to expedite the procedure after positioning to diminish anxiety brought on by fearful anticipation.

5. The nurse should ask a few more questions regarding the nature and characteristics of the vaginal discharge to differentiate between bleeding and radiopaque dye. If bleeding is not suspected, the nurse should reassure the patient that the dye used in the procedure causes staining when expelled from the vagina.

6. These findings are suggestive of a bacterial infection of the vagina (as opposed to candidiasis or trichomoniasis).

7. The high serum human chorionic gonadotropin level suggests that the patient is at approximately 2 weeks' gestation because these levels double approximately every 2 days for the first 9 to 10 weeks of pregnancy. (Normal levels in nonpregnant women are less than 5 mIU/ml).

8. a. C, b. H, c. S, d. C and G, e. C and G, f. S, g. H, h. C, i. S

9. a. vulva, b. Bartholin's, c. acidic, d. endometrium, e. luteinizing hormone, f. vas deferens, g. thicker, increases, h. does not (as long as ovaries are present), i. often

10. a. An elevated acid phosphatase level in this situation is not conclusive for the diagnosis of prostatic cancer. Acid phosphatase levels can be elevated after fever (patient recently had pneumonia) and after a rectal examination. Further evaluation is needed.
    b. Alkaline phosphatase is an enzyme normally found in bone. Elevated levels in conjunction with known prostatic cancer indicate increased bone activity and metabolism and possible bone metastasis.

11. a. Essential.
    b. Essential.
    c. Not essential. Obtains important data for health teaching, but not especially relevant to diagnostic process in this situation.
    d. Essential.
    e. Not essential. Could be important if tests are being ordered but not essential to the problem or diagnosis.
    f. Not essential. Important part of any sexual history but not especially pertinent to this diagnostic process.
    g. Essential.
    h. Essential.
    i. Not essential. Not of primary importance in diagnosing the problem but is significant regarding health history.
    j. Essential.
    k. Not essential. Worthwhile assessment data but not essential to diagnostic process in this case.
    l. Essential.
    m. Not essential. Again, not vital to diagnostic process but could provide data regarding lifestyle, stress.

CHAPTER 56

Female Reproductive Problems

1. a. Medium, b. low, c. medium, d. high, e. high, f. low, g. high

2. a. Correct.
   b. Further teaching is needed. Alcohol taken in conjunction with metronidazole can trigger an Antabuse-like reaction.
   c. Further teaching is needed. Some antifungal preparations for vaginitis are available over the counter; however, if she continues to have vaginal drainage, she should be instructed to return to her health provider for follow-up treatment.
   d. Correct.
   e. Further teaching is needed. Douching may reduce vaginal pH and normal flora. In addition, vinegar douches are not recommended for *Trichomonas* vaginitis.
   f. Further teaching is needed. The patient should refrain from intercourse during the infection to reduce the risk for reinfection.

3. Examples: deficient knowledge regarding prevention. Anxiety or fear related to effect on fertility and reproduction. Ineffective sexuality patterns. Other diagnoses are possible.

4. The teaching plan for prevention of toxic shock syndrome should include the risks involved in using superabsorbent tampons, douches, and contraceptive diaphragms during menstruation; prevention strategies for vaginal infections and *Herpes genitalis;* possible consequences of toxic shock syndrome; and signs and symptoms of toxic shock syndrome.

5. The nurse's role in this situation is as an educator. The woman should be advised of the possible consequences of continued strenuous exercise on reproductive health (e.g., endometrial cancer, dysfunctional uterine bleeding, infertility). The increased risk of osteoporosis should also be discussed. This information will help the individual make informed choices about long-distance running and the need for maintaining weight within normal parameters.

6. a. False. Symptoms must occur during the 5 days preceding menses for two consecutive cycles to confirm the diagnosis.
   b. True.
   c. True.
   d. False. Uterine prolapse is a severe uterine problem in which the uterus protrudes through the pelvic floor aperture or genital hiatus.
   e. False. Rectoceles cause chronic constipation and increase the risk for hemorrhoid development.
   f. True.
   g. True.
   h. False. Conservative care focuses on comfort and prevention of infection. Douching is contraindicated, although sitz baths are recommended.
   i. False. Endocervical polyps are purple to cherry red, smooth, soft growths that vary in size. Ectocervical polyps are pale or flesh colored, round or elongated, and often attach with a broad pedicle.
   j. True.
   k. False. Cervical cancer is asymptomatic during the early stages.
   l. False. Squamous cell cancers tend to be relatively unresponsive to chemotherapy.
   m. True.
   n. True.

7. a. As is common with many tumor markers, conditions other than cancer can be associated with abnormal values. Abnormal CA-125 values can be indicative of spinal cord and pancreatic tumors as well as ovarian cancer. Further information is needed.
   b. The patient had children relatively late in life (age 38 and 40) and began menopause at a late age.

These two factors have been associated with ovarian cancer, suggesting longer exposure to estrogen. Living on a dairy farm may suggest high consumption of animal fat and milk, but this should be validated through further assessment.

c. The patient should be given ample opportunity to express her feelings about the cancer. The nurse should acknowledge and validate the patient's feelings. The nurse should also explain the characteristics of the disease and the lack of effective screening tests make it difficult to detect ovarian cancer in its early stages.

8. Dos: cough, take deep breaths, ambulate frequently, increase intake of fiber and fluids, perform leg exercises. Don'ts: lift heavy objects, stand or sit for long periods of time, strain during defecation, engage in sexual intercourse until told it is safe to do so by health care provider.

9. Sterilizing a mentally challenged woman raises many ethical issues. Although the federal guidelines provided in the text do not specifically address this situation, they do imply that the person has the choice and understands the benefits and risks of sterilization. Important questions that should be raised include who requested the sterilization procedure? Was the patient involved in the decision? To what extent does the individual understand the procedure and possible side effects?

10. Many times the cause of infertility is unknown, in which case either or both individuals may place blame on themselves or their partner. During the process of infertility evaluation, both individuals may be highly anxious about the possible cause. Each may have guilt feelings for hoping he or she is not the one who is infertile. At the same time, each is hoping that his or her partner is healthy. The failure of one or both individuals to reproduce may have profound effects on masculinity or femininity. In addition, testing procedures may be viewed as degrading and humiliating and are often painful and expensive. The process of infertility testing may negatively affect the ability of the couple to enjoy sexual activity, which may further compound the problem. If one or both partners are infertile, the couple is faced with decisions regarding alternative approaches, such as in vitro fertilization. The nature of such options may force couples to look at each other's viewpoint, which may be in conflict. All these factors may affect every aspect of the couple's relationship.

CHAPTER 57

Male Reproductive Problems

1. a. Generalizations: all are commonly treated with antibiotics, require bed rest, and require careful assessment of their pain characteristics.

b. Differences: epididymitis requires management of scrotal swelling. Orchitis involves elevation of the scrotum and application of ice. In contrast, sitz baths are an effective treatment for prostatic inflammation.

c. Epididymitis: tenderness, scrotal pain, swelling, urethral discharge, urethritis (urinary frequency, burning). Orchitis: essentially the same as for epididymitis, in addition to nausea and vomiting, and pain radiating to the inguinal area. Prostatitis: urinary obstruction, fever, and hematuria.

2. Seminomatous tumors are highly responsive to radiation therapy, whereas nonseminomatous neoplasms are radioresistant. In the latter case, retroperitoneal lymphadenectomy or radical node dissection is generally performed. Chemotherapy may be indicated for advanced disease in both cases. Orchiectomy is generally performed for both conditions.

3. Because time is limited, the nurse should focus on testicular and prostate cancer. Teaching should include information on testicular self-examination and recommendations for annual rectal examinations after age 40 years. The program should also include education about sexually transmitted diseases, epididymitis, and the importance of using condoms and maintaining good personal hygiene.

4. a. Patient B is exhibiting signs of testicular torsion. The acute nature of the pain and the fact that positioning or elevation of the scrotum does not relieve the pain are characteristic of testicular torsion. Shortening of the cord by twisting, which causes the scrotum to raise, is also characteristic of torsion.

b. Testicular torsion interrupts blood supply, which can lead to ischemia and necrosis. Testicular gangrene could develop and require orchiectomy.

c. Cremasteric reflex is generally absent with torsion on the ipsilateral side. Measures to determine blood flow to the testis distinguish torsion from infectious or inflammatory processes such as epididymitis. An orchiogram or testicular scan can measure testicular blood flow. Urinalysis would show bacteria, and the white blood cell count would likely be elevated in the patient with epididymitis.

d. Antibiotic therapy is the primary treatment for epididymitis. Testicular torsion requires detorsion measures either manually or surgically (orchiopexy). Nursing care is similar: ice helps relieve scrotal swelling in both conditions. Monitoring for fever and signs of testicular necrosis is a primary consideration for testicular torsion. Both patients need to be counseled about safe sexual practices.

5. a. False. Prostate cell growth is stimulated by increased androgen and estrogen hormones and the enzyme 5-alpha reductase.
   b. False. Bladder pressure can cause hydronephrosis, but it results in kidney atrophy, not enlargement.
   c. True.
   d. True.
   e. True.
   f. False. Laser surgery causes little blood loss and allows for a quicker recovery than transurethral resection of the prostate.
   g. True.
   h. False. Retrograde ejaculation does affect fertility because it affects sperm viability.
   i. True.
   j. False. Surgical procedures for benign prostatic hypertrophy do not usually affect a man's ability to have an erection.

6. a. Questions: (1) "How long have you been having difficulty with starting or stopping urination?" (2) "How many times do you get up at night to urinate?" (3) "How often do you feel a sensation of not completely emptying your bladder?" (4) "Have you noticed dribbling after urination?" (5) "Have you noticed blood in your urine?" (6) "Have you had any discharge from the urethra?" (7) "Have you experienced fever, chills, fatigue, or low back pain?"
   b. Analyses of renal function, such as blood urea nitrogen, creatinine, and dip stick for hematuria. Prostatic enlargement impinges on the urethra, causing obstruction of urinary flow and potential backflow of urine into the kidney pelvis.
   c. Dos: drink plenty of water (approximately 2 L/day), empty your bladder frequently; Don'ts: Drink alcohol, perform heavy lifting or straining.
   d. Androgen antagonists such as finasteride (Proscar) often require significant time intervals for the therapeutic effects to become evident. Because side effects may include decreased libido and impotence, the patient may find it difficult to comply with the treatment regimen.

7. a. Prostate tissue is extremely vascular. Coagulation studies help determine the risk for bleeding during surgery.
   b. Radiation therapy. Advantage: potency may be retained, although impotence often develops as a result of scar tissue formation. Potential consequence: increased risk of urinary symptoms; deep vein thrombosis; pulmonary embolism with implants; immunosuppression effects.
   Hormone therapy. Advantage: patients may have a long symptom-free period; may relieve pain. Potential consequence: side effects such as nausea, impotence, and diarrhea.
   Orchiectomy. Advantage: decreases androgens and slows tumor growth. Disadvantages: sterilization and possible loss of sexual function.

   c. Staging refers to the degree to which cancer cells have spread or moved to other areas. Stage C indicates there is involvement of the urethra, bladder, and pelvic lymph nodes. Stage D indicates possible osseous involvement (explaining the patient's back pain).

8. Regardless of the surgical approach, indwelling urinary catheter care and urinary drainage are priorities. The risk of urinary obstruction from clot formation requires close assessment and possible bladder irrigation, either continuous or intermittent. Wound care for either approach requires meticulous skin care, although the risk of fecal contamination of the dressing is greatest for the perineal approach. Nursing care measures for perineal prostatectomy also focus on bladder and rectal continence.

9. The permanent nature of sterilization; possible conception immediately after vasectomy (not 100% effective immediately); possibility of wanting children at a later date (in the case of divorce, loss of spouse or child); alternative forms of birth control; possible psychological effects for both husband and wife.

10. The patient's blood pressure is elevated, which may be a function of anxiety. However, the patient's prescribed antihypertensive medications should be suspect. Impotence is a common side effect of many antihypertensive drugs and this area deserves further investigation.

CHAPTER 58

Problems of the Breast

1. a. I, b. I, c. N, d. L, e. N, f. N, g. I, h. I, i. C

2. a. 1, b. 0, c. 1, d. 0, e. 0, f. 1, g. 0, h. 0, i. 0, j. 1

3. The assessment findings are suggestive of a malignant growth based on lack of definite demarcation, firm and hard consistency, fixed mobility, and skin retraction with dimpling.

4. Example: although research is unclear regarding the value of breast self-examination in detecting cancer at an early stage, statistics show many breast lesions are first detected by women during self-examination. At virtually no cost to the patient or health care consumers in general, no good reason exists for not practicing monthly breast self-examination.

5. Example: silicone implants are soft sacs filled with gel. These are placed in a pocket under a large muscle beneath the breast area. The implant is sized and shaped in relation to the other breast. The procedure generally causes no more than minimal discomfort. The main disadvantage of the implants is the possibility of infection. Some dispute exists

450

regarding the safety of silicone implants, but the data are still not conclusive. Autogenous tissue flaps involve taking tissue from the upper back or lower abdomen to create a new breast. The main advantages of using a flap from the lower abdomen are that the tissue is similar to normal breast tissue and the abdominal scar can be easily hidden. The biggest disadvantage is the potential for wound separation.

6. Assessment questions should include: Does your breast tenderness vary with your menstrual cycle? Have you felt lumps in one or both breasts before? Have you noticed any nipple discharge? Physical assessment should focus on the shape and consistency of the lesion(s); whether the lesions have clear margins, are freely movable, or fixed; and whether skin retraction or dimpling is present.

7. The nurse should reassure the patient that the infant is not in danger from nursing on the involved breast. She should also be taught that continued breastfeeding can reduce pain. By decreasing the volume of milk in the involved breast, bacterial growth is reduced.

8. The nurse must refrain from offering personal advice regarding treatment options for breast cancer. The role of the nurse is educational and supportive in an effort to assist the patient in the decision-making process. The nurse should make every effort to be in attendance when the physician discusses treatment options with patients so that the nurse can evaluate the patients' understanding and clarify information.

9. Nurses can take a proactive role in health policy by writing legislators as advocates for access to breast cancer screening for all woman regardless of economic status, ethnicity, or sexual orientation. Individual nurses can lobby for improved health care access through their professional nursing organization. They can also serve as role models for relatives, friends, and patients by participating in screening.

10. b

11. b

12. a

13. c

14. b

CHAPTER 59

Sexually Transmitted Diseases

1. Chlamydia, gonorrhea, syphilis, chancroid, lymphogranuloma venereum, and granuloma inguinale.

2. Yes, the nurse can assist without violating the boy's confidence. He should be encouraged to contact the local health department as soon as possible. He can obtain treatment without parental consent. He should be praised for seeking help and assured that he is making the right decision in regard to his possible sexually transmitted disease. (Note: most states, but not all, allow for treatment of sexually transmitted diseases without parental consent.)

3. Examples: provide students with information about transmission, consequences, and prevention of sexually transmitted diseases. Solicit student assistance in disseminating educational materials or presenting programs aimed at addressing the problem. Encourage parents to become actively involved in student programs on sexually transmitted disease awareness.

4. Nurses are responsible for being knowledgeable about sexually transmitted diseases, community resources, and community programs aimed at disease prevention so they can provide accurate and timely information; for being actively involved in educating the public; for confronting their own feelings and attitudes about sexually transmitted diseases and helping other nurses confront their feelings.

5. a. Teach patient about self-care and medication schedules; advise patient to avoid sexual intercourse or to use condoms to prevent transmission or reinfection.
   b. Create an atmosphere of trust; remain nonjudgmental.
   c. Discuss sexual responsibilities in a nonthreatening manner; discuss the consequences of unprotected sex and teach about safe sex practices; discuss the proper use of condoms.

6. a. The patient may have gonorrhea. A Gram stain smear of the discharge from his penis needs to be obtained to confirm gonorrhea. In addition, cultures should be obtained. If the Gram stain is positive for gonorrhea, the patient needs to be treated with appropriate antibiotic therapy. The patient also needs to be counseled in a nonjudgmental manner about disease transmission.
   b. The woman's symptoms are not consistent with syphilis. Further information needs to be gathered about why the woman thinks she has syphilis. She needs to be assessed for fever, headache, and sore throat. Explain that a vaginal examination and further tests are required to determine which disease she has. Appropriate treatment for the symptoms she is experiencing may be necessary.
   c. Test results indicate previous or current syphilis infection. The patient needs to be counseled about disease transmission and asked to identify sexual partners so that they can be contacted for treatment. If an allergy to penicillin does not exist, the patient will be treated with 2.4 million units of penicillin administered intramuscularly.

451

d. Genital herpes should be suspected. Inform the patient that a smear of the lesion is necessary to confirm the diagnosis. Explain that genital herpes is extremely contagious and she should refrain from sexual intercourse while lesions are present and for 10 days after they heal. Teach her regarding the probability of future outbreaks. Treatment includes oral acyclovir and analgesics if necessary.

e. Chlamydia should be suspected. Explain that a cervical scraping will be necessary to verify that she has chlamydia. If chlamydia is confirmed, she will be treated with doxycycline 100 mg PO twice daily for 7 days. Her sexual partner will also need to be treated to avoid reinfection. She must have follow-up care and counseling because she is pregnant and could infect her infant during birth.

7. Syphilitic lesions are hard, pimplelike, or draining chancres that are painless and can appear on the genitals, lips, tongue, hands, or nipples. Herpes lesions are vesicles that appear on the genital area. The lesions may ulcerate, especially on moist surfaces, and are painful.

8. a. Chlamydia
   b. Syphilis
   c. Chlamydia
   d. Genital herpes
   e. Syphilis
   f. Genital herpes
   g. Syphilis
   h. Gonorrhea, chlamydia
   i. Genital herpes
   j. Chlamydia
   k. Gonorrhea
   l. Chlamydia

9. a. The patient may have contracted lymphogranuloma venereum.
   b. The presence of vesicular or papular painless lesions on the vagina, cervix, or rectal area; the presence of enlarged inguinal lymph nodes; bluish-red colored skin above any enlarged lymph nodes.
   c. She engages in frequent sex with multiple partners.
   d. Doxycycline or erythromycin.

10. Patients with both diseases may develop buboes; both diseases produce lesions that may cause edema of surrounding tissues; erythromycin is an effective treatment for both conditions; both may require lymph node aspiration.

11. a. Chronic trichomoniasis produces cervical erosion, which predisposes women to cervical cancer.
    b. Severe vulvular and vaginal itching; copious, frothy, green or greenish yellow vaginal discharge; inflammation of the vaginal area.
    c. Oral metronidazole (Flagyl) and vaginal metronidazole are most effective. Her sexual partner will also require treatment.

CHAPTER 60

Assessment of the Visual System

1. a. The purpose of aqueous humor is to nourish the lens and cornea.
   b. The shape of the eyeball is maintained by a liquid known as vitreous humor.
   c. Cones are concentrated in the macula near the center of the retina.
   d. The rods contained in the retina are receptors for dim (or night) vision.
   e. Visual information is transmitted to the brain by the optic nerve.
   f. The lens provides fine focus for light transmitted to the retina.
   g. The retina receives images from the lens and is the instrument of vision.
   h. The ability of the lens to adjust between far and near objects is known as accommodation.
   i. Pupils constrict when in bright light.
   j. The medial rectus muscles of the eyeball help turn the eye inward.
   k. During near vision, the lens is shortened (or thickened) to accommodate near objects.
   l. The cornea provides the main refractive changes for light entering the eye.
   m. The iris regulates entrance of light by contracting or dilating the pupil.
   n. Involuntary muscles within the eye that control the shape of the lens and pupillary size are known as ciliary muscles.
   o. Nutrients and antibodies are provided to the cornea by the conjunctiva.
   p. Tears drain from the lacrimal sac into the nasolacrimal duct.
   q. A problem with the right optic nerve is manifest by a problem with the left eye.

2. a. F, b. A, c. B, d. E, e. C, f. D

3. Age-related changes: deeper-set eyes related to decreased fatty tissue around the eye, reduced tear production, yellow discoloration and clouding of the lens (cataracts). Visual changes (farsightedness, astigmatism), need for more light (impaired night vision), decreased breadth of vision.

4. Interpretation: at 20 feet, the person can read what the normal eye can read at 60 feet.

5. a. Ptosis is drooping of the upper eyelid, which is often caused by neuromuscular disease. This finding should be accompanied by a thorough neurologic assessment.
   b. Ectropion is an eversion or outward turning of the lower eyelid that frequently occurs with normal aging from loss of elasticity in the eyelid. The nurse should asses for eye irritation.
   c. Entropion is an inversion or turning inward of the eyelid. It is caused by loss of elasticity or

skinfolds. The nurse should assess for eye irritation.

   d. An opaque lens occurs from cataracts. A thorough visual acuity assessment should be conducted.

   e. Decreased pupillary reflexes often indicate neurologic deficits. The nurse should conduct a thorough neurologic assessment.

6. a. Nearsightedness, or myopia. Light rays focus in front of the retina because of an abnormally long anteroposterior dimension of the eye, making it difficult to clearly see objects in the distance.

   b. Hyperopia or farsightedness. Light rays focus behind the retina, making it difficult to see objects clearly that are close.

   c. The term presbyopia is used when blurring of near objects is a result of decreased elasticity of the lens, which commonly occurs with aging.

7. Assessment: history of allergies, asthma, or hay fever. Ascertain that the patient has given informed consent. Teaching: explain the procedure and describe possible dizzy sensation from the camera flashes; transient nausea or vomiting; burning during dye injection; discoloration of the skin and/or urine from the dye. Discuss importance of oral fluids after the procedure and the need to avoid bright light after the procedure. Eyes will remain dilated for a few hours; therefore driving should be avoided.

CHAPTER 61

Problems of the Eye

1. a. E
  b. A, B, D, E
  c. G
  d. H
  e. A, D
  f. E
  g. A, D, F
  h. G
  i. H
  j. F

2. Additional assessment data: nutritional history because symptoms could be related to lack of vitamins A and B; alcohol consumption (vitamin B deficiency coupled with heavy alcohol intake can cause bilateral optic neuritis), diabetic and blood pressure history for hypertension.

3. Several treatment errors were made. The only correct steps were placement of the protective shield over the injured eye and covering the uninjured eye to prevent excessive movement of the injured eye. The eye should not be irrigated and under no circumstances should the penetrating object be removed.

4. Generalizations: nursing care is directed at promoting comfort and may include the application of compresses, administration of analgesics as prescribed, and decreasing visual stimulation (dimming lights and use of dark glasses), teaching patients about instilling prescribed eye medication, application of compresses or an eye shield, and measures to prevent spread of infection if present.

5. Discharge teaching: (a) importance of wearing the eye shield at night; (b) activity restrictions, including no driving, stooping, or bending; avoid sneezing, coughing, straining, and lifting; check with the surgeon regarding the length of restrictions; (c) avoid sleeping on the left side for approximately 3 to 4 weeks to avoid pressure on the left eye; avoid getting soap or water in the left eye; avoid rubbing or touching the eye; (d) teaching administration of eye medications as prescribed; and (e) notifying the physician if eye redness develops; eye pain, increased eye or green discharge develops, or vision decreases.

6. Open-angle (chronic) glaucoma is caused by an obstruction in the outflow of aqueous humor through the trabecular meshwork. It is the most common type and frequently involves no early signs or symptoms. Progressive bilateral loss of vision occurs with persistent but dull eye pain. Narrow, or angle-closure (acute), glaucoma results from obstruction to the outflow of aqueous humor caused by the following structural problems: narrow angles between the anterior iris and the posterior corneal surface; shallow anterior chambers; and thickened iris, causing angle closure. Onset is rapid and constitutes an emergency to avoid blindness. Symptoms include pain or eye pressure, pupillary dilation, blurring, photophobia, and colored halos around lights. This type of glaucoma may be unilateral.

7. a. The patient understands the importance of having medication available so that missed doses can be avoided.

   b. Peripheral iridectomy will help prevent further eye damage but will not restore lost sight. It will help prevent any further loss of vision. Further teaching is needed.

   c. Generally, eye restrictions are not required. Use of the eyes will not worsen glaucoma. Further teaching is needed.

   d. The patient is not clear about which signs and symptoms constitute a medical emergency. These include eye pain, sudden change in vision, and halos around lights. Further teaching is needed.

   e. The patient has a good understanding of the importance of consistent availability of eye medication.

   f. The patient does not realize that she will need to take the eye medications for the rest of her life. Further teaching is needed.

453

8 a. Degree of independence enjoyed before visual impairment; job that requires good visual acuity; decreased ability to participate in home projects, resulting in a feeling of inadequacy.
   b. The patient's own resources and position in the health care system, which may provide him with supportive relationships, assistance, and access to rehabilitative programs; and his wife's professional resources and support.

9. a. Examples of priority nursing diagnoses: Disturbed sensory perception (visual), related to diabetic retinopathy; Anxiety (moderate) related to knowledge deficit regarding treatment; Powerlessness related to uncertainty of the disease and degree of vision loss; Risk for ineffective health maintenance related to difficulty administering insulin caused by impaired vision.
   b. Examples of patient outcomes: The patient will describe how the disease process affects vision and the importance of controlling her diabetes; describe the rationale for the treatment modality and verbalize decrease in anxiety; identify factors that she can control (diet, insulin administration, regular eye examinations); identify alternative means of administering insulin injections (human resources, equipment options).

10. a. False. Progressive visual loss occurs in one area, not across the visual field.
    b. True.
    c. True.
    d. True.
    e. False. Adults are rarely able to compensate for double vision from new-onset strabismus.
    f. False. Botox, when injected into the extraocular muscle, interferes with the release of acetylcholine the neuromuscular junction. It improves strabismus by weakening the injected muscle.
    g. False. The retina, not the iris, must remain intact to restore vision.
    h. True.
    i. True.
    j. True.

CHAPTER 62

Assessment of the Auditory System

1. a. False. The top of the pinna would have to fall well below the eye-occipital line for the attachment to be greater than 15 degrees.
   b. False. The temporal bone has four parts, the three listed and the tympanic part.
   c. True.
   d. True.
   e. True.
   f. False. The findings listed are abnormal, except for the presence of ear wax, which is a normal finding.

g. False. Presbycusis begins in approximately the fifth decade and produces higher frequency hearing loss.

2. The needed surgery is both cosmetic and functional. The external ear is necessary to collect and direct sound as well as amplify some frequencies.

3. a. Mechanical transmission of sound vibrations.
   b. Facilitates entrance of sound vibrations into the inner ear.
   c. Allows sound vibrations to exit from the inner ear.
   d. Regulates pressure and ventilation within the middle ear.

4. Air conduction transmits sound vibration through the middle ear, involving the tympanic membrane and the ossicles. Bone conduction transmits sound vibrations through the skull to the inner ear. Both augment hearing.

5. a. Factors that precipitate or exacerbate pain; the presence or absence of itching, pressure, or facial weakness; and the presence of other clinical manifestations not related to his ear disorder, such as fever.
   b. The nurse moves 1 to 2 feet away from the patient and asks him to occlude one ear. Several two-syllable numbers are whispered by the nurse. If the patient is able to repeat the syllables correctly and hear equally in both ears, the test is normal.
   c. His bone conduction is greater than his air conduction; therefore he may have an air conductive hearing loss.
   d. The patient could have simultaneous impairments in two or more systems (vestibular, cerebellar, proprioceptive, or visual), or more than one system could be transmitting contradictory information.
   e. Blood tests, such as a white blood cell count, may be useful in detecting systemic abnormalities; however, ear cultures would be of little use because he does not have any ear drainage.
   f. A magnetic resonance imaging scan is useful for visualizing bony structures and soft tissues, such as blood vessels and nerves of the ear, which will be useful in establishing an accurate diagnosis.

CHAPTER 63

Problems of the Ear

1. a. Functional
   b. Sensory
   c. Bone conduction
   d. Air conduction
   e. Neural
   f. Central
   g. Sensorineural

2. The nurse is correct that the patient will have difficulty with word differentiation, responding inaccurately to oral communication and/or seeking frequent clarification. However, he will be abnormally aware of sounds. The nurse failed to demonstrate empathy by telling the patient not to worry. Hearing loss may significantly alter a person's life, causing depression and withdrawal. Treatment options should have been reviewed.

3. Approach patients from the front or walk into their field of vision; attempt to get their attention by touching them lightly if they do not see you; speak slowly and distinctly; use short phrases; do not shout.

4. The nurse should teach the patient to moisten the applicator in alcohol and insert it into the canal only to the length of the applicator tip. The nurse needs to further explain that he will effectively clean his ear canal by this method without the risk of ear injury. Cotton tipped applicators should not be used because they can injure the eardrum or push accumulated wax against the eardrum.

5. If the ear is not clean, the medication may not be able to reach the infected area; therefore, the infection may go unresolved. This places the patient at increased risk for more severe localized infection and possible systemic infection.

6. The nurse missed a few procedural steps: otic medication vials are generally warmed by hand or water to prevent dizziness from cold drops. The tragus of the ear should be pressed gently to ensure proper medication instillation, and the external ear should be wiped dry with a cotton ball or tissue after administering the medication to prevent skin irritation.

7. The nurse needs to assess for history of eardrum perforation. Perforation is a contraindication for instilling solution into the ear canal because leakage of the irrigation solution into the internal ear could occur.

8. a. Infection
   b. Infection
   c. Positive pressure in the ear
   d. Negative pressure in the ear

9. Similarities: both may have fever from inflammation or infection, ear drainage, and decreased hearing. Differences: patient A will have throbbing ear pain, whereas patient B will have ear pain coupled with tenderness over the mastoid cavity located behind his ear. Patient B may demonstrate protrusion of his pinna as a result of swelling over the mastoid, whereas patient A will not. Patient A's eardrum will show bulging and may perforate. Patient B's tympanic membrane is not likely to perforate.

10. a. F, b. B, c. H, d. A, e. E, f. C, g. G, h. D, i. A

11. a. Their diminished hearing caused by packing, swelling, or bleeding.
    b. The nurse can explain that hearing will improve after the removal of packing and as healing occurs.

12. Suggest that the patient attempt to mask the tinnitus with background noises such as soft music, the television, a fan, or a noise-making machine (sounds of waves, rain, etc.).

13. Onset of vertigo, precipitating factors, and associated symptoms such as nausea or hearing loss.

14. Answers will vary depending on the student's experiences and feelings.

CHAPTER 64

Assessment of the Skin

1. a. The outermost layer of the skin is the <u>epidermis</u>.
   b. The <u>dermis</u> is the second layer of the skin and is also called the corium.
   c. The purpose of the corium is to <u>support</u> the epidermis.
   d. The epidermis is composed of a layer of cells called <u>melanin</u>, which gives skin its color.
   e. Another common name for the epidermis is the <u>stratum corneum</u>.
   f. The major function of the stratum corneum is to protect the body against <u>bacterial</u> invasion.

2. a. C, b. F, c. E, d. D, e. A, f. B

3. Examples: *If* there is any break or weakening of the epidermal skin layer, *then* there is an increase in the potential for invasion of bacteria and other foreign substances.
   If ointments are applied to denuded skin areas, *then* excessive drug absorption may occur.
   If there is excessive moisture on the skin, *then* overgrowth of microorganisms can occur.

4. Usual skin condition and appearance; when changes were first noticed and other symptoms at time of onset; any change since onset, location of lesions, or new symptoms; recent use of prescriptions or over-the-counter medications or herbs; exposure to sun or other irritants; measures that have relieved the symptoms.

5. Expected changes: Skin: paleness (reduced blood flow and loss of cells giving skin color), brown spots (increased pigment associated with sun exposure), purple patches (blood leaking from fragile vessels), dry skin (decreased activity of sweat glands), thin skin (epidermis thins because of reduced blood flow). Hair: thinning (reduced hormones and blood

455

flow), facial hair in women (increase in testosterone, reduction in estrogen). Nails: brittle, thick, or yellow (because of decreased blood flow).

6. These areas of the body have less pigment; therefore color changes are more readily noticed.

7. Because the patient has a history of altered liver function, the nurse should assess the patient for jaundice. Because the patient is dark skinned, the hard palate needs to be assessed for jaundice. Yellow discoloration of the sclera is a normal finding in this population.

8. a. Although dark-skinned individuals have greater protection from the effects of ultraviolet radiation and do develop skin cancers less frequently, all dark-skinned people are not free of the risk for skin cancer.
   b. Light-skinned individuals do appear pale. However, dark-skinned persons exhibit a dull or grayish tone.
   c. This is an illogical deduction. Although the person may be dehydrated, dry skin is common in older adults. No data suggest that her mucous membranes are dry, and no finding validates dehydration.
   d. The patient could have hypothyroidism, and further evaluation may be warranted. However, these symptoms are commonly associated with the aging process. Without further data, this is a premature and possibly incorrect deduction.

CHAPTER 65

Problems of the Skin

1. a. Furuncle
   b. Erysipelas
   c. Impetigo
   d. Folliculitis

2. a. I: Reemphasize that at this time psoriasis has no known cure and that symptoms may recur.
   b. I: Reemphasize the need to wear long sleeves and long pants during all outdoor activities.
   c. I: Although cool temperatures may help reduce itching, extremes in temperature may cause skin trauma, which may facilitate the spread of psoriasis.
   d. I: Clarify the need to apply coal tar 2 to 3 times per day. Review the entire Goeckerman regimen.
   e. E: No further teaching needed.

3. a. False. The term premalignant suggests a tendency toward malignancy; however, not all premalignant lesions will become malignant.
   b. True.
   c. False. Poorly fitting dentures or rough-edged teeth can cause chronic irritation to the oral mucosa.

These factors do have an etiologic relation with oral leukoplakia.
   d. False. Not all moles cause malignancy in all individuals; many moles are relatively insignificant but should be monitored for changes.
   e. True.
   f. True.
   g. False. Early diagnosis is important and leads to a more favorable prognosis. Rate of growth is variable, and recognition of early changes in skin pigmentation and appearance of moles is essential in early treatment.
   h. True.

4. Similarities: each can occur when the immune status of the individual is compromised; both cause lesions that are painful and may pose a threat to the individual's body image; care must be taken to prevent spread of the virus, especially when lesions are draining. Medical management for both may involve administration of acyclovir (Zovirax). Differences: they are caused by different viruses. Herpes simplex is caused by the herpes simplex virus, and herpes zoster is caused by the same virus that causes chickenpox (varicella). Unlike herpes zoster, herpes simplex remains in the cells of the sensory nerves and can cause recurrent lesions. Herpes zoster can cause postherpetic neuralgia, especially in older adults, leading to chronic pain.

5. Phototoxicity occurs in some individuals after exposure to ultraviolet light after taking a drug that produces photosensitivity. Symptoms include a sunburn-type skin reaction (erythema, edema, vesicular formation). Photoallergy is a cell-mediated hypersensitivity reaction that occurs after several sensitizing exposures to photosensitizing drugs and sunlight. Skin reactions resemble eczema.

6. a. A generalized vesicular rash is the first clue of a systemic problem. This type of urticaria is commonly seen in an allergic reaction to drugs such as penicillin.
   b. The patient's recent history of an upper respiratory tract infection alerts the nurse to seek further information about the patient's current prescribed and over-the-counter drugs, especially antibiotics taken during her illness.
   c. Dermatitis lesions as a whole tend to follow a pattern that begins with erythema and localized edema. Vesicles then form with oozing, which is followed by crusting over of the lesions.
   d. Recent contact with external agents (new cosmetics, perfumes, deodorants, detergents or soaps, and poison ivy), onset of lesions, changes in temperature, stress, location of lesions, duration of lesions, and whether itching started before alterations in skin integrity appeared.
   e. Contact dermatitis: teach recognition of possible irritants (e.g., poison ivy). Teach need to wear

gloves if handling potential skin irritants and to wash linen and clothing with mild soaps.

Eczema: teach prevention of secondary infections. Teach need to avoid skin irritants, such as soap and rough fabrics (e.g., wool); to avoid drying agents and the cold; to rinse garments to remove residual soap. Teach skin hydration.

Stasis dermatitis: teach need for elevating the extremities; avoiding scratching and skin breakdown; increasing circulation and leg exercises; avoiding constrictive socks and tight shoes.

7. a. Intrinsic factors: decreased circulation related to diabetes and generalized edema; metabolic alkalosis related to hypokalemia; decreased hemoglobin level, which limits oxygen-carrying capacity; low albumin level, indicating protein deficit, contributing to poor wound healing. Extrinsic factors: bowel incontinence; skin exposure to diarrhea stool and excessive moisture; compromised mobility.
   b. Stage 3 involving full-thickness skin loss extending into the dermis and subcutaneous tissue.
   c. Promote adequate nutritional support; prevent further skin breakdown by frequent assessment, early detection, and meticulous skin care; determine causative factors related to incontinence (e.g., tube feeding); control exposure to moisture; enhance mobility through frequent repositioning; reduce pressure areas; promote circulation and venous return.
   d. Because of the exudate, a product that absorbs, such as Debrisan or DuoDerm granules, may be best. In addition, the wound should be protected by a dressing such as DuoDerm, which provides an optimal wound environment and enhances absorption.

CHAPTER 66

Burns

1. Treatment options vary depending on whether the mechanism of the burn injury was flame, contact with a hot substance, scalding by steam or a hot liquid, chemical, electric, or radiation. The mechanism of the burn injury allows for better estimation of the depth and severity of injury, including the potential for systemic effects, such as hemorrhage or cardiac dysrhythmias associated with electrical burns or inhalation injury caused by smoke exposure.

2. a. False. The amount and duration of flame, not chemical, determines the depth of injury. The severity of chemical injury depends on the chemical involved, its concentration, and length of exposure.
   b. True.
   c. False. Most exposures to radiation produce localized manifestations such as those listed.
   d. True.
   e. False. A total of 65% of burns occurring in children are from scalds, 20% are contact burns, and the rest are from flames.
   f. False. Superficial burns are also called first-degree burns. However, they involve only the epidermal layer of the skin, not the dermis.
   g. False. Eschar forms from surface dehydration, not blistering.
   h. True.
   i. True.
   j. False. Burns do stimulate the release of catecholamines; however, they decrease rather than increase cardiac output.
   k. False. Fluid loss and vasoactive mediator release can result in hypovolemic shock, not orthostatic hypotension.
   l. True.
   m. True.
   n. False. Infections are very serious in patients with major burns and can readily lead to sepsis and multisystem organ dysfunction.
   o. True.

3. a. The data suggest that the child has a major burn when compared with the woman, who has a moderate burn injury. Major burns have no healing potential and require grafting, whereas moderate burns should heal if infection can be prevented. Thus the woman has a better potential for healing without grafting, although healing time may be increased because of diminished inflammatory responses in older adults.
   b. The woman is at higher risk for developing serious complications than the child. The physiologic stress associated with burns may exacerbate latent disease such as chronic obstructive pulmonary disease, diabetes, or arteriosclerotic heart disease. This patient is at increased risk for cardiac complications such as myocardial infarction or heart failure. In addition, older adults are more subject to hypoxia, hypoventilation, and infection.

4. a. Persons sustaining burns to highly vascular areas, such as the face and muscle tissue, have a greater fluid shift than individuals with similar burns elsewhere.
   b. Vasodilation and increased capillary permeability cause fluid to shift from the vascular to the interstitial spaces. Although the fluid is still in the extracellular space, it is no longer in the vascular compartment and the body interprets the shift as an actual fluid loss. In addition, during this initial fluid shift, protein leaks into the burn area. The interstitial space becomes even more hypertonic, pulling fluids from capillaries and contributing further to edema. All these events lead to hypovolemia.
   c. Hypovolemia, hyperkalemia, and hyponatremia. Nursing actions: monitor for hypovolemic shock,

457

decreased renal function, elevated potassium levels, and resultant cardiac dysrhythmias and heart failure. Strictly adhere to the prescribed fluid replacement plan.

5. Water and heat loss from the wounds causes a dramatic increase in the body's metabolic rate, which promotes weight loss. Fluid loss during the diuretic phase and catabolic processes related to tissue damage also contribute to the patient's weight loss.

6. Generally, the normal daily protein requirement is 0.8 g/kg of body weight for the adult. This means that under normal, healthy conditions, this patient should receive approximately 60.7 g of protein (0.8 g × 75.9 kg) per day. After a major burn, protein requirements increase two to four times normal. Thus the patient may require between 90 to 195 g of protein based on the extent and depth of his burns, general nutritional status, and presence of underlying diseases. Caloric requirements can increase to 3500 to 5000 calories.

7. Patients undergoing skin grafting are often underprepared for the pain of both the graft and donor sites. The patient should be assured that pain management will be a nursing priority and that the pain at the donor site will subside within 1 to 2 days. Preoperative discussions should allow time for the patient to verbalize any fears and emotions and have questions answered.

8. a. B, b. C, c. A, d. A, e. B

9. a. Reentering a burning structure places the patient at high risk for an inhalation injury. The patient assessment should include observing the nose, oral mucosa, teeth, and gums for the presence of singed hairs or coloring; respiratory assessment to determine the presence of increased sputum, the color of sputum, cough or hoarseness, or other signs and symptoms of respiratory distress.
   b. Intubation is done prophylactically because of possible swelling of the upper airway, which can advance to obstruction. Hourly urine output is monitored to guide fluid replacement, and a nasogastric tube is placed to prevent gastric distention if an ileus develops.

c. The following formula is used to calculate fluid replacement for the first 24 hours after a burn injury: 4 ml solution × weight (kg) × % body surface area burned = milliliters for first 24 hours, or 4 ml × 77.27 kg × 23% = 7108 ml (first 24 hours). Because half of the total amount is generally administered in the first 8 hours, the patient should receive 3554 ml of lactated Ringer's solution in the first 8 hours, or 443 ml/hr.
   d. An isotonic solution does not alter the osmotic pressure in the intravascular space. Consequently, tonicity in the intravascular space remains isotonic, and fluid is not drawn out of the interstitial spaces. A hypertonic solution would be preferable because it creates an osmotic pull of fluid from the interstitial space back into the intravascular compartment.
   e. Colloids such as albumin are effective in generating an osmotic difference between the intravascular and interstitial spaces. Colloidal suspensions are helpful for pulling fluid back into the plasma from the tissues.
   f. Fluid replacement is inadequate. The patient's urine output needs to be maintained between 30 and 50 ml/hr. His vital signs and central venous pressure indicate fluid volume deficit (high pulse, low blood pressure, low central venous pressure), and his pH is acidotic, indicating less than maximal tissue perfusion (anaerobic metabolism leads to metabolic acidosis).

10. Many anxieties and fears occur as patients are readied for discharge from the hospital: safety, possible rejection or ridicule, ability to engage in activities of daily living to the same extent as before the burn. Thus part of the rehabilitation process involves getting patients ready to integrate back into home life, physically and psychologically.

11. Examples include: Emergent: risk for ineffective airway clearance; deficient fluid volume; risk for excess fluid volume. Acute: risk for infection; imbalanced nutrition: less than body requirements; risk for ineffective individual and family coping. Rehabilitative: risk for disturbed body image; anxiety. Nursing diagnoses common to all burn patients: acute or chronic pain (with partial-thickness injury); impaired skin integrity; anxiety and/or fear.